The Psyche and Schizophrenia

The Psyche and Schizophrenia

The Bond between Affect and Logic

Luc Ciompi

Translated by Deborah Lucas Schneider

Harvard University Press
Cambridge, Massachusetts
and London, England
1988

Originally published as *Affektlogik*, ISBN 3-608-95037-0
© 1982 Ernst Klett Verlage, Stuttgart

This book is printed on acid-free paper, and its binding materials
have been chosen for strength and durability.

Library of Congress Cataloging-in-Publication Data
Ciompi, Luc.
    The psyche and schizophrenia.

    Translation of: Affektlogik.
    Bibliography: p.
    Includes index.
    1. Psychoanalysis. 2. System theory. 3. Schizo-
phrenia. 4. Cognition in children. I. Title.
[DNLM: 1. Psychoanalysis. 2. Schizophrenia. 3. Systems
Theory. WM 460 C576a]
BF175.C5513   1988   616.89'82   88-6768
ISBN 0-674-71990-5 (alk. paper)

Contents

Preface

For many years I have been in the habit of making notes now and then to keep from forgetting new ideas and thoughts that occur to me in my daily work with psychiatric patients, most of whom are schizophrenics. Eventually these notes, jotted down in a fairly random way, grew into a whole edifice of thoughts; they seemed to contain material worth communicating to others. For a long time I hesitated to put them into book form, and they appeared to be too incoherent to be published just as they were. In the spring of 1979 I wrote up some of those ideas as a lecture on the connections between psychoanalysis and systems theory, which later appeared in the journal *Psyche*. This became the kernel around which the rest of the book grew as I began to write in the fall of that year.

I had thought at the start that I could see the path ahead of me clearly, or at least the main stages of the journey. Not until I had set out, however, did I realize that these were only the peaks of the mountains on the way, and not always even the most important peaks. I came to see that between them lay deep valleys full of obstacles but also full of hidden beauty. My aim was to create stronger links, in a broad sense as well as in certain details, between several areas of knowledge that can all contribute to our understanding of the psyche and psychosis. At times this seemed like a rash undertaking, but while I was at work on the manuscript various publications appeared pursuing the very same lines of thought. I saw more and more clearly that I was not alone or on the wrong track, but involved in questions about which many other researchers were thinking and to which some were finding quite similar answers.

My ideas are based primarily on twenty-five years of clinical work and research in classic psychiatry and psychopathology and on a love-hate relationship with Freudian psychoanalysis that has persisted since my student days. In reaction I became increasingly interested in modern forms of family therapy based on communications and systems theory as these new methods of treatment showed considerable success over the years. The apparent contrast between these two approaches was finally resolved for me when I acquired a deeper understanding of the monumental work of Jean Piaget. His structuralist version of the psyche and psychic differentiation, though almost exclusively cognitive, had anticipated central elements of current systems theory as early as the 1920s and seemed to me to be a valid model not only for affective phenomena but also for events in the family and society. When I encountered the ideas of the French structuralists, particularly those of Claude Lévi-Strauss, at about the same time, I felt confirmed in my conclusions, especially after it dawned on me that the concepts of a structure and a system were virtually identical.

All of these topics are discussed in this book. Simultaneously, however, something new developed into the central idea: the concept of "affect-logic." In my view, feeling and thinking, affect and logic, are interacting forces that together constitute the psyche and operate in conjunction; they *resonate* together. I became convinced that this perspective could lead to a new understanding of both normal and abnormal psychological phenomena. In particular I came increasingly to see the most important psychosis, schizophrenia, in a new light. Finally, quite significant therapeutic consequences became apparent that I had not foreseen, since my main concern had been to reach a better understanding, not to devise a course of action. Yet it is certainly no accident that these results resemble many recent efforts to introduce new forms of therapy based on very different theoretical principles.

The path of my journey is reconstructed in the following chapters. In Chapter 1 I discuss the relationship between psychoanalysis and systems theory, drawing on my original *Psyche* article. Here I argue that psychoanalytic thought and systems theory are not fundamentally incompatible, as is often claimed, but are rather, despite their evident differences, complementary in many respects. Recognition of this fact provides a solid basis for exploring the question of the existence of an affect-logic.

This question is the central topic of Chapter 2. A comparison of the most important findings from Freudian psychoanalysis and Piaget's genetic epistemology points to the conclusion that the psyche can be understood as a double system with affective and cognitive poles. These are inseparably connected and interact to form common structures in the course of development. Affect is associated predominantly with specific physical sensations, the cognitive functions with increasingly nonmaterial, abstract intellectual processes. Building on this foundation, we can recognize at least the beginnings of an affective structure of logic and a logical structure of affect—that is, of an affect-logic, in which both components develop together in shared structures.

In Chapter 3 I attempt to define and clarify the often confusing concepts of differentiation, structure, and system. The last two prove to be virtually identical: "the product of an invariance and a variance." These basic ideas lead finally to the central concept of affect-logic as a system of reference. Such affective-cognitive systems, which are to be thought of as equilibrated in Piaget's sense of the term, appear to provide the essential components of psychic structures on many different levels.

In Chapter 4 I investigate consciousness and its relation to language (or Piaget's "semiotic function"). Consciousness appears to be the result of a process of increasing consolidation (or abstraction) of information that in the end comes to be characterized by (linguistic) signs. From this perspective, in contrast to the traditional one, information is understood to contain both cognitive and affective components. It becomes evident that the continuing integration of new information into existing affective-logical systems of reference is an essential function of consciousness; the psyche can be regarded as a framework for processing information, or as a network of hierarchically ordered systems of reference extending between organisms and the external world.

In Chapter 5 I discuss the affective-logical structures of conflicts, paradoxes, and double binds in an attempt to answer the question: How does such a carefully equilibrated system for processing information arrive at a state of pathological tension and confusion? Recent ideas from the fields of psychoanalysis, family dynamics, and communications and systems theory are combined to produce the following hypothesis: In individuals at risk for schizophrenia, important affective-logical systems of reference are internalized on the basis of unclear and contradictory experience. As a result, they are structured in a vague and confused manner and are far more labile than in normal individuals.

Having traveled along many byways, in Chapter 6 I discuss a partially new understanding of the "dis-order" of schizophrenia, an understanding based on the perspective of affect-logic. I sketch a general theory of such disorders and try to relate it to our current knowledge of the disease.

Finally, in Chapter 7 I discuss some practical implications for the treatment of psychotic conditions, including general principles for treatment, the therapeutic setting, interaction with patients, and special techniques for altering systems of reference. Some of the points of view that emerge bear a startling resemblance to modern approaches to therapy derived from other theoretical traditions.

Although each chapter may be considered an independent entity and read separately, each is also an essential element of a larger whole; Chapters 1 through 4 are quite theoretical, and Chapters 5 through 7 focus on practical therapeutic questions.

One other question that I had to consider as I was writing and wondering what kind of vocabulary to use was, for whom was I in fact writing this book? At first I was mainly concerned with ordering and developing the ideas that I had hastily jotted down as notes, and I had a quite anonymous reader in mind, perhaps a kind of alter ego. In the process I became involved in an inner dialogue with those authors to whom I owe the most. Many of them are no longer alive: Jean Piaget, Gregory Bateson, Milton Erickson, and Albert Scheflen died while I was working on the manuscript. I also thought frequently about the experts and researchers in the various fields this book would touch on: the strict geneticists, medical practitioners, and biologists, on the one hand, and the proponents of classic psychoanalysis, family dynamics, and systems theory on the other. They were on my mind as I encountered unexplored territory in my "controlled speculations," as one of them once aptly described my reflections. In the end, what I had to say was determined by the questions I had posed and thus addresses readers in all these fields—an approach not without its difficulties. Nonetheless the emphasis is on psychoanalysis and social and family dynamics.

As I approached practical questions I also realized increasingly that I had other readers in mind who were much closer to me. I wanted to make my ideas clear to colleagues in the field of mental health—the doctors, psychologists, social workers, nurses, and hospital employees who spend their professional lives among the patients with whom this book is concerned. And then I saw that I was also writing for people like those with whom I have been fortunate to work for a number of years at the University Hospital for Social Psychiatry in Bern. It is a diverse, committed, and questioning staff; a microcosm of individuals with different backgrounds and training, but all united in one task: to understand what is going on in the people whom we call "mentally ill" or "schizophrenic," and to use this understanding to do the things that appear likely to help them, while leaving undone the things that do not.

My goal as I wrote was to be as clear and as simple as possible, and to combine "controlled speculation" with critical thought. Since the human mind is fortunately not the exclusive province of psychiatrists and their co-workers, I hope readers from other disciplines will benefit from my efforts to avoid technical jargon and abstruse medical terminology whenever I could. When this was not possible I have made every effort to explain such terms.

I wish to thank those people without whose assistance this book would not have been possible. First and foremost are Dieter Signer—psychiatrist, psychoanalyst, close friend, and partner in discussions since our youth—and his wife, Rita Signer, who has been a source of much hospitality and much information. I am also indebted to my teachers: Max Müller, an expert on psychodynamics and somatic therapy; his son Christian, a pioneer in psychotherapy for schizophrenics and in modern social psychiatry; the psychoanalysts Ernst Blum and Germaine Guex; my colleague Luc Kaufmann, a pioneer in family therapy; and Gottlieb Guntern, the systems theorist and therapist. Manfred Bleuler, though never my teacher in the strict sense, has been a model and inspiration to me not only because of his undogmatic scholarship, versatility, and integrity, but above all because of his commitment to and affection for his schizophrenic patients. I would also like to thank Kathrin Balmer, my loyal and untiring secretary, and my translator, Deborah Schneider, for such pleasant collaboration in the preparation of this book.

I do not mean to forget the most important people, about whom this book is written. I refer to my schizophrenic patients, those special people who—underneath their "insanity"—are not only more sensitive, acute, and vulnerable than many others, but also in many ways more authentic, original, and interesting. They have my warmest thanks for everything that association with them has given me, as well as my affection.

Caminante, no hay camino,
se hace camino al andar.

Traveler, there is no road,
We create the road as we travel.

—Antonio Machado
(1875–1939)

1 Psychoanalysis and Systems Theory: A Contradiction?

> A clash of doctrines is not a disaster, it is an opportunity.
> —Alfred North Whitehead,
> *Science and the Modern World*

This book is devoted mainly to exploring certain questions about the structure of the psyche and psychosis. There are several important reasons to begin with a discussion of the relationship between psychoanalysis and systems theory.

Only twenty or thirty years ago there existed just one theoretical model of the human psyche that was comprehensive, detailed, and therapeutically useful: psychoanalysis. Since then, however, new models have been created, some of which stand in sharp contrast to psychoanalytic doctrines. Among these new approaches are behavior therapy, which grew out of learning theory and behaviorism, and systems theory. First applied to physical and biological processes, systems theory was later introduced in the fields of psychology and sociology.

In recent years there has been a great deal of discussion among dynamically oriented psychiatrists about psychoanalysis and systems theory. The points of departure of the two methods appear contrary in many respects, and some people see them as completely irreconcilable. It is indeed the case that psychoanalysis has always focused on the intrapsychic processes of individuals; its main area of concern has been the emotions, the world of affect, whereas systems theory uses a different and broader approach. In the form of "general systems theory" it claims to be a universally valid theory of science, a new "paradigm," as T. S. Kuhn has called it, that embraces the various disciplines.[1] Over the past twenty years a concept of systems theory quite distinct from psychoanalysis (for example, Rüesch, Bateson, Haley, Minuchin, and Watzlawick) has played an increasingly important role in family therapy, although another trend in family therapy has direct psychoanalytic origins (for example, Lidz, Wynne, Searles, Selvini Palazzoli, and Stierlin). As we shall see later, systems theory is also quite consistent with Piaget's "genetic epistemology," the most profound and useful model of intelligence and cognitive functions available today.

The main criticism of psychoanalysis put forward by systems theorists is not new; several older schools of psychotherapy, including the so-called culturalists (such as Sullivan, Horney, and Fromm), raised similar objections that psychoanalysis concentrates in too limited a fashion on an individual's intrapsychic experiences and neglects the many forms of involvement connecting him with his environment, and in particular with his family. In addition, systems theorists accuse psychoanalysts of continuing to think in terms of a linear, Cartesian causality. This approach, they claim, is outmoded and fails to do justice to psychic and social processes that are in fact parts of systems of a circular nature. On the other hand, many psychoanalysts regard systems theory as intellectually one-sided and superficial; as they see it, it does not take sufficiently into consideration either the significance of an individual's particular history or the deeper motives for behavior rooted in human sexuality and other drives. Consequently—from the psychoanalytic point of view—systems theory misunderstands and manipulates the individual as a lifeless, unfeeling "element" of equally lifeless and abstract larger structures.

It is obvious that great disparities exist between the two theories in their points of departure, their perspectives, and above all in their practical approaches to therapy. Nevertheless, their fundamental relationship is not one of opposition. Rather, it is a *hierarchical* relationship, involving a general and a special theory, and thus consistent with the claim of systems theory to universal applicability. Given the fact that systems theory focuses on interpersonal and family dynamics, whereas psychoanalysis concentrates on individuals and intrapsychic dynamics, their relationship is *complementary* and corresponds approximately to processes in molecules and atoms. Thus the processes of family dynamics that can be expressed in terms of systems theory turn out to be in no way opposed to a psychoanalytic understanding of intrapsychic processes; on the contrary, these two aspects, perceived from two different standpoints, complement each other and can be combined to form a logical whole, in a manner quite similar to what naturally occurs in reality, where the events of individual and family life are combined. To make this point clearer, I shall first compare important elements of the two models on a rather theoretical level and then use two examples—the relationship of narcissistic and oedipal problems to family dynamics—to demonstrate how the two approaches can be fruitfully combined in a kind of psychoanalytic systems theory or systemic psychoanalysis.

Systems Theory

The origins of systemic thinking as we know it today go back to the work of the Austrian biologist Ludwig von Bertalanffy, who first formulated his ideas on the subject in 1928.[2] After various intermediate modifications he expanded them into a "general systems theory" in 1950. The central idea of this approach is that the observer must direct his attention away from single processes occurring in certain units (or individuals) and toward the entire systems of which these units form a part. J. G. Miller, a leading systems theorist, has defined a system as "a set of units with relationship among them," in which "the state of each unit is constrained by the state of other units."[3] The word *system* derives from the Greek verb *synistēmi*, meaning "to place or be placed together." The word has a tradition of use in philosophy since ancient times, and, in accord with its original sense as both an active and passive form, it has been used to mean both "an existing order of things" and "the free design of an order of things." In his article on the concept of systems in a handbook of philosophy, from which I have taken the preceding information, Zahn has noted that philosophers have never been able to agree on which definition should take priority; the term has sometimes been regarded as referring to a static state, at other times as denoting a dynamic process.[4] The fact that the same holds true for the concept of a structure suggests a close relationship between the two terms (discussed in Chapter 3). In fact quite striking correspondences exist between the perspectives of systems theorists and structuralists. Piaget, for example, in a short but crucial book on structuralism, described a structure in dynamic terms, as "a system of transformations according to specific principles";[5] and as the three most important characteristics of these principles he named wholeness, transformation, and self-regulation. In addition, clear links exist between systems theory and several other schools of philosophy that tend to think in terms of the dynamic interaction of opposites within a larger whole, from the Chinese *yin* and *yang*, through Heraclitus, to Hegel, philosophical and scientific phenomenology, and gestalt psychology. Modern scientific thought has been dominated by ideas of linear causality, deduction, and analytic attention to single phenomena, but before it there existed—and has continued to exist alongside and, as it were, "behind" it—an entirely different, global mode of thought based on the idea of balancing opposites. Modern systems theory represents only one of the possible forms of this kind of thinking; we might think of it as a secularized, scientific form.

Systems theory conceives of the entire universe as a hierarchy of concrete systems (and subsystems), of which biological and social systems represent special cases. It also distinguishes between open and closed systems. Living systems are always open and, according to Miller, consist of at least nineteen essential subsystems, including (1) those that ingest, distribute, convert, store, and extrude matter-energy (such as the digestive and circulatory systems); (2) those that process both matter-energy and information (such as the reproductive system and sensory organs); and (3) those that process only information (such as the input, coding, memory, decider, and output information subsystems of the central nervous system). A living organism provides the best possible example of an open system; another good example is the interplay among many organisms in a biological ecosystem such as can be found in any square yard of an untouched natural environment.

In addition to the global approach, several other concepts are central to systems theory:

- The relationships between the single elements (or individuals) of a system are *circular*, not linear; this view suggests that the cause-and-effect thinking of traditional physics or the stimulus-and-response thinking of classical psychology is too simplistic.
- Such circuits operate by means of feedback mechanisms, in which a transformation of element B caused by element A leads in turn to a transformation of element A. Thus:

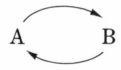

- A dynamic state of equilibrium, or homeostasis, is maintained in a system by means of *negative feedback;* the greater the effect A has on B, the more A is reduced, as in the case of a thermostat or the regulation of a water reservoir. Negative feedback prevents a continuous transformation of the system in one direction; otherwise it would finally reach a state of complete uniformity—that is, the point at which the system would disappear according to the second law of thermodynamics (the general tendency of all natural processes to entropy, a state of maximum disorganization). Negative feedback is thus essential for a system's continued survival.

  When we consider the mechanisms by which psychoses arise, we shall also see that in many areas of biology *positive feedback* also plays a decisive role. In this case certain processes are accelerated by an increase in the rate of another; that is, the more A is amplified, the greater its effect on B. Positive feedback also counteracts drift toward entropy, particularly in the development of increasingly complex forms of organization such as the evolution of living creatures.

- Systems theory is oriented primarily to the present and thus is ahistorical in its approach. It is much more concerned with the relationship of all parts to a whole at one particular time than in their development over time. Similarly, the importance attached by structuralists such as Ferdinand de Saussure and Claude Lévi-Strauss to synchronic rather than diachronic thinking in linguistics and anthropology has had a profound influence on both fields. The parallels between systems theory and structuralism are in fact so striking that they need no further emphasis.

These central concepts of general systems theory, to which one could add the notion of *equifinality* (the idea that the same final state in a system can be reached from entirely different initial states), have all been applied to a special field of psychotherapy: systems-oriented family therapy. Psychic disturbances in one member of a family are no longer regarded and treated as the expression of personal problems originating in that individual's life history, but rather as evidence of dynamic processes occurring then and there in the entire family constellation and regulated by (possibly pathological) homeostatic mechanisms. Haley and Hoffmann, Watzlawick, Minuchin, Selvini Palazzoli, and others have described such processes in detail.

Many connections also exist between systems theory and modern cybernetic information and communications theory. This is true not only of social and linguistic communication in the narrow or traditional sense, which takes place in specific communication networks such as a family, but also for a much broader definition of information. If every effect of one element of a system (be it abstract, mental, organic, or inorganic) on another element—that is, every kind of dynamic process—is considered to be a transfer of information, then it can also be regarded as communication in the wider sense. Thus systems theory always also implies modern communications and information theory.

Psychoanalysis

Several essential elements of Freud's psychoanalytic theory are of special interest for the connections between psychoanalysis and systems theory. First, Freud must be regarded as the founder of modern psychodynamics. He developed a view of the workings of the mind that went far beyond the limits of linear causality, such as those expressed in the doctrine of stimulus and response. For Freud, dynamic motion between two or more poles, the reduction of tension, equilibrium, and compromises resulting from the interaction of the most varied forces all played an important role. For example, he saw neurotic symptoms, parapraxis ("Freudian slips"), and dream content as compromises determined by the complex interplay of drives and defense mechanisms. Thus despite the fact that the language of psychoanalysis was originally borrowed from physics and mechanics (a feature that it shares with systems theory), psychoanalytic thinking is not "reductionist." Scientific thought in terms of simple cause and effect had ceased to exist anywhere in pure form by the beginning of this century.

The reductionist paradigm is monocausal, monofactorial, and one-dimensional. It is based on an all-or-nothing determinism that is often rigid and reduces the etiology of observable phenomena to a single factor ... The systemic paradigm rejects such reductionism as incorrect and explains the causes of behavior in terms of the here-and-now structure of a complex transactional field. This paradigm is multiconditional, multifactorial, and multidimensional. It replaces monocausal determinism with the theory of probabilistic determinism. Probabilistic determinism means that several factors, in summation and in their specific structural pattern, raise the probability of pathological behavior to the point at which it actually occurs.

As an example of the reductionist paradigm we have chosen Freud's theory of psychoanalysis, since its influence on psychotherapy has been particularly lasting.[6]

Anyone with more than a superficial knowledge of psychoanalysis will realize that it never propagated the kind of reductionist caricature attacked in the passage above, not even in its early stages, when it viewed sexuality as the single, direct cause of neurotic disturbances. The criticism applies even less to the later and much more complex concept of libido (in connection with aggression), and several decades of modern, multicausal scientific thinking have modified psychoanalysis still further, in particular the school that deals with narcissistic and psychotic disturbances and their relationship to the family. In this field the causes of mental illness have long been regarded as "multiconditional, multifactorial, and multidimensional."

Freud's original theory already contains elements closely related to the concepts of systems theory, even though they were formulated differently. Such relationships are particularly strong in the psychoanalytic theory of drives, psychoanalytic ego psychology, and the modern psychoanalytic doctrine of narcissism.

The Psychoanalytical Theory of Drives

The overall structure of the psychoanalytic theory of drives—as of psychoanalytic theory in general—is dualistic or polar.[7] Mental states, and drive states in particular, are regarded as the continually fluctuating results of dynamic processes occurring within a field of numerous poles or pairs of opposites. The most important of these are listed below (although various pairs overlap and the categories listed on the left and right may not correspond directly).

Conscious	Unconscious
Love	Hate
Life instincts (libido)	Death instincts (destrudo)
Object libido	Ego libido (narcissistic libido)
(object love or hate)	(self love or hate)
Pleasure principle	Reality principle
Tension	Relaxation
Stability principle	Nirvana principle

Bipolarities represent the simplest possible form of a "system"—a fact whose general significance has not been sufficiently recognized. Here, the feedback existing between A and B, illustrated as A ⇄ B, also indicates the existence of a simple system. More complex systems arise when several bipolarities interact. These bipolar structures, most especially the "stability principle" and "Nirvana principle," which Freud took over from Gustav Fechner and Barbara Low, correspond exactly to the concepts of homeostasis and entropy.[8] They indicate that, where intrapsychic events are concerned, the founder of psychoanalysis had in mind processes that are fundamentally similar to, if not identical with, those later explored and defined by systems theorists in the context of a different "whole" (such as the family or society). In this respect at least, we can hardly speak of a contradiction or opposition between the two theories.

Psychoanalytic Ego Psychology

As is well known, since Freud's death a number of authors (including Hartmann, Kris, Loewenstein, Jacobson, and Rapaport) have developed a psychoanalytic theory that places less emphasis on drives than on the ego. This "ego psychology," however, is based on some of Freud's own ideas, as well as on those of Anna Freud, involving the concept of defense mechanisms.[9] It regards the ego as a highly complex agency that mediates between the demands of drives (or the pleasure principle), on the one hand, and perception, experience, commands, and prohibitions (or the reality principle and the superego) on the other. The goal and purpose of this complex "psychical apparatus" (Freud), which governs motor activity, language, memory, and perception, is to maintain a state of equilibrium (homeostatis) between the numerous forces and stimuli to which the individual is constantly exposed. Such equilibrium is necessary to ensure survival. The concept of defense mechanisms was developed in this context; slightly modified to "coping mechanisms," it has come to play a central role in modern crisis theory, as well as in research on "life-events" (which investigates the connections between stressful life situations and psychic decompensation) and in the theory of under-, over-, and optimal stimulation in relation to a given "channel capacity."

The attitudes and formulations of psychoanalytic ego psychology do not appear to be any more fundamentally opposed to systems theory than does earlier psychoanalytic theory. On the contrary, it matches or even anticipates some of the ideas of systems theory:

We ascribe to the ego first of all the function of orientation and detection. Like a monitor or periscope it constantly scans the environmental horizons for possibilities and necessities, threats and opportunities. Simultaneously it remains in constant contact with the internal situation; it "listens" to many voices. It is aware of instinctual needs and urges, of states of somatic functioning, of standards and stipulations of the conscience and of various internal autonomies, including its own. The conjunction of internal and external details makes an infinite kaleidoscopic pattern; pressures sometimes coincide and sometimes conflict. An infinite number of reconciliations is achieved, most of them without any strain or stress. Like our breathing, the ego acts for the most part automatically. But circumstances can accelerate it or slow it or distress it to the very threshold of extinction.

. . . the ego may be described as a controlling agency which recognizes, receives, stores, discriminates, integrates, and acts by restraining, releasing, modifying, and directing impulses. It may be conceived of as an expression (and product) of basic biological tendencies toward organismic unity, synthesis, integration, and steadiness. At the same time the instincts, which are also expressions of biological tendencies toward survival and adaptation, are among the pressures which the ego has to mediate and manage. Thus the ego is the guardian of the vital balance.[10]

It is not possible to read such a passage and continue to believe in a basic opposition between psychoanalysis and systems theory, unless one specifically limits the validity of the latter to interpersonal and social processes, denying it for intrapsychic and individual ones. To do this, however, would contradict the claims of general systems theory to be universally applicable, claims that I regard as quite legitimate. Modern psychoanalysis does indeed regard the psyche as a dynamic system in which the ego serves as a balancing agent, maintaining equilibrium by constantly mediating between various internal and external influences. Clearly, a structural analogy exists here with social systems (such as groups or families) on a higher level, and with biological systems (such as organs or cells) on a lower one. Hartmann suggests such a parallel himself when he compares the "conflict-free sphere of the ego" to the peaceful hinterland of a country whose army is engaged in conflict with invaders at its frontiers.[11] All psychoanalysis is nothing but an attempt—which has its drawbacks, but for the time being is still indispensable—to understand the structure and functioning of this intrapsychic system, using the methods of introspection, empathy, and precise observation of an intimate interpersonal process, namely the analytic relationship itself. The results are, as Freud always emphasized, hypothetical constructs with a certain margin of error; nevertheless, no other theoretical model available today even begins to match psychoanalysis in its detailed understanding of intrapsychic processes.

The Modern Psychoanalytic Doctrine of Narcissism

Certainly one of the most important and fruitful developments in psychoanalysis in the last twenty years has been the expansion of the theory of narcissism by Winnicott, Balint, Grunberger, Kohut, Kernberg, and others. In general terms this theory focuses on the growth of a sense of identity and self-esteem in the first, "preoedipal" years of life and the possible ways in which such growth can be disturbed. In these early phases the object and partner relations that play a central role in the oedipal phase and still later in the neuroses of adult life are not yet possible.

The growth of a sense of individual identity is crucial to these early phases; the developmental task can therefore be identified as the formation of an independent psychical apparatus capable of functioning with sufficient stability and consistency. The child must develop a "self" or "ego" (a less precise term) separate from that of the mother, with whom it is at first inseparably connected.

I shall go into the issues raised by the theory of narcissism soon, particularly its application to psychotic conditions and thus also to the type of family constellation to which modern communications and systems theory has paid most attention. But first I want to point out that although the theory has been formulated in psychoanalytic terms, it can also be expressed in terms of systems theory. The question then becomes one of how to detach one system from another (in this case a psychic system) or how to construct a new system in a manner that allows it to form an independent whole with its own homeostatic laws while at the same time reproducing the pattern of an older system. This is an interesting process that occurs countless times in nature (as in cell division and sexual reproduction), and it is therefore of enormous general significance; however, so far as I know it has hardly been studied by systems theorists. In our particular context the process of separation and individuation is a good example of how certain psychoanalytical ideas can be formulated in terms of systems theory, and vice versa. It offers more support for the hypothesis that the two theories complement rather than contradict each other.

Even without citing further examples I feel justified in claiming that in principle psychoanalysis and systems theory are in close agreement on many points; I would even go so far as to say the Freud himself would probably have adopted systems theory and integrated it into his theory of psychoanalysis, had it been available in his day. No doubt we have to consider the possibility that "psychoanalytic systems theory" may represent a special application of the general theory; in that case it would apply to *intrapsychic* processes, which can be viewed as an open system *sui generis* in a hierarchy of higher- and lower-level systems and subsystems, such as cells, cell groups, organs, organ systems, and organisms, on the one hand, and individuals, families, groups, and societies on the other. There are indications that such a theory is being developed; an article by Otto Kernberg, though devoted mainly to other questions, has suggested that the internal world of object representations can be viewed as essential elements of an intrapsychic system controlled by the ego and limited by its boundaries. In Kernberg's opinion the primary task of this system is to fulfill the (object-oriented) needs of the id.[12] In my own view this concept is too narrow; I would prefer to consider the entire "psychic apparatus," including id, ego, and superego, as an intrapsychic system in the modern sense. Its function could then be defined as mediation not just between the needs of the id and external objects or their internalized representations, but rather between the needs of the entire organism (in psychoanalytic terms, the self) and all external and internal reality.

Kernberg's view of the world of internalized objects and its origins is of particular interest in connection with schizophrenic mechanisms, among other things (see Chapter 5). I hope also to establish, in the area of how internalized objects are formed, several more links between psychoanalytic and systemic concepts, and between intrapsychic and family processes. The two theories have used different methods and, not surprisingly, arrived at different conceptualizations; however, to conclude that they are therefore contradictory and mutually exclusive merely clouds our perspective, preventing us from seeing the possibilities that open up when we consider them together.

A striking example of such a possibility is offered in the field of cognitive functions by the genetic epistemology of Jean Piaget. Perhaps his greatest achievement was perceiving intrapsychic or psychological concepts (namely his "schemata") very early on as homeostatically regulated systems or structures in precisely the modern sense.

According to Piaget these systems accommodate themselves to the external world in a dialectical process as the child's intelligence develops (see Chapter 2), thereby permitting the child to deal with reality in the best possible way—as it is encountered. Partly for methodological reasons, Piaget paid little attention to the area of affectivity; but the possibility that analogous processes must also occur there is central to the idea of affect-logic that I wish to develop. Combining the approaches of psychoanalysis and systems theory appears to open the way to a better understanding of the interplay not only between the internal and external world but also between thinking and feeling.

The remaining two sections of this chapter present a preliminary outline of how such a synthesis might be structured, using two examples. These preliminary ideas will be refined and expanded in later chapters.

Narcissism and Family Dynamics

The major contribution of the modern psychoanalytic theory of narcissism to our understanding of human development consists in its identification of the problems of individuation and growth of a sense of self in early childhood. As the child detaches himself from his physiological and psychological fusion with the mother, a new and (within certain limits) autonomous psychic system is demarcated. Psychoanalysts have described what happens when this fails to occur—when no clearly defined, consistent psychic structure (or, in Piaget's terms, no equilibrated schemata capable of functioning effectively) comes into existence: a serious "ego weakness" is the result. The contours of internalized representations, both of the self and of objects, remain blurred; the weak ego boundaries, described so often in recent psychoanalytic literature on "borderline cases" and psychotics, manifest themselves in an insufficient demarcation between one's own feelings, thoughts, and opinions and those of others. Other manifestations include an increased tendency to various projections and introjections and a lower threshold of irritability (increased sensitivity and vulnerability). These occur in combination with a defective sense of identity and insufficient or inconsistent self-confidence (a tendency toward feelings of depersonalization, hypochondria, depressive self-deprecation, or manic self-aggrandizement). For the past thirty years both psychoanalysts and family therapists have been studying with an increasing degree of precision the conditions that can lead to such defective ego structures. They are completely agreed that these defective structures arise in dynamic interaction with the child's parents, especially the mother; the term *schizophrenogenic mother* was coined as a result. Although this overly simplistic concept has since been considerably refined and elaborated (the particular behavior of mothers of schizophrenics can be viewed partly as a consequence, and not as a cause, of her child's illness; similar constellations are observed in families without schizophrenic offspring; the term provokes hostility rather than insight and collaboration by relatives in practical work), one crucial insight has remained, although to my knowledge it has seldom been clearly formulated: mothers—or, as we shall see later, parents—of children with narcissistic ego defects often show similar narcissistic disturbances themselves. They tend to be insufficiently separated from their own mother or parents. Murray Bowen, Ivan Boszormenyi-Nagy, and others have gone on to develop the "multi-generational" theory of schizophrenia.[13] This kind of parent-child constellation produces as its most important consequence a pervasive *confusion*, which under some circumstances may persist into adulthood. Feelings, fears, needs, thoughts, opinions, and even perceptions are mixed together, or not properly distinguished, by parents and children.

In this field a wealth of observations by psychoanalysts and systems and communications theorists, working either independently or together, has converged to an astonishing degree. It is obvious that close links must exist between the blurring of generational boundaries by means of abnormal alliances across generations, such as has often been described by Salvador Minuchin,[14] Mara Selvini Palazzoli,[15] and other systems-oriented authors, on the one hand, and the psychoanalytic accounts of weak ego boundaries or insufficient demarcation between parents and children on the other hand. Parental conflict is usually present in such families, though in concealed rather than open form. Placed in a psychoanalytic framework, such conflict appears not only understandable but inevitable. The same applies to the often-described general inability of such families to endure open conflict (see, for example, L. C. Wynne's concept of "pseudo-mutuality"):[16] if the parents manifest narcissistic defects themselves—and it has been shown that there is a high probability that *both* parents will, since each will be attracted to this kind of partner on the basis of immature and "pregenital" idealizations—their object or partner relations will necessarily have a strongly narcissistic flavor. In other words, they will be looking above all for their partner to provide them with a sense of completion, a correction of the "basic fault" from which they suffer, which consists in essence in the lack of a sense of self-esteem and identity.[17]

It is just as inevitable that a spouse suffering from severe narcissistic disorders will be able to provide little or no "completion," since he or she is unable to give support to the other except to fulfill the need to get support himself or herself. The result, in the short or long run, is deep mutual frustration, disappointment, and alienation, a marital conflict that the partners cannot openly admit to or deal with, since in their narcissistic relationship every step toward genuine independence by one must be felt by the other as a great threat. (In narcissistic object relations the other is a part of myself; his function is to satisfy my basic needs, and if he becomes independent, I lose all hope of "completion.") Thus the reasons why such families have particular difficulties confronting each other face to face are deep-rooted. Spouses frustrated in this way tend to "solve" the problem by seeking a substitute partner in one of their children, especially if a child is particularly dependent and thus suited for the role of narcissistic object. (Since the child's lack of independence may be influenced by illness or a weak constitution, it is also possible that genetic factors may be involved in such a process.) When such mechanisms exist in both parents and in their children—the fatal chain in which children acquire the same weaknesses as their parents'—we have a system of powerful forces, activated by the needs of all participants. Every family member seeks to maintain the pathological constellation at all costs and to prevent any of the others from achieving real change by becoming independent. The participants' intrapsychic needs are understandable only in psychoanalytic terms, however. In this situation systems theory can merely register the factual existence of processes occurring in an "interpersonal system" (the family); the origin of the pathological homeostatic forces remains entirely unclear until psychoanalytic investigation of the dynamics of the "intrapsychic systems" (individuals) involved can shed some light on it.

Confusion pervades the communications structure in such families. In addition, both psychoanalysts and communications theorists agree that this structure is characterized by a number of special phenomena that appear designed to sabotage any autonomous impulse by a family member that might lead to a genuine escape from the pathological constellation. Since family researchers began to study this state of affairs twenty or thirty years ago, ever subtler forms of such sabotage have been described, including devaluation, contradiction, denial, splitting, disqualification, and mystification. The psychoanalyst H. F. Searles was the first to show that such constant acts of sabotage can create so much confusion and tension in one of the participants that it finally "drives him crazy."[18] The family member with the weakest ego, either generally or at a particular moment, will then retreat into his own system of reference—a system of feeling, thinking, and functioning that is accessible to normal understanding only with great difficulty or not at all. (Chapter 6 deals with the mechanisms of this disorder in more detail.)

Our insight into the confused forms of communication that often prevail in families with psychotic or prepsychotic members was greatly improved by the introduction of the concept of the double bind—the paradoxical and painfully confusing simultaneous communication of contradictory instructions, rules, feelings, or "definitions" of interpersonal relationships on different levels of logic or expression.[19] Although double binds (affective-cognitive dilemmas) are difficult to pinpoint in practice and are not limited to families with psychotic members, most family researchers concur that the phenomenon is an important aspect of severely disturbed affective-cognitive communication.

This particular process suggests another possible synthesis of the two general theories under discussion here. Everything indicates that we can advance our understanding of the double bind as an interpersonal phenomenon only by taking a psychoanalytical approach and studying the intrapsychic constellations of the participants, particularly the mother and child. Initially the mother-child relationship is characterized by the child's narcissistic and physical needs. If, however, the narcissistic needs are *mutual,* and the child represents a narcissistic object to the mother (and possibly to other family members as well) in psychoanalytic terms, then this relationship must have the following structure: The mother would like to love the child for his own sake only, just as she loves her husband and the other family members. She pretends (without being aware that it is a pretense) that she is prepared to promote the child's growth toward strength, adulthood, and autonomy according to *his* needs, just as selflessly as a gardener must take care of a plant according to the laws of its own growth if it is to flourish—and the family goes along with this pretense. But this apparent love is in a deeper and unconscious sense something else: the mother in fact loves the child not mainly for his own sake but for hers. She wants him to fulfill her own (unconscious) need to be whole, intact, and loved. She forces him to carry out this function in her life, and above all she cannot permit him to grow away from her and become independent.

This tragic and irresolvable paradox defines the double bind. Although it may take countless different forms—crass or subtle, open or concealed—the same basic phenomenon can always be found at bottom, which is no less serious for being so simple. The paradoxical, simultaneously positive and negative message can be summed up as:

I (don't) love *you* $\rightleftarrows$ I (don't) love *myself.*

The description above was limited to the mother-child relationship only for simplicity's sake. In reality an equally narcissistic child-mother relationship must also exist, one which is created and which transcends the infant's normal physical needs for care; there must also be a narcissistic relationship between the child's mother and father. It has not been sufficiently emphasized in the literature on the subject that the double binds in such a family are *mutual,* not one-sided. Regular, periodic observations of families in which psychotic patterns of communication prevail have shown that the children as well as parents constantly present their own needs, thoughts, and feelings as those of the others. They, too, negate those of other family members and send double-bind messages such as

I (don't) love you $\rightleftarrows$ I (don't) love myself

or

I am doing this only for you $\rightleftarrows$ myself.

This is only logical from the point of view of both systems theory and psychoanalysis: the children necessarily suffer from the same fundamental problem as their parents. A simple learning process is certainly involved; beyond that, however, on a deeper level the children have no other choice. They have to communicate their own situation as it really is, and the only possible response to a double bind may be a double-bind answer. The child must continually confirm and simultaneously deny the mother's love for him (and his love for her). The systems theorist would describe this situation as one in which the alteration of one element (here an element in a communications system) must necessarily lead to alteration of all other elements.

This analysis makes it easier to see that often—as family researchers have come to recognize more and more clearly, especially in the case of schizophrenics—guilt and shame (which are essentially transgressions against life), real and not merely imagined psychological rapes, and archaic forms of cruelty such as being mentally invaded and destroyed play a major role in disguised forms. (See also Boszormenyi-Nagy's concept of "debit and credit accounts.")[20] Such things usually remain hidden far below the surface, and routine exploration in family sessions rarely brings them to light. In certain cases even a therapist who has known the family of a schizophrenic patient for decades may be able to catch only some glimpses of them. All the participants "know" of their existence, although this knowledge is rarely conscious; beneath the surface, however, such mechanisms dominate their behavior. I suspect that an additional and highly effective motive to maintain the "family homeostasis" lies in the participants' panic at the thought of their "debit account" being exposed, since this may have existed for decades and be virtually unpayable in objective terms. The two following case histories may help to suggest how the debit account can function.

A talented thirty-year-old man, the son of a wealthy and authoritarian farmer, was raised from an early age, much against his own inclinations, to take over the farm and carry on the family tradition.[21] His father prevented him from getting the kind of education that might "lead him astray." From the age of eleven on* the boy became increasingly withdrawn and "strange." He experienced an outbreak of severe, catatonic psychosis accompanied by mutism at eighteen, on the very day he had passed the examination for the school of agriculture to please his parents. The patient's condition became chronic immediately, and he spent several years in a psychiatric hospital, until the father finally was forced to sell the farm and take a job as a traveling salesman. From that moment on the patient began to improve! He acquired a startling degree of insight into his own illness, and in individual therapy sessions he was able to grasp at once that he had "come out the winner" in the end; he had forced his father to give in. The father

* *Translator's note:* The age at which, in Switzerland and many other European countries, children move from primary to different types of secondary schools, only one of which prepares for college or university entrance.

then took to preaching to everyone at meetings for patients' families that one must give the children a free rein.

A married woman had been in her early childhood the adored only daughter of a patriarchal businessman. At age eight, however, she was completely dethroned by the arrival of the longed-for son and heir and later a younger sister. At about age thirty, shortly after her father's death, she became psychotic (a chronic paranoid-catatonic psychosis that lasted until the end of her life). The relationship with her entire family was characterized by strong tensions at this time, particularly in the case of her sister. Not until long after her death were the facts surrounding the outbreak of her psychosis brought to light. It transpired that when the patient was pregnant, and following the birth of her child, her younger sister had succeeded in winning the affections of the patient's husband. These events were hushed up by the entire family for decades, so that they remained unknown to the younger members. The patient's occasional references to them and her outbursts of rage were simply ascribed to her "craziness."

In the first case the combination of personal and family difficulties is evident, at least on a superficial level. This is also true for the second case, after a little psychoanalytic interpretation (made easier by additional information). The sensitive girl's dethronement by her brother, whom she had treated ambivalently from the time of his birth, both spoiling and protecting him while also aggressively rejecting and dominating him, had clearly led to a severe identity crisis. This was later exacerbated by the arrival of a younger sister. It is not difficult to imagine the unbearable complications and "fluctuations" (discussed further in Chapter 6)—both familial and intrapsychic, real and experienced in transference—that arose when the father's death coincided with both the birth of a child and the husband's infidelity, with this younger sister. Everything fits together like the pieces of a jigsaw puzzle, but a full understanding of the case requires the points of view of both psychoanalysis and family dynamics.

Oedipal Problems and Family Dynamics

The problems of the later oedipal stage, like those in the stage of primary narcissism, occur both intrapsychically and within the family.

It again appears evident that a synthesis of psychoanalysis, systems theory, and family dynamics can lead to insights that one theory alone cannot provide. However, this area so central to psychoanalysis has received surprisingly little attention in research on family dynamics.

Two aspects of the oedipal stage appear particularly significant for our topic from a psychoanalytic point of view. First, it is a dynamic process that—as is becoming more clearly recognized today—can occur in the form originally described by Freud only when all the participants, children *and* parents, have previously reached a certain degree of psychological maturity. They must have achieved sufficient narcissistic consolidation and demarcation to make genuine object relations between two (relatively) autonomous people possible. The primary narcissistic ties between mother and child described above (which include the infant's physical needs) must have been loosened enough to permit both to perceive themselves as relatively independent "centers" capable of feeling desires. Thus the mother and father, at least, must possess clearly determined identities with regard to their own sex, age, and role, and definite boundaries must exist between the generations. Second, it is structurally important that the problems and dynamics of the oedipal stage are specifically concerned with *three* participants. The original symbiotic unity between mother and child has become dramatically expanded and complicated by the appearance on the scene of a third party, the father. He, for his part, can emerge from the original foggy undifferentiation of all the partners (or systems) in the constellation and take on clear contours only to the degree that the mother and child succeed in demarcating and separating themselves. Freud, followed by Jacques Lacan in particular, repeatedly stressed the importance of this "hinge" on which the further development of psychological maturity depended. Some ideas from systems theory—or in this case its close relative, structuralism— can help to explain why this is so. The expansion of a dyadic system (which in fact strongly resembles a single-element system for a considerable while) to a triadic system involves an enormous gain in combinatory possibilities. Not only do many more possible relationships and combinations of relationships exist between three partners than between two, in the purely mathematical sense, but also in a certain sense the expansion from two to three is for the child like escaping from a prison. The opening of the door to a third person represents the child's first experience of the possibility that someone or something else exists at all. Thus he leaves the confinement of the exclusive mother-child relationship for true freedom. *Everything* else—every number larger than two, every conceivable constellation—is implied and experienced intuitively by the child as possible, for the first time.

It is no wonder that Lacan has drawn a connection between the entrance on the scene of the father, the *third* element, with the first flashes of intellect, language, and symbols in general, a structuring element of the most dramatic kind (here it should be stressed that no sexist implications are intended). A large number of combinations and "games" in the family relationships, in both the mathematical and the psychological sense, becomes possible, and at least some of them are experimented with in practice. These combinations involve both feeling and thinking; that is, to they occur in that area of total affective-cognitive experience which I call affect-logic and which without any doubt makes up our actual psychological reality much more than either aspect on its own. These games could be considered as a kind of "psychoaffective gymnastics" of exploration, practicing, and maturation, with immense power to structure experience. Once the protagonists in the triangle have been isolated and defined, all the possible oedipal constellations described by psychoanalysts—positive, negative, and hybrid—can be played out in a ballet of attractions and rejections, approaches and retreats, sympathies and antipathies, accompanied by feelings of rivalry, jealousy, guilt, castration, and failure, on the one hand, and gain, affirmation, wholeness, and success on the other. This process establishes fundamental functional systems that are both psychoaffective *and* cognitive, systems that, once established, must be used or run through repeatedly at later times, like associative or semantic channels or networks of meaning.

In the next chapter we shall see that such affective-cognitive systems of reference have a structure analogous to Piaget's schemata in the purely cognitive area, and that this structure is arrived at by similar processes of assimilation, accommodation, and equilibration. This means that they are essentially accessible through the concepts of systems theory and structuralism, so that once again, as in the case of narcissism, more profound insight into the actual psychic events of this decisive phase of development can be gained from a synthesis of psychoanalysis and systems theory.

There is yet another area in which systems theory can shed light on oedipal constellations, although to my knowledge it has hardly been explored yet. Clearly, the psychoaffective gymnastics of possible combination described above must proceed in widely differing ways, depending on the degree of maturity (firmly established identity, independence, and ability to recognize the "separateness" of others) attained by the parents, and thus also depending on the general quality of their relationship. If the parents' narcissism makes them too preoccupied with their own emotional needs, or if they are in conflict for other reasons, then the games and combinations cannot be experimented with freely to produce the best possible structures. Instead, sudden fixations will occur, as well as excessively painful or pleasurable incestuous ties or complexes laden with affect or guilt; these are certain to work themselves into functional systems of reference as they are established. The normal process of grief, for example, so essential for the establishment of identity and maturation, which the child must go through at the end of the oedipal stage, is rendered impossible if the child is not permitted to experience clearly the limitations of his sex and age, and if because of their own narcissism the parents take an ambivalent stance and encourage the child's incestuous hopes.

It appears likely that later neurotic constellations are connected with such (potentially) pathological behavioral fixations; it is also theoretically possible that an analysis of family structure and dynamics with an orientation toward systems theory could uncover these important interpersonal behavior patterns and modify them in the family more easily than could an individual psychoanalysis.

We now arrive at the question of how relevant these largely theoretical observations may be to practical therapy. At this point I can do no more that sketch the outlines of an answer, for we have only just begun to investigate the connections between the two theories. The psychoanalytic point of view as presented here may perhaps contribute to a refinement of systems theorists' therapeutic techniques; it has already had a clear influence on the sophisticated techniques of Mara Selvini Palazzoli, the former psychoanalyst who now practices a radical form of systems-oriented therapy (see Chapter 7). Likewise, the insights of systems theory and family dynamics can certainly broaden the conceptual horizons of psychoanalysts. It is entirely conceivable that an understanding of both approaches could lead therapists in future to choose one or the other form of treatment in accordance with the particular situation. Thus in instances of explosive, narcissistically determined guilt in the type of psychosis described in the case histories above, the psychoanalyst might recognize the advisability of a systemic approach, whereas in the case of, say, a neurotic schoolteacher, personnel manager, or family head, systemic reasons might lead to the choice of a psychoanalylic treatment, since changes in one person's intrapsychic situation could be expected to lead to a number of changes in the whole system. In this way crucial considerations of the most efficient way to achieve the ultimate goal could determine the choice of treatment, rather than unclear preferences, which today often resemble articles of belief more than objective criteria do. A careful and fair comparison will remain impossible, however, as long as both theories continue to be seen as irreconcilable opposites.

A discussion of the specific therapeutic consequences arising from these considerations will be reserved for the last chapter, but for the time being I hope to have shown that a combination of the two approaches is not only theoretically possible but also probably promising in practical terms, even if we keep their fruitful differences in mind. We must now take a closer look at the possible structure of affect-logic, continuing all the while to take into consideration both the psychoanalytic and systemic points of view.

2   On Affect-Logic

The writer's joy is the thought which can become all emotion, the
emotion which can become all thought.

—Thomas Mann, *Death in Venice*

In the preceding pages I used the term *affect-logic* several times to
describe the coexistence of feeling and thinking, or affective and cognitive functions, in an inseparable whole that characterizes the way
our minds experience reality far better than either aspect taken on its
own. This chapter explores the question of what this affect-logic actually is or might be: The logic of feelings, and the feelings of logic. I
must say right at the outset that the answer is by no means certain,
either for me or, so far as I know, for anyone else. We are confronted
here with a genuine scientific problem, the solution of which would
no doubt take us a long way toward a better understanding of the
human psyche. It will not be possible to offer complete answers to
such a difficult question, and my aim is much more modest: to define
the problem clearly and to map out the general area of possible solutions.

The Problem Defined: A Postulate of the Unity of the Psyche

The problem poses itself in the following manner: As soon as we
attempt to study the human mind, we are accustomed to approach it
through the various scientific disciplines that concern themselves with
this subject. Because each of these has its own particular point of
view, however, we possess many pieces of information about different

aspects of the mind and brain that have little or no apparent connection with one another. We have academic psychology on the one hand and the most varied schools of psychoanalysis on the other; anthropologists, neuropsychologists, communications and systems theorists, and researchers in other areas all construct their own specific picture of the psyche. Each field takes a slice of the pie, so to speak, the slice that looks most promising for investigation with its methods; but it soon appears that we have lost sight of the phenomenon as a whole, which it was our original intention to study.

The fact that scientists choose particular aspects of phenomena to study is obviously a methodologically necessary and efficient procedure, and I have no general quarrel with it. But in our context it is striking that this division has occurred in the case of affect and logic. They have tended to become the subjects of very different and unrelated disciplines. This is true for psychology and the study of affectivity in general, but especially for the two fields of research which have specialized in these phenomena and with which we will be particularly concerned here: Freud's psychoanalysis for affective phenomena and Piaget's genetic epistemology for the cognitive functions. In the more than fifty years that these disciplines have existed side by side, they have undergone simultaneous and parallel development and gained in both depth and breadth; nevertheless there has been surprisingly little integration of the two theories. Affective factors play a very limited role in genetic epistemology, cognitive factors represent only a very small part of the psychoanalytic picture of the human mind.

At the same time, however, there is no lack of evidence that both Freud and Piaget originally had the *totality* of the mind in view. In two early works "Project for a Scientific Psychology" (1895)—which remained unpublished until recently—and *The Interpretation of Dreams* (1900), Freud was concerned with fundamental questions about the connections between feeling and thinking, between the mechanisms of drives and affects, on the one hand, and of cognition on the other.[1] (Freud theorized that thought developed from substitute "hallucinations" when a drive was not directly satisfied; he also differentiated between "primary processes," governed by drives and affects, and "secondary processes," structured by rationality and reality. Then for many years psychoanalysis focused on drives and affects, until Freud's work on the ego and the id (1923) led to the development of ego psychology and a renewed interest in the connections between affective and cognitive functions. A few psychoanalytic authors—among them de Saussure (1933), Rapaport (1950), Gressot (1955), Gouin-Décarie (1962), Escalona (1963), and Haynal (1975)—attempted to establish explicit links with Piaget's genetic epistemology. The brief survey below is based in part on their work.[2] In addition, a recent study by Henri Schneider contains a number of ideas that often bear a striking resemblance to those discussed here.[3]

As a young man Piaget was so interested in psychoanalysis (and therefore in the affective aspect of the psyche) that he undertook a training analysis, treated several patients, and actively participated in psychoanalytic congresses. In 1923 he published a study of symbolic thought in children in which he devoted much more attention to affective factors than in his later publications. There he uses the term *affective logic,* which he does not define precisely, however, and to my knowledge never used again. This work of Piaget's resembles Freud's "Project for a Scientific Psychology" in that it outlines many themes of the author's later work: Piaget mentions here the concepts of assimilation and accommodation, reversibility, the role of mental imagery, and the structure of the unconscious. It is in fact a veritable storehouse of interesting ideas. In 1933 Piaget addressed a congress of French-speaking psychoanalysts on the relationship between psychoanalysis and intellectual development; this paper was the counterpart of de Saussure's 1933 article. In 1970 Piaget addressed the American Psychoanalytic Association on "The Affective Unconscious and the Cognitive Unconscious."[4] Still, the amount of space devoted to affective as opposed to cognitive functions in Piaget's immensely wide-ranging work is extraordinarily small. Not until 1966, with the publications of *The Psychology of the Child* (coauthored with Bärbel Inhelder), did signs of an actual synthesis appear.[5] The following passage is found in the conclusion:

> As we have seen repeatedly, affectivity constitutes the energetics of behavior patterns whose cognitive aspect refers to the structures alone. There is no behavior pattern, however intellectual, which does not involve affective factors as motives; but reciprocally, there can be no affective states without the intervention of perceptions or comprehensions which constitute their cognitive structure. Behavior is therefore of a piece, even if the structures do not explain its energetics and if, vice versa, its energetics do not account for its structures. The two aspects, affective and cognitive, are at the same time inseparable and irreducible.[6]

My reflections on the nature of affect-logic below are based—in complete accord with Piaget and Inhelder's findings—on the assumption that in our experience there is no real and clear distinction between affect and intellect (or between affective and cognitive functions, between feeling and thinking; this also means, as I shall go on to show, that there is none between the more "physical" and the more "intellectual" aspects of the psyche). I use the term *affect-logic* merely to indicate that logic and affects are closely connected and indeed, just as Piaget emphasizes, never occur independently of each other. This term also is meant to imply something that represents a certain deviation from Piaget's lines of thought, namely that both possess a similar basic structure pointing in turn to a similar and common genesis. And insofar as the affective and cognitive areas can be regarded as the two most important manifestations of psychological activity (meaning that taken together they represent something quite comprehensive), the concept of an affect-logic postulates a structural unity for the mind as a whole. The idea of affect-logic aims at a "unified field theory of the psyche," with "psyche" to be understood in the broadest possible sense, including not only affective and cognitive phenomena but also social, cultural, scientific, and artistic phenomena. The final goal of a fully developed theory of affect-logic would thus be the ambitious one of understanding the affective and cognitive components of *all* possible psychological processes and manifestations, not in isolation, but in their close and constant interaction. This theory should finally enable us to understand the workings of affect-logic in the narrower sense, that is, the logical structure of affects and the affective structure of logic.

I shall first summarize some of the central elements of the two theories important for this task, psychoanalysis and genetic epistemology, then attempt a synthesis.

Affect and Intellect in the Psychoanalytic View

The psychoanalytic doctrine of affect is extraordinarily complex and far-reaching, since all psychoanalysis deals with hardly anything but affect. On the other hand, there is a paradoxical but significant sense in which this doctrine is in fact simple, since beyond the two main affects or drives of love and hate (also referred to, approximately synonymously, as pleasure and unpleasure, libido and destrudo, sexuality and aggression, or eros and thanatos, depending on the stage of development of psychoanalytic theory and the particular context), there remain virtually only fear, grief, and melancholy; all the many other affects and fine gradations between them have not been systematically integrated into the theoretical framework. Love and hate appear as the two central opposing forces in our emotional life; grief and melancholy, like affect-laden obsessions and compulsions, hysterical phenomena, and other neurotic symptoms, represent merely specific transformation of feelings which were originally erotic or aggressive but which are prevented by unconscious repression from entering the higher levels of the mind. Fear is a signal of external danger, but perhaps even more an indication of internal danger threatening from the possible eruption of forbidden and repressed feelings. The most important regulators of our emotional life are the pleasure principle and the reality principle (the striving for pleasure, avoidance of what is not pleasurable, and the necessary adaptation to reality). In addition the dynamics of emotional life are governed by the "Nirvana principle," which constantly seeks to equalize tension and reduce it to a minimum.

Several other aspects of psychoanalytic doctrine are also of importance for our topic. Libidinal and aggressive affects (which are not clearly distinguished from drives or instincts in psychoanalysis) develop from birth throughout childhood in a regular progression. Each phase is marked by a particular dominant drive and centers on the corresponding erogenous zone. Thus the major stages are the oral phase, with a focus on the area of the mouth and the intake of nourishment; the anal phase, with the processes of excretion and retention in the foreground; and, finally, the phallic and genital stage, in which sexual organs and feelings predominate. Each of these major stages, however, provides a matrix for a large number of much subtler emotions whose underlying connection with their origin is no longer immediately obvious (see the discussion of sublimation below). Tamed, modified, and equilibrated by the regulators mentioned above, both libidinal and aggressive impulses undergo a process of increasing differentiation in the course of maturation, culminating in the oedipal conflict of the genital phase. Somewhere between the ages of two and four the child experiences most intensely the triangular situation existing between himself or herself and the parent of the same and opposite sex. If the child can pass through this phase and resolve the conflict under favorable conditions, a differentiated and stable equilibrium of affective forces results. This lays a foundation for the later development of a harmonious personality. In less favorable circumstances disharmonious, pathological, or pathogenic states of tension and "fixations" develop, in which psychoanalysts see the seeds of neuroses and other psychological disturbances of adult life.

This description of affective development should make it clear that even psychoanalysts do not see it as occurring in an abstract intrapsychic space, but rather in interaction with those closest to the child, usually beginning with the mother but later including the father, siblings, playmates, and so on. Initially, of course, the infant is not able to perceive these partners as independent objects separate from himself; he is thus equally unable to cathect them with particular feelings. The perception of objects, the creation of internal object representations, and, parallel to this, the growth of a sense of a defined self with its own identity all undergo an important process of development in the first years of life. This process is inseparably linked to affective development and, like it, reaches a preliminary culmination during the oedipal phase.

Since psychoanalysts see cognitive as well as affective factors at work in the creation of adequate internalized representations of both self and objects—as Kernberg in particular has stressed in the last few years—psychoanalytic theory contains an implicit recognition of the inseparability of affect and intellect.

The following concepts in connection with *thinking and intellectual functions* are also of importance in our context.[8] Ever since Freud's early formulations in his "Project for a Scientific Psychology" and *The Interpretation of Dreams*, psychoanalysis has located the origin of intellectual functions in the differentiation between primary and secondary processes that begins in the first year of life. These are primary drives in need of immediate gratification that obey the laws of the unconscious; and the secondary cognitive processing of these drives, which leads to consciousness and rationality. These secondary processes arise from the necessity, repeatedly imposed by reality, of accepting a delay in the gratification of primary drives. Psychoanalysis thus sees the origins of thinking in a hallucinatory or imagined gratification, which anticipates and acts as a substitute for the actual gratification. This substitution during the period of delayed gratification is made possible by memory traces in the brain. To start with, therefore, thinking represents a detour to the gratification of primary drives. Even though the reality principle structures thought to an increasing degree, contributing to the development of the secondary processes, thinking is governed indirectly by the pleasure principle. According to Freud, thought is to be understood primarily as a *trial action* using small quantities of displaced energy, developed in conjunction with internalized representations of the objects that provide drive gratification (in early childhood usually the mother). Piaget's formulations are quite similar. Psychoanalysis clearly sees the driving force behind all thought in internal, instinctual needs—that is, in something either pleasurable or not pleasurable and thus affective, whereas the content of our thoughts derives from external reality as perceived by our sensory organs.

This is the general model on which psychoanalytic understanding of cognitive functions and their development is based. The content changes according to the various phases of libidinal development—that is, the oral, anal, and genital stages and their different objects. But the impetus, though affected increasingly by the reality principle and proceeding to higher stages, remains the same striving for pleasure or avoidance of pain. With time the child learns to sublimate his undisguised drives in many ways, so that sexual curiosity, for example, may take the form of intellectual curiosity, or the sexual rivalry of the oedipal phase become the self-assertiveness and competitiveness of the adult.

The ideas of Heinz Hartmann are especially interesting in our context of the interplay between affective and cognitive factors. In 1939 he introduced a concept in ego psychology which he called the "conflict-free sphere of the ego" ("neutralization," "deconflictualization") and which is connected with the process of sublimation.[9] This theory states that motor, sensory, or cognitive functions such as walking, sensory perceptions, speaking, and thinking are originally laden with emotion and therefore with conflict as well. They originate in sexual, aggressive, or other affective impulses (such as the striving for pleasure or power, the hope of winning someone's love, identifying with and imitating important persons, and feelings of rivalry or inferiority), but because they are under the control of the ego, these functions can come with time and under favorable conditions to operate in an increasingly affect-free and conflict-free manner. In the end an almost total affective neutralization and automatization can be reached, although affective cathexis and conflict can surface again at any point. One good example is the experience of driving a car; almost every driver can recall the strong emotions associated with learning to drive, and the way in which driving became an "automatic" activity only occasionally interrupted by strong outbursts of renewed conflict.

Both orthodox psychoanalysts and modern ego psychologists agree that affective elements are involved in *all* motor, sensory, and cognitive functions, in either this or a similar way; they diverge only in their opinions as to how far these elements can be neutralized and over the question of whether—beyond such secondary, deconflictualized components of the ego—there exists from birth a primary, conflict-free sphere of the ego (possibly taking the form of innate potentials for motor, sensory, and cognitive development differentiated according to their own laws). Ego psychology has thus made an important contribution to the *affective* side of a possible affect-logic that is consistent both with the psychoanalytic doctrine of affect and with academic psychology.

Nevertheless, ego psychology and other schools of psychoanalysis take the cognitive functions into account in only a cursory manner. As yet there has been no genuine attempt to integrate into psychoanalytic theory the results of research on the origins and structure of intelligence.

Intellect and Affect in Piaget's Genetic Epistemology

"I believe that questions concerning the cognitive unconscious are similar to questions concerning the affective unconscious ... I am convinced that one day cognitive psychology and psychoanalysis must merge and form a general theory, which will improve and correct both cognitive psychology and psychoanalysis." Jean Piaget made this avowal before the American Psychoanalytic Association in 1970.[10] Piaget, his colleagues, and his students have been systematically investigating the structure and development of cognitive functions in children, both in minute detail and on a monumental scale, for more than fifty years. We can thus expect important insights into our topic from his life's work, which represents a counterpart to psychoanalysis both in its broad scope and in its tendency to exclude affective factors.

Like psychoanalysis with respect to affectivity, genetic epistemology has established the existence of *a regular pattern of development for human cognitive functions* from birth to adolescence. There are four major stages in this development.[10]

1. In the *sensorimotor* period, which lasts from birth to about eighteen months, a purely practical and concrete "intelligence" is formed,

focused exclusively on very small distances and very short time spans. Six developmental steps follow one another in smooth transition: spontaneous reflexes and movements; first habits; secondary circular reactions; coordination between means and ends; discovery of new means; and invention of new means through internal coordination and sudden insight. Nevertheless, this early "logic of action" contains clear structures of order and relationship created through the combination of simple schemata. The most important of these are the realization that objects are permanent (as the child grasps the continued existence of objects and people who appear and disappear again), the creation of a first continuous structure of space and time, and the practical grasp of simple relations of cause and effect. These represent the foundation of all later thought processes.

2. In the next stage, which lasts from about eighteen months to age seven or eight, the child acquires a *semiotic or symbolic function* in a slow, progressive transition from concrete action to intellectual operations. The child becomes able to reproduce objects, events, or concepts with the aid of symbols and signs (differentiation between de Saussure's "signifier" and "signified"). Imitation, symbolic play, drawings, memory, the construction of mental images (ideas), and, above all, the acquisition of language play a central role in this process. It is crucial to this stage that the simple diachronic intelligence of the sensorimotor stage, which operates only one step at a time, gradually become able to condense successive actions into a representative synchronic whole. Repeated actions generate a schema—the elements of the action that can be repeated and generalized. Schemata thus represent *internalized actions*, just like the "operations" of a later stage.

In a first subphase (lasting until about age four), *symbolic thought* takes the form of *preconcepts* without the formation of general classes and without reversibility (see below). These represent an intermediate stage between general logical concepts and the purely individual action schemata of the sensorimotor stage, with all the limitations of such an "imaginative empiricism." In the next subphase, *intuitive thought* (which lasts until about age seven or eight), a mixture of two kinds of thought occurs. One kind is still largely connected with actions; it is subjective, egocentric, partly symbolic and partly logical, but without the full conservation of a whole, without reversibility, and without an objective concept of time. The other kind of thought shows the beginnings of generalization and objectification or "decentration," which lead to the stage of actual intellectual operations.

> Two small glasses, A and A₂, of identical shape and size, are each filled with an equal number of beads, and this equality is acknowledged by the child, who has filled the glasses himself, e.g., by placing a bead in A with one hand every time he places a bead in A₂ with the other hand. Next, A₂ is emptied into a differently shaped [e.g., thinner and taller] glass B, while A is left as a standard. Children of 4–5 years then conclude that the quantity of beads has changed, even though they are sure none has been removed or added . . .
>
> Suppose a child estimates that there are more beads in B than in A because the level has been raised. He thus "centres" his thought, or his attention, on the relation between the heights of B and A, and ignores the widths. But let us empty B into glass C or D, etc., which are even thinner and taller; there must come a point at which the child will reply, "There are fewer, because it is too narrow." There will thus be a correction on centring on height by a decentring of attention on to width . . . Now this transition from a single centring to two successive centrings heralds the beginnings of the operation; once he reasons with respect to both relations at the same time, the child will, in fact, deduce conservation.[12]

3. The period of *concrete operations*, which begins at about age seven and lasts until eleven or twelve, brings about a highly significant and often quite sudden change: relationships in the most diverse areas, which had previously been grasped only intuitively, are now brought into balance by a process of equilibration and are clearly recognized. The decisive step forward consists in the child's finally "grouping" several single aspects of a system into a related whole, as in the example with the beads cited above. This whole (the quantity of beads) is now preserved despite all transformations, such as being shifted to different containers. The operations performed on it become *reversible* (inversion, or negation and reciprocity); at the same time the abilities to classify, list, and order (from one group to another, from one to many), acquired separately in earlier stages, now come together to form a coherent whole. Among other things this permits the child to grasp the ideas of general time and space, measurement, and the system of whole numbers. All these operations remain limited to concrete objects and actions, however; the child's intelligence is not yet ready to grasp abstract ideas if they are presented as purely verbal propositions.

4. At eleven or twelve the child reaches the stage of *formal or propositional operations*. His thinking grows increasingly free of the need for direct and concrete actions through a kind of "literal" (that is, having to do with letters as symbols) reflection on a higher level ("reflective abstraction"; the performance of operations on operations). The basic operations such as classifying, ordering, counting, measuring, placing, and displacing in space and time, which formerly had to be connected with actions, can now be completely internalized and performed on purely verbal propositions (for example: Edith has lighter hair than Susan; Edith has darker hair than Lily. Who has the darkest hair of the three?). The child has acquired a maximum of formal mobility, a freedom and reversibility of thought that conforms to the laws of axiomatic, symbolic, and algorithmic logic. He now has at his disposal a new ability to perform logical operations not only on objects but also on ideas or hypotheses. These operations include implication (if . . . then), disjunction (A or B; A or also B; A and B), exclusion (either . . . or), incompatibility (neither . . . nor), and reciprocal implication. Both concrete and abstract wholes are conserved despite all transformations; the concepts of space and time extend generally and to infinity; thinking goes beyond the here and now. In contrast to the younger child, the adolescent enjoys using his newly acquired hypothetico-deductive abilities to form and discuss theories about everything imaginable, beyond the present moment and his own immediate experience. A fundamental process of *decentration* has occurred, decentration being the capacity to go beyond one's own actions and experience. This capacity begins to be acquired with the first sensorimotor schemata and grows clearer with each successive stage of development. The fact that an adolescent can group whatever he or she encounters within the framework of a coherent whole implies more generally the ability to take into consideration eventualities and abstractions as well as what is factual and real. It is obvious that with the acquisition of these formal abilities in adolescence possibilities open up for new and further decentration, not only for the individual but also for society. Insight becomes less egocentric and more allocentric, that is, inclusive of others' points of view.

It is significant for the topic that concerns us here that Piaget places this development toward decentration in a broader biological context. In various experiments he repeatedly demonstrated that cognitive processes of decentration bear a close resemblance to certain biological processes: they grow out of a dialectical interaction between *assimilation* (the organism's integration of external elements into existing internal structures, as in digestion) and *accommodation* (the organism's modification of existing internal structures under the influence of external elements, as in the adaptation to new kinds of food or the acquisition of immunities). The adolescent has reached an optimal level of decentration, and thus reversibility of thought processes, when a balance establishes itself between egocentric processes of assimilation (centered in one's own actions and experience) and allocentric processes of accommodation (centered on external elements). In functional terms this balance is not achieved until the stage of formal operations; before this, assimilation outweights accommodation, just as action outweighs thought. The development of intelligence is directed toward this balance from the very beginning; intelligence in its entirety can be understood only in relation to this striving toward equilibrium. In a fascinating synthesis Piaget shows how the seeds of the final stage of fully equilibrated reversibility of formal intelligence are already contained in (1) the dual rhythms of inborn instinctual and reflexive schemata of action, that is, biological processes; and (2) the agonistic-antagonistic regulations of the sensorimotor period. They become increasingly internalized and finally fully differentiated in the balanced "groupings" of the highest stages of development.

It thus appears that the equilibration of more and more complex systems plays as decisive a role in the psychological sphere, in the creation of a single schema and also in cognitive development as a whole, as it does in the biological sphere. In his crowning concept of "optimizing equilibration" ("équilibration majorisante") Piaget demonstrates how this continuing development toward higher levels can be understood in cybernetic terms: the appearance of "interference" or "incongruities" in existing schemata or conceptual systems forces their integration by means of assimilation or accommodation; this process is set in motion by each interference over and over again.[13] Piaget's entire theory is fully consistent with modern communications and systems theory; the powerful homeostatic forces that affect cognitive systems at all levels—just as they do all other types of open, equilibrated systems—explain why intellectual progress is time-consuming for individuals, for groups, and for society as a whole (or ontogenetically as well as phylogenetically, so to speak). It must repeatedly overcome considerable resistance within the system and can take place only when major disturbances occur. These must lead to enough tension and disharmony to force a change in the entire system by their integration.

At just this point the question arises again as to what role *affective* factors play in this magnificent theoretical framework of Piaget's. I have already noted that he considers them only in passing and, it must be added, in a strikingly undifferentiated fashion. There are indications that he might have had personal, as well as scientific and methodological, reasons for doing so.[14] In many of his studies affects are not mentioned explicitly at all, although they are implicitly omnipresent, as when he illustrates how "object permanence" is acquired with an account of the pleasure—which he certainly must have shared!—shown by his nineteen-month-old daughter Jacqueline on finding a pencil hidden by her father under cap A, handkerchief B, or jacket C: "I then show it to her a third time before putting it under C, where I leave the pencil and afterwards show her my open hand, repeating 'cuckoo the pencil.' Jacqueline immediately looks for the pencil under C.; she finds it and laughs."[15]

Not even in Piaget's work on the development of moral concepts and systems[16] is there any direct recognition of the role played by affective factors, despite numerous references to feelings of pleasure and pain, admiration, sympathy, respect for elders, fear, and so on. (One instructive example is his account of the game of marbles, the rules of which are internalized by the child step by step in a pattern matching that of general cognitive development.)

Not until 1966, when Piaget and Inhelder summarized their work in *The Psychology of the Child,* did they pay detailed attention to the significance of affect as the "motor" or force behind cognitive development. However, they emphasized here in a not very clear manner that affects were neither the cause nor the effect of cognitive structures. Even for the early sensorimotor period they postulated a parallel but independent development of cognition and affect, citing the studies of Spitz, Gouin-Décarie, and Escalona:

> The cognitive schemes which are initially centered upon the child's own action become the means by which the child constructs an objective and "decentered" universe; similarly, and at the same sensorimotor levels, affectivity proceeds from a lack of differentiation between the self and the physical and human environment toward the construction of a

group of exchanges or emotional investments which attach the differentiated self to other persons (through interpersonal feelings) or things (through interest at various levels).[17]

In their view, affects are at first completely centered on the child's own body and actions; only later are they directed toward other persons in a manner parallel to the first decentration processes that lead to the cognitive grasp of object permanence. At the beginning these persons represent merely particularly active, unpredictable, and therefore interesting objects; for just this reason the child reacts to them in an increasingly specific way, constructing systems of exchanging gestures and facial expressions as communicative schemata. An important difference between inanimate objects and people lies in the fact that the child can establish a direct relationship between the behavior of persons and his own actions.[18] Once the child acquires the concept of object permanence, and especially once he acquires the semiotic function (internal images, memory, language), the affective object "may be present and active, even in its physical absence. [At one point Piaget and Inhelder use the expression "sensorimotor-affective object," which is particularly interesting for the line of questioning pursued here.] This fundamental fact results in the formation of new affects in the form of lasting sympathies or antipathies toward other people and of a permanent awareness and valorization of oneself as regards the ego."[19] It is evident that such formulations are fully consistent with psychoanalytic theories on the same stage of development.

For later phases the authors place more and more emphasis on the *social* aspect of affective reactions. Play appears as "an area of interference between cognitive and affective interests."[20] In games with rules such as the game of marbles mentioned above, a child learns behavioral norms by imitating older children and internalizing their instructions. (The authors refer here specifically to the Freudian concept of the superego.) As the child gains a better understanding of the reasons for the rules themselves and is less influenced by the authority of the older children, these behavioral norms develop into a "moral consciousness" centering on the idea of justice. This creates mutual respect and enables the children to cooperate. The school of Piaget sees in these reciprocities a phenomenon paralleling the reversibility of thought in the cognitive field and occurring at approximately the same time.

Convergences and Divergences between
Psychoanalysis and Genetic Epistemology

Before we discuss further the nature of affect and intellect, and an affect-logic embracing them both, it will be useful to clarify the similarities and differences between psychoanalysis and genetic epistemology.

1. Both psychoanalysis and genetic epistemology are strongly "historical" and "constructivist" in their orientation, since both understand the adult psyche as the result of a long developmental process, either affective or cognitive, beginning in earliest childhood. Both distinguish between different phases in its slow growth; however, these phases coincide in the two theories for only about the first eighteen months of life. Thus psychoanalysis sees the decisive steps toward affective maturation in the oedipus conflict (at the age of three or four) and, to a lesser degree, in the phase of puberty after a latency period. According to genetic epistemology, the most important progress in cognitive development is made precisely in this "affective latency period," between the ages of seven or eight and eleven or twelve—a view that psychoanalysis shares. If both theories are correct, what we have is thus not a case of completely parallel development (apart from the first few months of life), but rather a case of *characteristic alternation*. Affective and cognitive maturation would then occur in only partially overlapping phases, a phenomenon that makes great sense if we assume that progress in one area provides the basis for progress in the other.

2. Both psychoanalysis and genetic epistemology consider affect and intellect to be inseparably connected yet basically different. Although cognitive factors play only a marginal role in psychoanalytic thinking, like affective factors in genetic epistemology, both arrive at virtually identical views of development in the first year of life, using virtually identical terminology. For later phases of development there exists a kind of general correspondence, but it does not extend to details. However, this may merely appear to be the case because of lack of research on the subject.

In particular both theories are agreed that during the first year of life "all actions show an interdependence between the subjects and the objects, which are bound together with no pre-established frontier separating them. There are as yet no objects independent of the subject (object permanency starts at only around nine to ten months) and reciprocally, the subject does not know himself as such, but only in reference to his successive actions."[21] The results of research in both fields lead to complete agreement that the first permanent object is a *person* and not a thing, as Gouin-Décarie was able to demonstrate in specific experiments.[22] Piaget's view that such persons become lasting, internalized sensorimotor affective objects with sympathies and antipathies attached to them corresponds fully to the psychoanalytic concept of internalized object representations. Similarly, the remarks of Piaget and Inhelder quoted above on the ego and self-awareness in relation to affects could just as well be taken from the modern psychoanalytic theory of narcissism. Not only can the partner as an independent object be viewed as a general cognitive-affective concept in Piaget's sense, but reciprocally so also can the self, as H. C. Shands in particular has shown.[23] This self takes on increasingly clear and stable contours as it is "reflected" in another person during childhood (or perhaps later in a psychotherapeutic relationship).

Both theories seem to be more or less agreed that affect is primarily energy, whereas intellect is mostly structure. The (developing) structure of cognitive functions has been explored in detail by genetic epistemology; psychoanalysis has either tacitly accepted it or, as psychoanalytic ego psychology, identified it explicitly as "neutralization" or the "conflict-free sphere of the ego." The situation is far less clear in the case of affectivity, however. The two theories do agree that the energy inherent in affects originates in biological drives, which manifest themselves in human behavior as a permanent striving for what is pleasurable and avoidance of what is not. Piaget occasionally makes a global reference to the positive or negative feelings with which objects are cathected: "On the one hand, affectivity is characterized by the distribution of positive and negative object cathexes. On the other hand, the cognitive aspects of behavior are characterized by their structure, be they elementary action schemes, concrete operations (seriation, classification), or propositional logic."[24] Yet how affects are structured remains unclear. For psychoanalysts, all affective development represents nothing other than a growing structuralization; Lacan's remark that even the unconscious is "structured like a language" has often been quoted.[25] When genetic epistemologists speak of affective energy at all, they sometimes present it as a kind of counterpart to cognitive structuralization. Thus Piaget: "Affective and cognitive mechanisms are inseparable, although distinct: the former depend on energy, and the latter depend on structure."[26] At other times, however, Piaget follows Pierre Janet and speaks of the existence of "affective regulations," in one instance (at a psychoanalytic congress)[27]—even of "affective schemata," which in principle are structured in the same way as cognitive schemata. In this case they would correspond to the important analytic concept of complexes.[28] Since to my knowledge Piaget never went on to develop this idea, which is of the greatest interest in our context, we must probably conclude that a certain divergence exists between psychoanalysis and genetic epistemology on this point. *One* fundamental area of agreement should still be stressed, however: in both theories all the countless nuances and shades of feeling existing in affectivity clearly arise between only *two* basic poles, pleasure and unpleasure, "positive" and "negative" feelings.

3. No fundamental divergence, but rather a significant convergence, emerges in Freud's view of thought as "trial action" with small quantities of energy and in Piaget's concept of cognitive schemata and operations as "internalized actions." According to Piaget, all developments of intelligence can be understood as "a step-by-step process of performing actions which are then internalized" as a child matures. Cognitive schemata and operations—and I would add affective operations—appear to be a kind of "program of action" stored in the brain, not unlike a computer program. They take shape as the child acquires experience, and become equilibrated in a continuing process of assimilation and accommodation.

4. The all-important concept of the unconscious is an area in which the two theories show interesting convergences as well as certain possible divergences. In "The Affective Unconscious and the Cognitive Unconscious" Piaget recognizes the existence of the unconscious as fully defined by psychoanalysis but doubts the existence of unconscious representations or images. In the cognitive unconscious, at least, which he compares and contrasts with the affective unconscious, no representations of objects are stored, but rather schemata and operations, or *relations* in the sense of the programs of action mentioned above. "There are no concepts in representational form in the cognitive unconscious. The idea of 'unconscious representation' seems contradictory to me. The cognitive unconscious is made up of sensori-motor or operatory schemes already organized into structures. The schemes express what the subject can 'do' but not what he thinks. The subject also has affective and personality schemes, i.e., tendencies, drives, etc."[29] Psychoanalysis has paid little attention to

such a cognitive unconscious, even though the latter could certainly have a place in the theory of the unconscious components of the ego. In all probability no real contradiction exists on this point, however, since even Freud expressed the opinion that it was not representational elements, but rather the relations between object-impressions and their images, that were unconscious.[30] Both theories seem to converge in the idea that both an affective and a cognitive unconscious exist; Piaget sees the determining characteristic of the unconscious as a lack of abstraction and conceptualization: "The affective unconscious is only a special case of the unconscious in general. This unconscious includes everything which cannot be made explicit because of the lack of reflective abstraction, conceptualization, etc. The unconscious is everything which is not conceptualized."[31] This postulate corresponds to the psychoanalytic idea of the primary unconscious, but not to the idea of the secondary (repressed) unconscious. We shall return to this important difference in the chapter on language and consciousness.

5. Within a larger framework further significant similarities exist between the psychoanalytic view of narcissism and Piaget's concept of egocentricity, although to my knowledge they have never been directly compared. The former recognizes a general developmental tendency from primary (and secondary) narcissism, with its fusion of subject and object, to mature (oedipal or genital) object relations between autonomous partners. The latter sees a development from the egocentricity of early childhood, which is centered on the child's own body and actions, to the stage of optimal decentration and cognitive reversibility in adolescence. Both schools of thought ascribe central importance to the idea that object permanence occurs on increasingly higher levels; this proceeds from the beginnings of clear distinction between self representations and object representations to a capacity for genuine mourning (from the psychoanalytic point of view) and to the capacity for cognitive grouping of similar phenomena (in genetic epistemology). Both the affective and cognitive lines of development finally converge in the ability to participate in a cooperative partnership governed by the notion of justice, which Piaget studied in children's games and in the formation of moral values.

In addition to these various points of convergence between the two theories, there are two striking contrasts. As in the case of so many other apparent differences, however, these seem to have a complementary rather than a truly contradictory relationship.

6. The basic structures of affective and cognitive functions are governed by obviously different polarities. In the case of affect there is the clear opposition of love and hate (libidinal and aggressive feelings, pleasure and unpleasure, eros and thanatos). In the area of cognition, however, the polarity is much more abstract and consists in the reciprocity of logical operations, such as addition and subtraction, multiplication and division, implication and exclusion, affirmation and negation. All these operations are characterized by reversibility, that is, the possibility of returning to the point of departure. They make *freedom of thought* possible, including the transformation of diachronic action into synchronic thinking, and vice versa. Without going into the matter more deeply here, we can conclude that both such differences and their underlying similarity might be important with regard to the structure of affect-logic. The significant point of resemblance is that both theories imply a fundamental binary and polar structure for all psychic activity.

7. Whereas psychoanalysis concerns itself not only with affect but also with relationships between people (or their gradually internalized representations of others), genetic epistemology concentrates not only on cognitive functions but also on the child's relationship to the world of *inanimate objects* and concepts (such as materials, space, time, logical relationships, and categories). This is certainly no accident. We need only remind ourselves that, according to Piaget and Inhelder, a small child reacts to other people—who represent objects of a very special and active kind—in an increasingly specific way, by constructing a system of communication based on imitation and interaction. It is clear that such a system of communication with active participants provides the child with intense experiences of pleasure or pain from the very beginning and is sustained by *affect*. Affects represent *the* basic means of communication between living creatures, whereas cognitive functions remain secondary for a considerable time. Exactly the opposite seems to be true for dealings with the world of inanimate objects.

From this comparison we can draw the preliminary conclusion that research in psychoanalysis and genetic epistemology has described two different aspects of the human psyche, aspects that both disciplines consider to be inseparably connected, although one or the other aspect may predominate in a given situation: psychoanalysis concerns itself with the world of *persons and feelings,* genetic epistemology with the world of *inanimate objects and ideas.* The extensive convergences between the two lead us to suspect more than ever that fundamental similarities of structure exist—in other words, that both are subsumed under a broad affect-logic that forms the reality of our daily experience more than either area alone. Before exploring the possible structure of this affect-logic, we should consider how these two aspects of our mental life are likely to interact.

"Affective-Logical Schemata": The Logic of Feelings and the Feelings of Logic

As Piaget and Inhelder suggested in passing with their term *sensori-motor-affective object*—and as psychoanalysts would agree—there must exist not only cognitive schemata but also cognitive-affective, that is, specifically *affective-logical,* schemata in which "feelings" and "logic," the affective and cognitive components, are inextricably linked in the manner postulated by both schools of thought.

Indeed I would go so far as to claim that in reality *all* schemata are affective-logical and not merely affective or cognitive. According to Piaget internal schemata arise from the sensorimotor actions of the organism as these grow more regulated, coordinated, equilibrated, and internalized; however, it is clear that these actions always contain an emotional element, particularly in the case of dealings with other people, but not exclusively so. The goal or result of action is, broadly speaking, pleasure or its opposite, or, in more precise terms, all the possible shades of feeling existing between these extremes. The biological function of pleasure and unpleasure is to indicate to the organism what is useful (for gaining or conserving energy and maintaining life) and what is not useful (dangerous or destructive). The fact that it is often important for an organism not to seek such pleasure directly, but rather to use various detours in delaying the gratification of drives, does not alter the basic situation. It remains essential that information concerning feelings of pleasure or pain be securely integrated into the internalized actions and "instructions for action" of which the schemata (and later operations) consist, since this information can be vital to life. When a child acquires a cognitive schema about fire, for instance, from his own actions and experience, it is certainly of the greatest importance that this schema contain the possible unpleasurable feelings and dangers connected with fire in the form of signals for both fear and caution. This is precisely what occurs, and a multitude of observations both from everyday life and from scientific studies confirm it. The panic of Pavlov's dogs at the sight of water after the great flood in St. Petersburg, when they barely escaped drowning in their cages, is another example, and still more can be found in the studies of conditioned reflexes and anxiety neuroses in human beings. The same must doubtless apply to all the other possible schemata or instructions for action, especially those for interpersonal situations (involving a mother, father, siblings, playmates, persons in authority, strangers, and so on). Psychoanalysis has provided an impressive demonstration of how efficiently such affective components determine our actions in the workings of the phenomenon of *transference,* the more or less automatic repetition of patterns of behavior and emotional response with a person (such as a boss) who resembles the original model of one's early childhood, usually a parent. Clearly, all cognitive schemata thus acquire a particular affective stamp or imprint that is gained from active experience, exactly like the cognitive components. Looking ahead to the terminology of a later chapter, we can say that this imprint represents a condensation (or an "abstraction") of the affective invariance (*and* its possible range or variance) of what is experienced. The goal of this process is to extract a most appropriate and efficient pattern of action. Thus the affective structure in fact appears to be truly inseparable from the cognitive structure, because they have been formed together in a largely analogous manner. The built-in affective component gives all our intellectually determined actions and operations a specific emotional color. Although this can be weakened and neutralized over time, it can also be reactivated at any point, and it provides our actions with their general orientation and motivation, that is to say their energy.

This assumption is fully compatible with important ideas presented some years ago by Miller, Galanter, and Pribram on internalized plans of behavior;[32] it is also supported by corresponding results from research in brain anatomy and physiology. Thus, for example, there are an extremely large number of neuronal links between certain parts of the paleocortex (the rhinencephalon, hypothalamus, and limbic system) that are closely related to moods and feelings such as fear, aggression, and pleasure when basic drives are satisfied, and the areas of the neocortex (particularly the central and prefrontal regions) that regulate such typical cognitive functions as the perception and the processing of sensory data on higher levels of thought, and of judgment. The well-known brain researcher and Nobel laureate John Eccles has written on this subject:

> the hypothalamus and the limbic system modify and colour with emotion the conscious perceptions derived from sensory inputs and superimpose on them motivational drives. No other part of the neocortex has this intimate relationship with the hypothalamus ... So one can think of the prefrontal cortex as being the area where all emotive information is synthesized with somaesthetic, visual, and auditory to give conscious experiences to the subject and guidance to appropriate behaviour.[33]

Basically in agreement with this view is the following passage by the psychoanalyst Otto Kernberg:

> various inborn physiological, behavioral, affective, and perceptive structures are internalized jointly as a first unit of intrapsychic structure. Cognition and affect are thus two aspects of the same primary experience. Although the neurophysiological structures responsible for affective experience and for (cognitive) storage capability of this experience are different, their integration in the earliest affective memory establishes, in my opinion, a common structure (pleasurable or unpleasurable primitive experience) out of which cognition and affect will evolve in diverging directions. This has relevance for psychoanalytic instinct theory.[34]

One cognitive-affective circuit that has been especially well studied is the so-called Papez loop, a circuit now regarded as the morphological basis for emotions and moods. Kerberg also refers to the long-standing postulate of an "affective memory," through which affective elements, particularly pleasurable and unpleasurable experiences, are related to ideas.[35] Although research on affective-cognitive links at the neuronal level is still far from complete, their existence can no longer be doubted. From recent studies it even appears that they are constantly expanded in a network of fine dendritic connections reflecting the experiences undergone. Much suggests that such circuits function as open systems, just as psychological affective-cognitive schemata or systems of reference can form open systems equilibrated in response to experience. According to Schneider, for example, it is useful "to formulate empathic, introspective experiences in terms of [the development of] psychological systems according to Piaget's theories.

These systems would correspond to neurobiological findings on the elaboration of neuronal networks.[36]

We can use these results in our search for the structure of affect-logic. On the one hand we can begin to recognize *affective components of logic* and on the other *logical components of affect*. About the former we can conclude that if all cognitive schemata really do contain an affective imprint, then it must have played a crucial role in their formation. Just this appears to be the case, even though genetic epistemology has not pursued a number of observations pointing in this direction. Consistent logical operations are intensely *pleasurable* at every level of development, if only for the reason that they reduce tension. They are more economical and harmonious than what they replace; they correct a "disturbance," create a more pleasant balance, and thus open up entirely new possibilities for understanding the world and acting in it. Even the recognition of a regularity—for example, in the form of an event that repeats itself—is (usually) pleasurable in and of itself. This can be observed easily in the case of children, and as adults we experience a similar pleasure when we encounter a familiar person or object in a strange environment. This pleasurable component is surely essential to a highly important constructive principle, namely the desire to create *continuity*. From the very first days of a child's life, continuity leads to the formation of positively cathected habits. Generally speaking, the child's genuine pleasure in rhythms, repetition, and recognition of events plays an essential part in the development of intelligence, from the formation of cognitive (or cognitive-affective) schemata to the later operations of classification and grouping. A positive affective coloring is always present when something is "right" or "the answer comes out," that is, when we discover agreement or harmony in things. This may occur as the confirmation of an implicit hypothesis on a very early level of development; examples are the pleasure shown by Piaget's small daughter on finding where a pencil had been hidden, and the satisfaction a first-grader feels on grasping basic reciprocal rules such as $1 + 1 = 2, 2 - 1 = 1$; or $2 \times 2 = 4, 4 \div 2 = 2$. It may also occur as the euphoria of the adolescent who becomes capable of new mental operations on a higher level, sometimes quite suddenly. Piaget has described this feeling vividly, though without incorporating it into his theories. The joy of discovery felt by a researcher when the pieces of a puzzle fit together all at once, after a long and often far from pleasurable search for a solution, is basically no different from the other instances of pleasure. One famous example is James Watson's account of the discovery of the double helix, the structure of DNA.[37] We may at least conjecture that this pleasure in harmonizing things—which always means both a reduction of tension and a gain in economy— plays an important part in all human intellectual and affective development and may contribute to all structures, even on a biological level. We can find hints along these lines in Piaget's work as well as in some psychoanalytical writings; Gressot, for example, has surmised (quite plausibly and with far-reaching consequences) that achieving a balance between assimilation and accommodation in Piaget's sense is a pleasurable experience.[38] If this is correct, then the claim of psychoanalysis that a striving for pleasure is the driving force behind all cognitive development can be understood in new and more precise terms. W. G. Cobliner writes along similar lines: "It is clear that learning without the involvement of feelings is artificial . . . The process of learning is set in motion by affective processes and experiences, and is related to them. These intrapsychic forces exert an enormous influence on learning, affect intellectual growth, and in general contribute as much to ontogenetic development as external influences do." [39]

Although the original pleasure derived from discovering that something "fits" decreases significantly with time, the discovery retains its positive affective label. Even the apparently unemotional or "cool" pleasure experienced by the mathematician when an equation comes out represents a new and specific label that becomes attached to the whole system of mathematical derivations. That is why one may speak of the "elegance" of a mathematical solution. This hidden aspect of pleasure becomes apparent at once when we feel its opposite, the annoyance when a proof fails to work out. In this sense we can say that mathematics and the exact sciences are systems of reference that contain a pervasive and quite uniform emotional quality as an "invariance" (see Chapter 3).

Concerning the possible *logical components of affect* many questions undeniably remain open, despite the fact that Freud provided an impressive demonstration of the degree to which our emotional and instinctual lives are determined, thereby implying the existence of an underlying logic. In addition he described most interesting affective "operations," such as reaction formation, negation and denial, splitting, condensation and displacement, projection and introjection. In all of these operations there are clearly structural and dynamic analogies to the logical operations of reversal and negation, implication and exclusion, and so on. Many phenomena that can be observed in the realm of feelings resemble the logical reversibility of intellectual operations. Thus the well-known fact that in the area of cognition one part requires a counterpart to form a complete whole (an operation is always associated with its reverse operation) can easily be demonstrated to apply to the field of emotions as well:

A patient in psychoanalysis spends hours describing his feelings of being small, worthless, and insignificant. Only later do the corresponding grandiose fantasies and hopes come to the surface which had been present from the beginning and completed the total picture.

Another patient claims emphatically: "I don't want to subordinate myself to my boss." As treatment continues, it becomes obvious that all possible opposites of this sentence apply equally well to him:
—"I want to subordinate myself to my boss."
—"I am afraid of subordinating myself to my boss."
—"I am afraid of dominating my boss."
—"I want to dominate my boss."

It is evident that the analysand cannot understand the feelings in question in their entirety or become fully himself until he is able to grasp his fundamental ambivalence. He must recognize the hidden counterparts to what he is saying and become able to feel and integrate them. It thus clearly follows that in the area of the emotions, precisely as in the area of cognition, insight into the basic reversibility (or duality) of every situation represents an immensely important step toward maturity.

Psychoanalysis has long been aware of the complementary nature of love and hate, pleasure and unpleasure, joy and pain, aggression directed toward others and toward oneself, hopes and fears, frustrations and their corresponding forms of overcompensation, and so on, often continuing for long periods. As was suggested in the first chapter, we can generally recognize a network of polarities that limit and determine the affective field of an individual and combine to create a typical "system." Beyond this a polar or binary structure of affect now comes into view, similar to that shown by Piaget to exist for the cognitive field and having origins that can be traced back to basic biological processes. When we consider that even the inorganic world of physics appears to possess such a polar structure—consisting as it does of positive and negative electrical charges, the duality/identity of mass and energy, matter and antimatter, and so on—then we arrive at the conclusion (to be investigated further in the next chapter) that all the phenomena described may reflect a ubiquitous principle of our universe.

For the moment we can summarize our findings as follows: Logic undoubtedly has affective components, and it seems equally clear that affect has logical components, or components at least similar to logic in their form and structure. Both appear to share a structural principle of polarity, of part and counterpart, statement and counterstatement. At the same time thinking and feeling themselves seem to represent fundamental and complementary counterparts. We appear to be on the track of some interesting general principles, without yet being able to formulate them clearly enough for the exercise to be entirely "satisfying" (harmonizing and pleasurable). We do not yet have enough insight into the dynamic interplay of affect and intellect. Thus we must take a closer look at how we in fact experience thinking and feeling in combination.

Feeling and Thinking, Body and Mind

We must now ask what kind of "reality" is hidden in the concepts of feeling (or affect) and thinking (or intellect), and what relationship these two realities have to each other.

If we attempt to grasp the meaning of these two concepts by asking what distinguishes them from each other, we realize that "feeling" is something connected with the body and physical experience, whereas "thinking" clearly belongs to a less material sphere, located more in the brain than in the rest of the body. Emotions or feelings are expressed mainly in physical sensations and reactions, such as blushing or paling, faster or slower breathing, and a tightness or relaxation in the chest. We may assume certain postures with corresponding facial expressions and gestures to express joy, sadness, or rage; we may tremble, or tighten or relax certain muscles. Popular expressions place feelings unequivocally in regions of the body—in the heart, the pit of the stomach, or the gut; they "run down our spine," we go "stiff with horror," shake, or "could burst with rage." Fear can make our hair stand on end; we go weak in the knees, or joy can make our heart pound. These old sayings have been confirmed by Hans Selye's work on the effect of stress on the endocrine system. We now know that feelings affect the body's chemistry, since hormones such as epinephrine (adrenalin) and norepinephrine are released into the bloodstream in different situations. These can cause a great variety of changes in some or all parts of the body, including blood vessels, smooth and striated muscles, and all organs and organ systems.

Nothing at all similar is known in the case of cognitive functions. If physical reactions do occur in connection with them, these can be traced back to the affect accompanying the supposedly "pure" thought processes: our pupils may dilate when we recall a frightening experience, our hearts beat faster when we think about an attractive person, or our muscles may tense involuntarily if we talk about a fight that took place. However, these physical symptoms are much weaker during recall than during our actual experience of such events. They represent only a reflection or a shadow of the original reaction, and they disappear almost entirely when we turn our minds to mathematical or philosophical problems, the emotional components of which have been largely neutralized. Popular expression once again confirms this: we may "rack our brains," or a problem may "go round and round in our heads," but otherwise we have no language to describe intellectual processes that would bear any resemblance to the "body language" for feelings.

Affects are thus psychic phenomena that influence the body directly and concretely, whereas thinking is largely immaterial, indirect, and not physical. Thinking is a "mental" process that takes place mainly in the brain, in ways we must now investigate more closely.

To understand better the nature of intellectual processes we must consider the phenomena of abstraction and relation (or operations with relations), since in my opinion they are what constitutes intellect. The word *abstraction* means a kind of condensation or consolidation of information; in cybernetic language one could also say that abstraction means "to extract an invariance." *The basic process of abstraction consists in discovering some common element in a number of different phenomena,* that is, discovering a single unifying element that includes them all and thus constitutes a whole of a larger order. The central Piagetian concept of "reflective abstraction" can certainly be understood in this way. In what follows we shall often be concerned with processes of abstraction (in the next chapter we shall see that extracting an invariance leads to recognition of typical structures; in the chapter after that I shall discuss the connections between abstraction and the beginnings of consciousness). The intellect operates less with direct, concrete bodily sensations (including those of the sensory organs) than with something that goes beyond these sensations and is thus more abstract and essentially mathematical. This is the set of connections and relations between these sensations.

A particularly simple case of operation with relations that leads to a first extraction of an invariance—and thus to abstraction and a grasp of typical structural and mathematical totalities—consists merely in observing the (repeated) occurrence of certain pieces of information. On a higher level, we abstract from abstractions and grasp the relation of relations to each other.

Obviously, intellectual processes or cognitive functions use this same principle of abstraction to grasp ever-new relations between ever-new wholes in an endless process. Thus, thinking differs from feelings in that the latter have to do above all with physical sensations in various parts of the body, even though feelings are of course registered in the brain and are even influenced by the brain to some extent, as in the pituitary regulation of hormonal processes. Thinking, on the other hand, consists largely of mediated processes occurring in the higher levels of the central nervous system; these processes deal much less directly with concrete physical or sensory phenomena than with grasping totalities and the relations between them.

One further circumstance is worth emphasizing: If it is really true that feelings can be located primarily in the peripheral areas of the body, and thoughts primarily centrally, in the brain, then they also occur in very different organic settings. This notion could help to explain the important differences in the forms in which they manifest themselves. As already mentioned, affective "messages" are transmitted to the body mainly by hormones released into the bloodstream, that is, by complex organic macromolecules that flow through the body at the same relatively slow rate at which blood circulates.[40] Hormones cause global chemical changes in the body that last a considerable time; even though hormones can be effective in low concentration in the blood, these changes require much larger quantities of chemicals than those needed for thought processes. It is well known that brain processes can transmit information with incomparably greater speed and efficiency by means of minute electrical currents. These are created by transporting simple sodium and potassium ions tiny distances. In addition, as Eccles emphasizes repeatedly, these currents flow within the most highly differentiated system ever devised for organizing matter in the universe, namely the human brain, which has a complexity far surpassing all technology invented by human beings. We could thus compare the physical processes associated with affect to crude and cumbersome machinery, whereas cognitive processes have a highly refined form of neuronal "microelectronics" at their disposal. Freud anticipated this circumstance to some degree when he referred to thought as "trial action with small amounts of energy." Such a comparison is obviously an oversimplification and fails to take into account the fact that some affective reactions are transmitted via neuronal pathways; they thus also make use of the refined "machinery" described. Nevertheless this comparison helps to make clear a truly significant difference between affect and intellect—namely that feelings tend to be registered more globally and with less speed and differentiation than thoughts. By comparison thoughts are much more mobile, subtle, and varied.

These differences have important consequences for the possible structure of an affect-logic. On the one hand, feelings clearly form a relative invariance, upon which the more variable cognitive data are built. Affect thus characterizes entire complex affective-logical systems of reference as typical moods or "states of feeling." Kernberg must have had the same idea in mind when he referred to affects as the basic "organizers" of psychic structures. On the other hand, the psyche now appears to be a specific kind of *double system* constructed of two different components. The emotional component is anchored in material, physical, and concrete phenomena directly tied to perception and action (that is, it is sensorimotor); its origins lie deep in our animal and biological nature. The other component, which is intellectual or cognitive, continues to differentiate the structures anchored in the biological and sensorimotor realm, as Piaget has shown, and thus reaches far beyond factual, material events. As the intellectual component abstracts and internalizes these events, there is an immense gain in mobility, efficiency, and possibilities for expansion and differentiation. In other words, we gain freedom, although at the same time there is a certain loss of information

An affect-logic uniting these two spheres must, then, possess a double structure to an even greater degree than expected: it has not only an affective and a cognitive side, but also both a physical-material and an intellectual-immaterial side. Two poles or counterparts combine to form a whole that in a highly peculiar fashion appears to be both "dual" and "nondual." It thus seems possible that we might be dealing here with a particularly significant instance of that paradoxical polarity that has been postulated over and over again as the fundamental structure of the human mind and the entire physical universe, from the time of Heraclitus up to our own. The reason for this could lie in the central role of the idea of equilibrium in modern scientific thinking, and in systems theory and cybernetics in particular: the simplest possible way to create an equilibrium is (as was emphasized in Chapter 1) to establish a bipolarity and to balance one part with a counterpart. It is thus hardly surprising that such bipolar wholes appear repeatedly as the building blocks of more complex structures.

We shall take up these ideas again in the next chapter. Let us now consider the interaction between the two poles of feeling and thinking in that affective-logial unity of all psychic experience for which we have been searching from the start.

The Possible Structure and Dynamics of "Affect-Logic": A Preliminary Synthesis

Feeling and thinking, or affective and cognitive experience, must be regarded as truly inseparable but also as fundamentally different. Feelings are more connected with the body and thus with concrete material experience; thinking is more connected with the brain and the intellect, and thus with a much more abstract network of relationships. Together they form a kind of double system, or rather *one* unified system with two poles. This system represents the instrument by means of which we deal with our environment, that is, take it in (perception) and express ourselves (communication). Both aspects are formed in common and combine to create more and more complex affective-logical schemata or "circuits." It is possible that the growth of these two aspects does not proceed in a perfectly parallel or symmetrical way; instead a characteristic alternation of phases may occur so that the differentiation achieved in one area can become the basis for differentiation in the other. (One example of this is the enormous affective development of the oedipal phase, which is followed by a period of affective latency. During this latency period important steps in cognitive maturation are taken.) One indication that such alternation of phases exists may lie in the fact that phylogenetically the "feeling system" developed much earlier than the "thinking system."

Quite simple animals have primitive "feelings"; perhaps their origin even goes back to the global reactions of one-celled creatures to various environmental stimuli, such as light, warmth, touch, and chemotactic stimuli, from which the complex hormonal regulations of higher creatures gradually developed. The centers and pathways associated with feelings are located in the hypothalamus and limbic system, both extremely old regions of the brain. By contrast, the cognitive functions—and especially those that are specifically human, such as thought, language, and self-awareness—are clearly associated with the most recently evolved areas of the necortex, to the extent that they have been localized. In particular, as we shall see later, they are associated with the left hemisphere of the brain. Feelings thus represent a much more archaic form of perception and communication with the environment, a form that is also more direct and comprehensive than the intellect. By conveying first nonverbal and largely global "impressions" or "expressions" (moods, directedness, intentions), feelings provide a rough orientation that the intellect can then improve upon and refine. For this reason our emotional life probably has a more direct connection to the right hemisphere of the brain, with its nonverbal and more global functions, than to the left hemisphere, which controls more analytic activities such as thought and language.[41] We still have a great deal to learn about such brain functions, but we are able to say that emotions provide a foundation, a (relative) invariance upon which cognitive variance builds. We shall see in the next chapter that the combination of two such elements must necessarily lead to the formation of a typical "structure."

We are now in a position to describe some aspects of the basic structure of affect-logic, or those cognitive-affective circuit systems, extending from the cortical regions of the brain to the subthalamic centers, that we assume to be the cerebral substrate of affect-logic. We can distinguish between a gross and a fine structure, the former of course being easier to recognize than the latter.

Broadly speaking, we have seen that a very similar principle determines both affective and cognitive development—that fundamental polarities govern all feeling and thinking from the most primitive to the most complex stages. In the area of affect these are pleasure and its opposite (or love and hate, libido and destrudo). In the cognitive area a polarity can be comprehended correctly only as an abstraction, as something like "positivity" and "negativity," when the concretely experienced polarities of here and there, up and down, forward and backward, before and after, black and white, thick and thin, and so on are generalized.

The orignal, very broad opposites of pleasure and unpleasure (or love and hate) become refined and sublimated over time into all the nuances of attraction and aversion, sympathy and antipathy, which psychoanalysis has described and which form the foundations of our systems of values, our goals, and our motivations. The simple sensorimotor polarities gradually grow into that complex system of abstract mathematical reversibilities that Piaget places in the center of all intellectual development. Both meet in the phenomenon of decentration, the recognition of a fundamental difference between the self and the external world. This leads to a growing ability to understand the world allocentrically rather than egocentrically. An excellent example of how this occurs can be found in the differentiation of internalized representations of oneself and others (in the psychoanalytic sense of self and object), which should be understood as broad schemata (or systems of reference) with a typical affective-logical structure. The precondition for forming these inner constructs is integrating the recognition that they are fundamentally different and reciprocal. Not until they are distinguished do genuine object relations, that is, relations between demarcated affective-cognitive entities, become possible.

The cognitive side of the fine structure of affect-logic is identical with the network of increasingly complex and differentiated reversible operations studied by Piaget that is the result of experience. It culminates in formal logic, the universal "intellectual grammar" containing an infinite number of varying specific propositions. The affective side of affect-logic is by its very nature less accessible to scientific objectification; however, it does reveal structures corresponding, at least in broad outline, to hypotheses put forward long ago by Freud: specific affects become attached to specific mental images (such as the self and human "objects," but also inanimate objects, places, and situations). These have sometimes been labeled "complexes," and although they are certainly less structured than the analytical intellect, they do possess a high degree of complexity and specificity. They are also to be understood as the result of experiences that have left their mark as programs or "instructions for feeling." Piaget occasionally refers to them as "affective schemata" without describing them further. In combination with cognitive elements they form the basis of those (sometimes pathological) reactions so important for psychoanalysis, in particular reaction compulsions and the phenomenon of transference. Such a view can also without difficulty include the ideas of fixation and regression.[42]

It should not be necessary to emphasize once again that the affective and cognitive elements of the fine structure of affect-logic must always be regarded as closely linked, even though I have spoken of them separately here. One could even hypothesize that the fine structure of the psyche must be generated by the alternation of an affective and a cognitive element, since a quantity of emotional (unpleasurable) tension is probably always required to produce the energy to integrate a new cognitive element. This view would certainly fit very well with Piaget's concept of optimizing equilibration, which states that further development of cognitive schemata depends on the tension created by a disturbance of some kind.

Here, however, we are far more concerned with the *dynamics* of affect-logic than with its origins or structure. What we would most like to know is how the affective-logical structure of the psyche *functions*. To answer this question properly, we would need the results of studies and experiments as exact as those carried out in the field of cognition by Piaget and his school, but based on the ideas about affect developed here. These experiments would certainly be more difficult to conduct, and at this time they do not exist at all. We are thus forced to turn for an answer to a few general considerations and the partial results that psychoanalysis has to offer on the subject of affective-logical psychodynamics.

In principle every (psycho-)dynamic can be seen as an "actualization" or mobilization of a structure, just as every structure represents the condensation of a dynamic process. The analogy to a computer program is obvious. One could even say that a structure is a diachronicity that has become synchronic, and a dynamic is a synchronicity that has once again become diachronic. Structure is the result of dynamic processes, and dynamic processes are the result of structure; the two unite to form a whole in which each part is determined by the other. Of course, their dialectics are closely related to the alternation of assimilation and accommodation in the process of psychic differentiation. This means that the dynamics of affect-logic are as much determined by its structure as this structure is determined in turn by psychodynamics (or "action," according to Piaget). Affective-logical dynamic processes must always be "run through" the very schemata or circuits that were previously set up by processes connected with the same or similar problems, situations, or persons.

Another question may help us to understand the nature of affective-logical dynamics, namely what basic dynamic would additionally be possible in the kind of affective-cognitive and physical-intellectual double system I have sketched. This double structure in itself gives rise to a series of possible dynamic processes in which we can recognize any number of familiar phenomena, both normal and pathological. Two small examples may clarify what I mean.

> I am skiing cross-country through a forest covered with snow and bathed in sunlight. My body is working rhythmically and feels strong, with warmth pulsing through it. My mind registers the play of light and shadow on the glittering fir trees, sees their beauty, and at the same time regards my own self, in connection with the chapter of this book that I am engaged in writing—as I follow the track, both an intellectual and a physical being, who thinks and feels. I recognize and feel clearly a sense of well-being and harmony; I am wholly present, both whole and present in the moment.

An example of the contrary:

> Once a week I play a kind of soccer-volleyball with a colleague at work. This is an entertaining game that we have invented ourselves, using a net in a hall full of odd angles and corners that sometimes provide us with very comical surprises. We appear to be enjoying ourselves as usual—but something is wrong. A short time before, we have had unexpected and painfully harsh professional disagreement; it continues to affect us although neither of us has admitted it. Our thoughts are more occupied with this confrontation than with the game, so that on this occasion it does not have its usual relaxing effect.

It is evident that (physical) feeling and thinking are largely in harmony in the first example, but not in the second. I think that the first example is the norm, the simplest and truly "right" way in which affect and intellect work together; the second case represents one particular variant of a large number of possible complications.

Normally, feeling and thinking, the physical and intellectual aspects of our being, "say" the same thing, both to ourselves (in perception) and to others (in communication). They strengthen and validate each other, with the result that in both our perceptions and our communications we become "whole"—unified and unambiguous. Feeling and thinking work together like two lines (for taking a sighting) that meet at one and *only* one point. Like our binocular vision they enable us to locate with great precision what is meant. When feeling and thinking coincide, an optimal clarity and harmony and a particular Zenlike serenity (efficiency, minimal tension) result, even in situations in which the content of what is perceived or communicated is itself not harmonious, as in an athletic competition or the experience of grief after a painful loss.

It is obvious that if a child experiences the harmony of affect and intellect in this manner from an early age, then very clear affective-logical schemata and internalized instructions for action (or systems of reference) will be formed. As we shall see later, these probably coincide in large measure with the psychoanalytic concept of ego strength (or with what Erik Erikson has called "basic trust"). It seems obvious also that in this case *both* affective *and* cognitive functions must have a single, combined structure, or, put another way, that certain affects must be connected to certain cognitive schemata in a particularly stable manner.

The situation looks very different if there is a disharmony between thinking and feeling, as in the second example presented. Here, these two modalities of perceiving and communicating do not strengthen and validate, but weaken and refute each other. The result is an uncomfortable tension, a sense of uncertainty and uneasiness; there is dissonance in the total mind-body system. As we shall see in detail in the chapter on paradoxical contradictions and the double bind, such lack of harmony can rise to levels at which constant fear and psychotic confusion prevail. We can find many examples of mild and fleeting distortions between feeling and thinking in everyday life; when they become permanent states or attitudes, however, they appear to be central elements of neuroses, psychosomatic afflictions, and even possibly of all functional mental disturbances.

Psychoanalysis, in combination with the concepts developed here, can do much to elucidate the structure and dynamics of such conditions. Thus it becomes clear that the prevailing tendency toward balance and reduction of tension makes it necessary to adjust contrary thoughts and feelings until at least an appearance of equilibrium is achieved. All the "operations with affect" described by psychoanalysis, such as repression, negation, denial, splitting, reversal, projection, and introjection, can be seen in this light. A striking disconnection between thinking and feeling, or rather a replacement of "normal" connections by pathological ones, seems also to be the source of the peculiar annulment of apparently unambiguous cognitive perceptions occurring in cases of depression, mania, or delusion. A depressed person in the grip of fears of poverty, for example, may deny having any possessions in the face of obvious evidence to the contrary, or a person suffering from delusions may simply ignore all perceptions and thoughts that contradict them.

The ideas presented here ought to provide some fundamental clarification of psychosomatic disorders too: human beings appear, in a much more clearly defined way than before, to be psychosomatic creatures par excellence. Using mathematic terminology from group theory, we could say that feelings and thoughts, body and mind (or brain), have the relationship found in "bijective mapping": every element in one group (or whole) is linked to an element in another group. Together these two interlinked systems form an instrument with complementary parts that correspond to each other and work in harmony—rather like the manual and pipes of an organ—as long as everything is functioning correctly. However, this is precisely what has gone wrong in typical psychosomatic disorders. There is a gap between thinking and feeling; the body "says" and expresses something very different from what the mind is conscious of. The body may be full of blocked affects—such as rage, fear, the need to be loved, or the desire to dominate or be submissive—for which no paths to cognitive experience, awareness, or verbal expression seem to be open. This view corresponds fully to the modern psychosomatic concept of *alexithymia* (the inability to become aware of feelings) and the *pensée opératoire* of French theorists, which is defined as a mechanistic, largely nonverbal form of thinking cut off from feelings and bodily sensations.[43]

The general picture at which we arrive is thus a complex system of possible dynamic relations between the areas of thinking and feeling. These range from the simplest and most "normal" or "healthy" harmony between both aspects through various distortions of a cognitive and/or affective kind (negation, displacement, rejection, reversal) to complete contradiction or the disruption of every connection, as in splitting or annulment. It seems entirely possible that the whole spectrum of normal and pathological mental states, including abnormal reactions, neuroses, psychosomatic disorders, depression, mania, and schizophrenia, can be subsumed in such a system of constellations or dynamics between affect and intellect.

The extent to which these processes are *conscious* or *unconscious* is such an important question that I wish to reserve a more extensive discussion of it until later and will go into it only very briefly here. We have already seen that both psychoanalysis and genetic epistemology regard it as established beyond doubt that essential parts of such a psychodynamic process remain entirely unconscious or are repressed. The ideas discussed above suggest the interesting possibility—which has been supported by much clinical evidence—that in certain circumstances only *one* part of an affective-logical bipolarity may be repressed. The affective component may be missing for certain thoughts, such as memories of traumatic situations, while the cognitive component may be missing for certain affects of which a person is aware, such as attacks of anxiety or rage. The unconscious thus appears to be primarily a "set of structures and functions," as Piaget said—in other words, a set of instructions for action and thought with a typical affective-logical configuration, in which single bits of information are less important than the dynamic processes and relationships existing between them. Upon close inspection, however, this theory leaves major questions unanswered: Is the unconscious really highly "structured like a language," as Lacan believes, or is it on the contrary largely unstructured, the repository of everything "that cannot be made explicit because of the lack of reflective abstraction and conceptualization"? [44] The latter view might apply to the primary unconscious, but hardly to the secondary unconscious of psychoanalytic theory, which contains material repressed after a previous phase of awareness. A huge category of structured processes and abilities also belongs to the secondary unconscious. The ability to walk, write, or play the piano, for example, is acquired with difficulty and conscious effort, becoming automatic only at a later stage. The circumstances are obviously quite complex, but affective-cognitive schemata can definitely become conscious only under favorable conditions, which appear to be connected with their degree of abstraction as well as with many other aspects. [45]

Not much more can be said about the dynamics of affect-logic at this stage. However, we have come a step closer toward understanding something about the structure and dynamics of affect-logic, even if what has been achieved so far resembles a framework or set of rough coordinates in which many pieces of data based on specific experiments still remain to be entered. The most important features of this framework can be summarized as follows.

1. We have established that an affect-logic exists—that our psychological reality or our experience includes both affective and cognitive elements at every moment; they are inseparably connected and form a common structure.

2. Much evidence from both psychology and brain physiology supports the hypothesis that these elements are combined in affective-cognitive schemata (or programs for thinking, feeling, and behaving; systems of reference). They are based on action and experience and have a largely unconscious foundation.

3. The thesis that no fundamental obstacle stands in the way of combining the approaches of psychoanalysis and systems theory is confirmed quite strikingly by the almost pervasive convergence of psychoanalytical and genetic-epistemological views on the interaction of affective and cognitive functions. Many psychoanalytic insights into affect can most usefully complement the findings of systems theory for cognition, and vice versa. This is especially true for the central concept of optimizing equilibration, the process behind all intellectual development, since here disturbances causing tension are experienced as unpleasurable, while the harmony associated with reduced tension is experienced as pleasurable.

4. This last point, which represesnts the key link between Freud's theory of drives and Piaget's genetic epistemology, we owe to Piaget's recognition of internalized psychological concepts, schemata, and operations as "open systems," long before the formulation of an explicit systems theory. The extraordinary brilliance of this discovery has not been sufficiently appreciated. Piaget realized that the progressive differentiation of these open systems follows the same principles as the differentiation of biological and physical structures. Assimilation and accommodation, the two opposed but complementary regulatory principles of this development, can thus be seen as particularly complex forms of the ubiquitous feedback mechanisms that play such a central role in modern scientific thinking.

5. If we envision a polarity as existing between affective and cognitive experience, and if we associate the former with predominantly physical and concrete events, the latter with intellectual abstraction,

we gain some promising clarification. This hypothesis enables us to pursue several interesting and fundamental ideas both about the interaction of two poles in an affective-logical double system and about possible disturbances in it; the theory also leads to an expanded, more precise view of psychosomatic phenomena.

Finally, this last point raises once again the question of the potential value of the concepts developed here for practical therapy. Although it is still too early to present a detailed answer, I would like to make some general points, as I did at the end of the last chapter. From the point of view of affect-logic the overall goal of therapy must be to harmonize thinking and feeling, to remove the incongruencies and contradictions that create tension between these two poles. Points at which to undertake this suggest themselves in both the intrapsychic and interpersonal fields; the goal of therapy with an intrapsychic focus must be to clarify, stabilize, and valorize the affective-cognitive representations of the self, objects, and their relations to one another. Exactly the same goals would exist in the framework of family or social therapy for interpersonal communication and transactions. In both areas one should strive to attain more clarity, order, and unambiguity, which would lead in turn to a gain in reliability, security, and economy. Collaboration in striving to achieve more harmony and to set priorities in the event of contradictory wishes and goals need not mean simply avoidance of conflict. On the contrary, under certain circumstances it could mean conflictualization at the right time and place, with the ultimate goal a creative resolution of conflicts.

It thus seems likely that the relative merits of various methods of therapy can be determined only by a comprehensive study of both psychoanalysis and systems theory, and of both the intrapsychic and social fields. The resulting insights into the relationship between affects and the body could open the way to integrating somatic and psychosomatic forms of treatment as well.[46]

3 Differentiation, Structure, Systems, and Systems of Reference

The aim of this chapter is to define the concept of an affective-logical system of reference as clearly as possible. In order to do this we must continue some rather theoretical discussion, since the terms *system* and *structure* overlap to a considerable degree. In addition, it will be useful to include some thoughts on the nature of "difference" and "differentiation," for structure and systems arise as the result of differentiation. We must therefore ask in what relation these many-faceted terms stand to each other.

There are two reasons for understanding affective-logical systems of reference in terms of the internalized affective-cognitive schemata described in the last chapter. First, they represent typical carefully equilibrated systems as defined by systems theory; and second, they function as a framework or set of coordinates (largely acquired rather than inborn) that determines all our feelings, thoughts, perceptions, and behavior, by using the experience stored in them to bring these feelings, perceptions, and so on together in specific relations and patterns.

Let us begin with a general investigation of how such differentiations come to exist.

Differences and Differentiation

We may regard a differentiation as a framework of differences. The definition of a "difference" has become an important question for communications and information theorists in recent years. In the context of binocular vision Bateson has this to say on the subject: "Of all these examples, the simplest but most profound is the fact that it takes at least two somethings to create a difference. To produce news of difference, i.e., *information*, there must be two entities (real or imagined) such that the difference between them can be immanent in their mutual relationship; and the whole affair must be such that news of their difference can be represented as a difference inside some information-processing entity, such as a brain or, perhaps, a computer."[1] C. E. Shannon defines the basic unit or "bit" (a contraction of "binary digit") as the quantity of information necessary to dispel uncertainty (or make a decision possible) between two equally probable alternatives, in other words, a "difference." Every differentiation begins with the appearance of differences in what was previously undifferentiated and uniform. The simplest imaginable differentiation occurs when an entity or unit (a whole) is divided into two halves, or into a part and its corresponding counterpart.

This basic fact may at first appear so banal that there seems to be no reason to concern ourselves with it. It has far-reaching consequences, however, if we consider that it leads straight to a fundamental binary or polar structure of thesis and antithesis for every conceivable differentiation. The general reason for this lies in the fact that the number 2 is the smallest number larger than 1: any larger differentiation (of 3, 4, or 5 things, and so on) can always be split into at least two subdivisions ($2 + 1$ or $2 + 2$), whereas a binary differentiation cannot be divided any further. Before or after it there exists only something completely undifferentiated. We have already encountered a number of phenomena suggesting that the fundamental structure of the human mind is a binary one, including the polar structure of all affects as understood by psychoanalysis. Piaget posited a binary structure for all cognitive processes, such as a loss of equilibrium and a return to it. These ideas, as well as the fact that a bipolarity represents the simplest possible system, now appear in a new light. They have also been supported by much evidence from psychology and the physiology of the senses. The famous figure-ground problem is a good example: we can perceive something only when we can distinguish at least two components based on a "difference"—in this case a shape and a background. In fact every perception—but also all behavior, every relationship, and every "size"—is located on a scale between two opposites (large/small, bright/dark, hot/cold, and so on).

These considerations remain entirely valid if, remaining on an abstract level, we now move on to the further differentiation of a first "difference." Once again the simplest division of each of the two parts created by the first differentiation is into two more components; every more complex differentiation can be reduced, in the last analysis, to a polarity (but no further). We now have a total of (at least) four differences or forms of differentiation; after another division of each component into two parts, we have 8, then 16, then 32 differences, and so on. The simplest possible differentiation, the principal or basic framework of every differentiation, can thus be illustrated by the familiar "decision tree," shown upside down (Figure 1). We shall see that this fan-shaped construction, resembling roots or branches that continue to divide, reveals upon closer inspection several further characteristics of every differentiation that are of interest for our problem.

Such differentiations can occur in any number of concrete cases—in the development of organic or inorganic forms in nature (such as rocks, plants, or animal species), in objects designed by human beings (houses, churches, cars, washing machines), and also in ideas, theories, and forms of organizations and behavior. To illustrate a typical differentiation process, let us consider a simple object such as a table.

A table represents an extremely simple principle: the combination of a horizontal surface with one or more vertical supports. We may assume that it was discovered more or less by accident in prehistoric times, when human beings noticed stones arranged like a table in nature or perhaps playfully arranged stones on top of one another and realized that the result could be useful. In time they varied this principle by using larger or smaller, round, square, or many-sided surfaces, by using wood instead of stones, several supports instead of one, and so on. The discovery of the "principle" behind a table began as the perception of the first difference (in the sense described above)

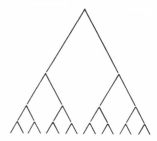

Figure 1.   The principle of differentiation.

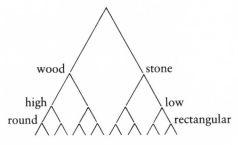

Figure 2. Differentiation of the table principle.

in the natural arrangement of stones previously seen as undifferentiated and lacking in any order. It marked the beginning of a process of differentiation leading to the almost inexhaustible variety of tables to be found today: tables of wood, metal, glass, or plastic, round or rectangular, wide or narrow, high or low; tables with one, three or four legs; tables that go as far to one extreme of emphasizing either the horizontal or the vertical element as the principle will allow and still remain tables. The primitive principle has fanned out in precisely the manner illustrated above. Every new element introduced into the differentiation process (every new idea, every "approach," every "bit" of information) leads to a doubling of the possibilities and variation. The diagram in Figure 2 shows that the number of kinds of tables that primitive man was potentially capable of building doubled as soon as he realized that he could use wood as well as stone, make them with high and low supports, with round and rectangular surfaces, and so on.

We can differentiate in this manner not only concrete objects but *all* developments, including the motor, mental, and social development of human beings. We can differentiate forms of dance, religious rites, linguistic modes of expression, and when scholars and scientists make inventories of them, they are in fact setting up a system, not only of the forms actually observed but also of all those possible in theory. This represents a typically "structuralist" approach, such as was first used by Lévi-Strauss in his analysis of social structures (for example, eating habits, marriage customs, and linguistic phenomena).[2]

If we look at the illustration of the decision tree again, its characteristics lead to further insights. It is evident that every such diagram represents a whole with all its parts; the unity of the whole is provided for by the fact that all the elements contained in it have a common feature—or an "invariance," to use a term now popular in many disciplines. In our example this invariance consists of the fact that every element is a table. However, every pyramidal subgroup that can be removed from any place in the diagram also represents a smaller whole with its own invariance. We can, for example, take the pyramid of stone or wooden tables after the first step in differentiation, or we can take the pyramids of high stone tables, low stone tables, high wooden tables, or low wooden tables after the second step. A differentiation thus proves to be a construction in which wholes of different orders are contained within one another in a complex manner.

One further characteristic of these wholes and invariances should be emphasized: to every invariance in the diagram there clearly belongs a corresponding variance, which arises through modification of the shared principle. Both of them *together* are necessary to form the whole of the specific differentiation. The whole of all tables consists of the totality of all stone, wooden, high, low, round, rectangular, etc., tables. The same is true for all the subgroups of only stone, wooden, high, or low tables. In other words, we are now in a position to recognize that *every* differentiation consists of *a combination of an invariance and a variance*. This concept provides us with a simple definition of structure that has both universal validity and a useful clarity.

Structure

Despite the fact that the use of the term *structure* has greatly increased in all fields of scholarship in the last fifty years—or perhaps *because* of this—it is not at all clear just what a structure is. In 1962, at the height of the structuralist movement in France, Roger Bastide published a collection of essays titled *Senses et usages du terme "structure"* (The meanings and usages of the term "structure"), in the introduction to which he wrote that this concept had as many meanings as there were writers who used it, and that in many cases the different usages could not be reconciled.[3] Twenty contributions from the fields of biology, linguistics, ethnology, economics, law, psychology, and sociology by such eminent specialists as Claude Lévi-Strauss, Daniel Lagache, and Raymond Aron tended to confirm this pessimistic judgment. However, the ideas presented above make it possible to discover a common denominator after all, and we shall see that it fits very well with the definition of the term just given.

The word *structure* comes from the Latin verb *struere,* meaning "to form layers, put together, build, or erect." As its root shows, a "construction" is a process that creates structure. E. Wolff mentions in his contribution to Bastide's book that architects, anatomists, and biologists consequently define structure simply as "the manner in which a building is built," or as "the manner in which the parts of a whole are arranged in relation to one another."[4] Dictionaries frequently include this meaning of the word.

In virtually all definitions one finds in addition the following elements: "The concept of a structure has to do with (1) a whole, (2) the parts of this whole, and (3) the relationships between these parts. Over time the last aspect, which is definitely more dynamic than the first two, has gained in importance. By the 1950s mathematicians were defining structure as "a specific system of relationships or laws describing the functions of a phenomenon that can be represented by a model."[5] Bastide himself describes a structure as "a system of connected elements, in which a change in one element necessarily leads to changes in other elements."[6] This tendency emerges clearly in Piaget's thinking. In his book *Structuralism* he describes a structure very generally as "a system of transformations," naming as its most important characteristics *wholeness, transformation,* and *self-regulation.*[7] For our context it is particularly interesting that in his chapter on mathematical structures Piaget mentions the phenomenon of invariance in connection with that of transformation; he emphasizes that they are "linked in solidarity" and that invariance is a constituting element of a structure.[8] Lagache makes a strikingly similar statement with reference to psychological and psychopathological structures, when he speaks of a *unitas multiplex,* a unity in diversity.[9]

We can see that in the use of the term *structure* by structuralist thinkers in many fields an invariable basic principle or element keeps appearing in new variations. Both components—both what remains the same (the invariance) and what changes (the variance)—are necessary and sufficient to create a structure.

There is no better place to recognize structures—and what constitutes the essence of structures—than in the visual realm, especially in what we can see from an airplane: cities, road systems, planted fields, the shapes of buildings, mountain ranges, the patterns in clouds or water as we fly over them. We find the simple rule everywhere confirmed that a typical structure occurs when an element is repeated but always varied slightly, such as square or rectangular blocks or ring patterns in street grids, characteristic curved lines in hedges and paths in hilly countryside, specific patterns of shape and color in farmland,

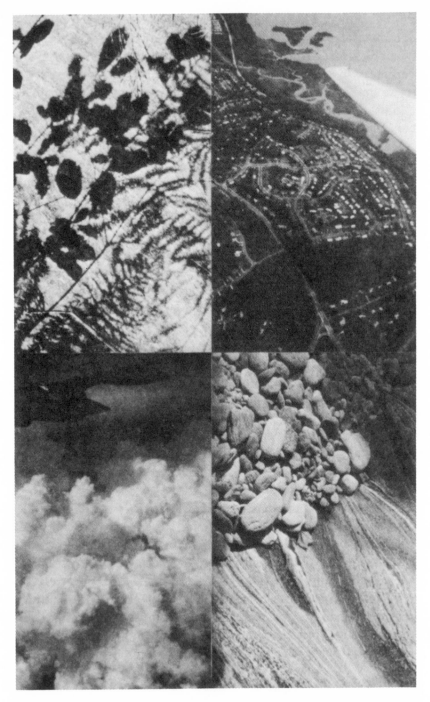

Figure 3. Examples of typical structures.

particular types of erosion in mountain formations, streaks or diamond patterns in the ocean or clouds (see Figure 3).

Obviously our eyes have a great deal of practice and skill in recognizing structures—and this means that the brain does, too. A formal element need only be repeated in three or four variations, and immediately we perceive both the invariance and the variance in the phenomenon and combine them into a structured whole. However, we do not perceive such a whole if there is only variance without any order or common element, or if there is only invariance without any variations or modifications. In the first case we register merely a disordered confusion, and in the second merely monotonous sameness. However, we have a strong tendency in every situation to structure things that are in fact structured only slightly or not at all. Thus we very quickly perceive the slightest similarities in what appears to be a street of totally dissimilar houses (perhaps they share the same type of roof), or we involuntarily group monotonously repeated sounds (such as those made by the wheels of a train) into rhythmic sequences. Gestalt psychologists discovered years ago that this "structuralizing" urge to give "good" or "economical" form to things conforms to definite principles and most probably represents a fundamental and innate quality of human perception. Today we can add to this insight the findings of modern neuropsychology and neurophysiology, which suggest that extracting the invariance while at the same time recognizing the variance is precisely the main task of central clusters of nerve cells associated with the sensory organs. It has recently been discovered that certain groups of brain cells register only special kinds of information; in the ocular region some cells register only horizontal, only vertical, or only diagonal forms. Platt considers the search for invariances to be a general organizational principle of all cortical processes.[10]

In addition, the fascinating studies made of so-called split-brain patients (whose two cerebral hemispheres have been severed by surgery) in recent years have shown that synthesis and the recognition of wholes (that is, invariance) tend to be a function of the right hemisphere, whereas analysis and the recognition of single elements are more a function of the left hemisphere.[11] According to Eccles.

The dominant hemisphere is predominantly symbolic and propositional in its function, having specialization for language with syntactical, semantic, mathematical, and logical abilities . . .

The minor hemisphere on the other hand is superior in pictorial and pattern sense and in musical sense, its synthetic abilities matching the analytical abilities of the dominant hemisphere . . .

We do know that you get a quicker judgment about the recognition of a face which has already been presented and which can later be picked out from an ensemble of faces by the *gestalt*-like mechanism of the right temporal lobe. This is much quicker than the more verbal analytical operations on the left side, so this is a sign that there is some specially organized, very efficient machinery in parts of the brain just to get out quick picture recognition in a *gestalt* manner.[12]

The dominant hemisphere (usually the left) thus appears to be occupied mainly with recognizing details, while the right hemisphere recognizes wholes. The definition of a structure arrived at in the preceding section therefore not only fits very well with the recent findings of neurophysiology but can also contribute something to these findings from a different perspective. The definition ran:

A structure is a product of an invariance and a variance.

This simple definition does in fact seem to take into account all the important characteristics of a structure:

It includes the element of *wholeness,* since all the elements of the structure as defined above contain a feature in common (namely the invariance) and thus together form a whole. (A whole can exist only on the basis of shared qualities.)

It includes the phenomenon of *transformation* in the element of variance, which is coupled with the invariable element.

Finally, it includes the important element of *self-regulation,* insofar as the required combination of an invariable with a variable component establishes a framework or principle; only within its limits is variation possible and permitted.

Two minor difficulties remain to be clarified. The first concerns the fact that completely regular structures, such as chessboards or honeycombs, do not seem to combine an invariance with a variance, since the recurring elements are exactly the same. If we consider, however, that in these cases the topographical position varies from element to element, then our definition remains valid.

The other point involves the objection that structure is frequently understood to mean only the invariance, the underlying sameness (in our example, the "table" principle), and not the variance, or many concrete modifications of the single, unvarying principle. This point of view is correct, and it arises from the basic ambiguity inherent in the concepts of structure and system from the beginning: they have been used in both a static and a dynamic sense at different times. The definition of a structure aimed at here is a dynamic one, corresponding to the prevailing usage of the term today, in which *structure is regarded as a system of transformations,* just as Piaget called for. Such a system includes variance as well as invariance.

Further reflection makes it clear that the three characteristics of a structure considered central by Piaget can all be reduced to a single principle, so that the definition is actually redundant: the phenomenon of self-regulation, that is, the operation of a law or principle, already includes the phenomenon of wholeness, since wherever a principle operates, regularity, similarity, and repetition (invariance) occur; therefore, a whole or totality is automatically implied. The operation of a principle also implies the presence of transformation—that is, variability or variance—since a principle embraces a multiplicity of different phenomena under a common rule. It thus transpires that, in the last analysis, the most general definition is: *A structure is the expression of a law or principle.* Although this statement is correct, however, it is also so much broader than the definition "a structure is the product of an invariance and a variance" that it ceases to be of much use for our purposes. Incidentally, we see in this case that both a law and a structure require a certain redundancy for us to be able to recognize them and find them useful in practice. The structure (or principle, or "law") of a table could certainly be deduced from a single specific example of a table, but it becomes much clearer if we place a whole series of different tables—high and low, round and square, wooden and stone, with one leg and with several legs—next to one another; then we can grasp both the variety and the unifying features of the phenomena (*unitas multiplex*) that constitute the table principle. Obviously this circumstance has great significance for the way in which the human mind operates.

The example of the table should remind us of our point of departure, the idea of differentiation. We can now see clearly that every differentiation "creates structure" or "has a structure" or must "be structured," since we have realized that a differentiation consists in a modification of something shared or held in common (for example, the table principle) by the introduction of new variations. According to our definition the new whole that is thereby created always combines an invariable with a variable component. All imaginable tables together form the total combinative differentiation, or the "system," of tables. If we depart from the invariable table principle, then we no longer have a table, but perhaps a chair or a lectern instead. Every other differentiation we can think of—the system of chemical elements, plant and animal species, works of art, household objects, or intellectual constructions such as religions, scientific theories, and all forms of social and political organization—is structured in precisely the same way and consists of an invariable and a variable component.

In this context several interesting characteristics of creative processes become apparent: it is evident that different levels of creativity exist, which can be divided into at least three main categories. The first and most spectacular kind of creative act consists in discovering a radically new fundamental principle (such as the table principle). The second level consists in varying this principle by discovering new combinations of elements, such as new materials or forms to which the principle can be applied. The third level consists in exploring all the possible combinations of these elements that have been introduced by creativity at the second level, such as different forms of tables in different materials. These three levels are exemplified in the kaleidoscope. The most creative person was without doubt the inventor of this magical toy (anonymous, so far as I know); the second step was taken by those who found new elements, such as bits of colored glass or metal, beads, and seeds, to put in the tube. Finally, we perform the third step every time we turn a kaleidoscope to produce the ephemeral combinations of all these elements, combinations which appear to be infinite, but which in fact are not. Analogous levels of creativity can easily be found in all the forms created by nature or human beings (crystals, chemical compounds, plant and animal species, forms of houses, fashions in dress, tools, and so on). Another line of creativity, which can sometimes lead to the discovery of entirely new structures, consists in varying the basic principle. Today, for example, new kinds of kaleidoscope exist, based on a system of lenses rather than on the original three mirrors. Similarly the "abnormal" variation of the fish principle may have led to the evolution of reptiles or birds, or the variation of the table principle to the discovery of the chair or the chest of drawers.

Creativity in this sense—the sphere of artists and philosophers, inventors, and visionaries much more than the sphere of technicians—

resembles the exploration of pioneers, who are constantly impelled by their curiosity to seek out the unknown, just as an ant colony sends out its scouts in all directions. They open trails, create links, build bridgeheads, and bring new information back to the familiar terrain of home and daily routines. Many, perhaps most, of these intellectual adventurers lose their way and come to grief; for this reason the stay-at-homes and dry scholars view their doings with great suspicion. But sometimes the paths upon which they set out are followed by organized groups, which strengthen the bridgeheads, place warning signs and railings along the cliff edges, and in time expand the most useful routes into a network of new roads. The masses do not follow until much later, when the critical junctions begin to appear secure and the (intellectual) connections that not long before had looked impossible begin to seem routine. Then the multitude comes along, bringing an arsenal of scientific instruments and laboratories for measuring, weighing, registering, and cataloging. The area of the known, be it in science or other fields, can thus be compared to a well-built network of roads, large and small, highways and byways on the periphery of which creative intuition is constantly seeking in all directions for new paths into the unknown.

It appears more and more likely that these road systems correspond to certain cerebral networks of associations formed through experience. We ought, incidentally, to include not only artists and philosophers among these "intellectual pioneers," but in a certain sense also the "insane," those borderline personalities and schizophrenics whose surprisingly unconventional associations and combinations of ideas are sometimes creative and fruitful. If we consider the millions of experiments occurring in nature in the almost inexhaustible multiplicity of forms of plants, marine life, and insects, then we must realize that the unceasing playful exploration of new combinations and possibilities by the human mind—whether we label it diseased or healthy—represents only a special case of a ubiquitous phenomenon. Far beyond the realm of living creatures all nature is at work creating new combinations. Nature itself is nothing other than a continuous, gigantic, combinative process of creation.

But let us return from this digression—although it is not so much of one as it may appear—to our subject. In the next section I will try to show that all the structures discussed above as the result of creative processes can also be understood as systems in the sense of modern systems theory.

Structures and Systems

In many academic disciplines the terms *structure* and *system* are often used synonymously. It is most revealing that Ferdinand de Saussure, the founder of modern structuralism, never referred to "structures," but always to "systems," as Benviste remarks.[13] At the beginning of the twentieth century, when all linguistic scholarship was devoted to the diachronic *history* of language, de Saussure's revolutionary approach treated language, with all its elements, as a whole synchronic system.[14] If we now compare the definitions offered for the term *system* with those offered for *structure,* we see that the similarities are striking, especially for the newer, dynamic understanding of structure. According to Miller, a system is a whole consisting of several elements, its main characteristics being wholeness, transformation, and self-regulation—just like a structure.[15] And in a system, just as in a structure, a "solidarity" exists between the constituent elements: a change in one element causes changes in others. The whole is not just the sum of its parts, but rather a framework of *relations* governed by certain principles. In the chapter on psychoanalysis and systems theory we encountered the idea of circular rather than linear causality and the idea of homeostasis achieved by means of feedback mechanisms (negative feedback in particular). These are also important characteristics of a system in the view of systems theory. All these characteristics have also been connected with the concept of structure, in particular in Piaget's theories and in mathematics.[16]

Since the definition proposed above for a structure contains the phenomena of wholeness, transformation, and self-regulation, this definition must be applicable to both concepts in the same way. Is it therefore permissible to equate "structure" and "system" and to use them as synonyms?

The answer is yes and no! Yes, if we take the virtually identical definitions into consideration; no, if we consider the finer nuances of usage. The word *structure* definitely contains a historical or diachronic component. A structure is a construction, something with a history; the arrangement of its parts reflects its development. From a crystal, a honeycomb, geological formations, and even social or intellectual structures we can gain a sense of how the whole has been formed by a process of combination and differentiation. The decision tree illustrates the abstract schema of a structure very well.

The same is not true of a system in the usual sense of the word. We do not usually become aware of the diachronic formation of a system, but only of its synchronic balance; in other words, we grasp a system as a dynamic process of homeostatic adjustment of "tensions" (to use a very general term) among a number of elements that are present simultaneously but whose origins do not appear to be of any particular significance. For this reason the best abstract illustration of a system is not the decision tree, but rather a closed shape containing a number of elements, such as ripples in a pool, a living cell, or the works of a larger clock with many big and small cogwheels that together make up the whole.

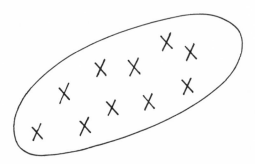

Obviously the concepts of structure and system do not denote exactly the same thing, despite virtually identical definitions and considerably overlapping usage. Nevertheless, as our intuition has told us all along, it is a matter of the same phenomenon in principle. This principle is seen from two different perspectives, however, and is therefore not described in totally synonymous ways.

In order to make this clearer I must return to my remarks on the concept of differentiation and to the polar structure of every single difference on the basis of which differentiation occurs. I have indicated that the fundamental constitutive element of every structure is a *bipolarity*. If we recall that the bipolarity $A \rightleftarrows B$ is also the simplest possible system, and further that every more complex system than that can be seen as a combination of a number of bipolarities, then we have established a virtually direct connection between the two concepts or, we might say, between the two systems of reference. A bipolarity—consisting of one positively and one negatively charged particle, or of two cognitive counterparts such as "large" and "small," or affective counterparts such as "love" and "hate"—represents the simplest of all conceivable systems; it forms a whole. In it a dynamic balance prevails between two diametrically opposed extremes. A large number of complementary variants is possible in this

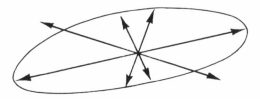

system—in other words, a whole series of transformations. In short, a bipolarity has all the fundamental characteristics of a system or structure. If a single bipolarity is expanded into a more complex formation, or whole, by the addition of several other bipolarities, then its overall condition is the result of an equilibrium among all the bipolarities contained in it, and we have arrived at a typical *system* as illustrated in the drawing. Examples on various levels are the previously mentioned living cell, the individual psyche, or the family—in all of which a number of (real or potential) opposites are equilibrated to form a whole.

These considerations reveal the complete identity of the terms *structure* and *system*. Both arise diachronically from a number of diametrically opposed bipolarities that ultimately form a whole of elements existing simultaneously in a variable but interdependent—that is, *ordered*—manner, as one might imagine a system of connected pipes. However, in the concept of structure the diachronic aspect or genesis is visible, in a system the synchronous aspect, the "stasis" or condition.[17] Nevertheless the phenomenon as a whole, which has a diachronic-historical-formative aspect and a synchronous-ahistorical-momentary aspect, is the same in both cases. This phenomenon is essentially an abstract one: *Structures as well as systems are in fact equilibrated networks of relationships.*

It is especially interesting to note that in the end the factor of time becomes irrelevant: both structures and systems can be either synchronous or diachronic. The simplest diachronic system, which corresponds precisely to a bipolarity, is the pendulum. The "pendulum of history" is a well-known example from the social sciences, and in psychoanalysis we are familiar with diachronic compensatory mechanisms, some of which may last for an entire lifetime (such as an insatiable lust for power after a previous painful experience of helplessness). Another example is the system of family "debit and credit accounts" studied by Boszormenyi-Nagy.[18] *Diachronic* means "historical," "a longitudinal section," and *synchronous* means "the present," "a cross-section," but clearly they are not irreconcilable opposites. It appears to be more a case of two different aspects of one and the same phenomenon or principle, the nature of which probably consists above all in *equilibrium*. One fact that supports this view is the impossibility of making a sharp distinction between them; they merge into each other without any clear line of demarcation: depending on the context and our point of view, we may consider entire years, centuries, or even millennia (in an evolutionary or geological framework: as "the present," or nuclear physicists may mean by "the present" mere fractions of a second.[19]

There will perhaps be an opportunity later to return to some of these ideas. However, before we turn to the specific question of affective-logical systems of reference, we must take a closer look at the virtual or functional identity that exists between the concepts of a system and a system of reference.

Systems and Systems of Reference

It is obvious—and clearly implied in the term itself—that all systems of reference are "systems" in the specific sense of the modern theory. It is not nearly as evident whether the reverse if true—that is, whether all systems also function as systems of reference.

We need only recall, however, that all complex systems may be regarded as combinations of a large number of bipolar elements, which must of necessity lie somewhere between two extreme positions or states. Organic cells, for example, which clearly represent the kind of (open) system we have been discussing, can survive only within specific limits of pH, temperature, relation of total mass to surface, electrolyte composition, water content, and so on. The total cell system is a combination or result of all these bipolarities. Bateson writes in this connection: "The whole network of biological values depends on upper and lower limits. There are no variables which an organism can safely maximize. Too much of the best thing becomes toxic. Too little of the worst thing is likely to become toxic, too."[20] The same applies, though in a less obvious manner, to cognitive, affective, or social systems. Since value systems, for example, have both affective and cognitive components, we are certainly justified in calling them "affective-logical systems"; they consist of a complex combination of thoughts, feelings, and corresponding types of behavior, all of which fluctuate between two extreme positions. The value system that governs our behavior when we enter a church, for example, permits a series of moderate variations within "permitted" (= "good," "correct") limits, between extremes of two many or too few clothes, too much motion and immobility, speech and silence, extremely intense contact with others and no contact at all, and so on. All variations of behavior approaching too closely to one extreme or the other are considered inappropriate, "bad," or "wrong." If someone chooses to behave in one of these ways, we consider him "crazy," that is, removed from a middle range felt to be the norm. This norm is like a familiar, customary safety zone, one that does not cause an excess of disturbance or tension, one that conserves energy and thus seems pleasant.

We could describe any other value system in similar terms and also—as Piaget has so clearly demonstrated—any single cognitive concept or schema. Consider our example of a table. Contrary to our first impression, this concept does not represent a static, single element, but rather a dynamically equilibrated system. What is a table and what is no longer a table (but a chair, a chest of drawers, or a cupboard) is determined within a wide range of outer limits by the possible dimensions of legs and top surface, the relationship of one to the other and the angle at which they meet, the materials used, and so forth. We have seen that this typical *unitas multiplex* is experienced by a child as he acts, in a process of learning and interaction with the environment characterized by assimilation and accommodation. In the end the child acquires a (functional) schema of what a table is. Thus the concept "table" also represents a norm or mean value within specific limits. Whoever oversteps these bounds, by using the term in an inappropriate manner (that is, using too broad or too narrow an interpretation), begins to disturb and unsettle other people, and in the short or long run they will consider him "crazy."

This analysis should have made it clear that concepts are systems and that at the same time such systems are *systems of reference,* and why this is so: Every concept, every value system, and, what is more, all concepts and value systems in combination are equilibrated, customary, and economical norms and mean values, comparable to a system of good roads in rough terrain. They are constructed with the aid of experience (trial and error) and direct our thinking and feeling into certain paths or channels in a manner that grows increasingly automatic with time—in other words, in a manner that causes less and less friction and tension. These channels grow deeper and wider with frequent use; conversely, they will dry up if they are not used. They draw our thoughts and feelings into them as a canal system draws water; they function as a preexisting network and after a certain point will not be altered except in the case of massive disturbances that cannot be dealt with in any other way. In the light of current understanding these networks are probably neuronal systems of associations created by experience. They are what we call our personal "truths" or "reality," or vice versa: so-called truths are actually relatively customary, efficient systems of reference, formed through interaction with the environment and functioning with a minimum of tension and effort. This implies at the same time that the affective-logical truths of an Amazonian Indian must necessarily be quite different from those of a New Yorker, and the truths of an American will not resemble those of a Russian or West European. Systems of reference are able to function as structuring networks or truths and to provide guidelines for perception and behavior only if they possess a certain minimal amount of coherence and clarity. We shall see later that this circumstance is of great importance in understanding schizophrenic confusion and ambiguity, and especially in understanding that collision and interlocking of incompatible systems of reference or truths usually known as the double bind.

We may even go so far as to assume that in fact *all* systems function as systems of reference in this sense: since they are equivalent to states of equilibrium between several extremes, states with a minimum of tension, they have to "pull" their elements in a particular direction. In other words, systems are states or constellations in which objects, circumstances, and so on tend to dispose or arrange themselves as they do for reasons of economy, just as the pieces of glass in a kaleidoscope form patterns that, although they can vary enormously, are still dictated by the existing framework. Every differentiation in organic and inorganic nature (not only atoms and molecules but also tissue, organs, organisms, and social and intellectual structures) must be understood as equilibrated systems within a given framework. This discussion has thus led us to a unified structuralist view of a number of different phenomena; in this view the human mind and social conditions represent merely special cases. It is with them, however, that we must now concern ourselves in greater detail.

Conclusions about the Nature of Affective-Logical Structures and Systems

The question is to what extent the theories discussed so far can contribute to a more profound understanding of the nature of the mind in general and of affective-logical systems of reference in particular. It is already clear that we can draw a number of conclusions, and several more suggest themselves in outline.

We can obviously regard psychic differentiations and every type of affective or cognitive concept as typical structures with a variance and an invariance, and also as systems and systems of reference in the sense described above. This may even apply at the level of neurons. An important example of a comprehensive affective-logical system of reference, albeit a complicated one, would be the internalized schemata determining our object relations (and thus also our *behavior*)— that is, our relationships to important people in our lives, as defined by psychoanalysis. We can reconstruct the genesis and structure of such a system of reference with the largely overlapping insights of psychoanalysis and genetic epistemology as follows.

The inborn sucking reflex is activated by hunger (an unpleasurable sensation) and certain sensory and tactile stimuli; its activation brings about pleasure, and it is halted by satiety. This reflex acquires additional elements within a few days of birth, including better-coordinated movements of the mouth, head, and eyes, grasping movements of the infant's hands, and increasingly differentiated affective "moods" or experiences of pleasure or its opposite. As it comes to include ever more precisely perceived elements (certain temporal rhythms, tactile stimuli, temperatures, sounds, faces), it quickly develops into a quite complex sensorimotor and affective "program." After several months of development these simultaneously occurring affective and cognitive elements (with respect to the mother and other important caretakers) fuse to form demarcated "objects" or wholes. The child finally grasps their permanence and the fact that although they may disappear for a time they will reappear. At the same time the child also begins to acquire a first sense of the continuity of space and time with regard to his immediate surroundings, as well as the seeds of self-awareness.

Internalized affective-cognitive wholes of this kind continue to increase in differentiation until clear, gestaltlike representations of the objects encountered are formed, particularly of personal objects (mother, father, siblings, and others) and the child's own self, all of which have particular basic affects attached to them. The child finally experiences a large number of dynamic relations between these now well-demarcated figures with particular intensity in the oedipal phase, and internalizes them. As more time passes the child accumulates more experience and expands the original mother figure (and possibly a sister or sisters) into a picture of women in general. In the same way the father (or earliest and most important male figure) contributes decisively to the child's picture of what a man is, along with the ac-cumulation of attributes experienced in other men. Eventually men and women are habitually perceived in the affective-cognitive frame-work thus established. There is a great deal of evidence for the view that schemata of this kind, equilibrated over the course of years, are typical affective-cognitive systems of reference in the sense described above; in addition to many psychological theories I would cite partic-ularly the phenomena that psychoanalysis has gathered together under the heading *transference:* it demonstrates in all clarity that we relate people whom we encounter to a particular schema because they remind us of other people encountered before. Depending on how our internalized representations are designed, we perceive—and sometimes *deform*—people in the same way, over and over again. For example, someone may experience all men bearing some resemblance to father figures stereotypically as authoritarian, aggressive, and dan-gerous. Not only will all his thoughts and feelings correspond to this schema, but also all his behavior. Therapeutic experience has taught us that such schemata possess a high degree of resistance to change and will be re-formed only with considerable expenditure of effort, as genetic epistemology has demonstrated.

From this perspective it appears probable that the entire "psyche" consists of just such hierarchically organized affective-cognitive sys-tems of reference, or instructions for feeling, thinking, and acting; once activated by certain contexts or precipitating factors, they affect our behavior. These equilibrated, synchronous systems reflect the es-sence of all diachronically acquired experiences at every stage of life. Every person, every age group (and, generally speaking, every epoch, every country, and every group of people with a common history) thus possesses its own truths, which correspond to the truths of other people or age groups (or epochs, countries, peoples) only to the extent that this experience is shared.[21] This indicates what philosophers have long been claiming, namely that no "objective" truth exists. There are only more or less general, "interpersonal" and conventional "accuracies," which function because people have accepted them on the basis of the same experiences.

I now return to the interesting question of whether the psyche has a polar structure throughout, a possibility that has suggested itself in several different ways. Although the preceding discussion does not permit any definite conclusions, it does provide several indications that polar structures are ubiquitous, one such indication being the fundamental role of differentiation and the potential polarity of every differentiation. In addition, we have seen that both cognitive and affective perceptions are always located on a continuum between at least two poles: The figure-ground problem shows that without a corresponding counterpart to a part we are incapable of perceiving anything at all. In the same way every intense emotional experience (be it love, joy, pleasure, pain, sadness, or fear) is possible only against the background of its opposite; the one determines and constitutes the other. Without some swings of the pendulum (differences) toward *both* sides, we would end up experiencing nothing. It is especially interesting in this connection that such regularities exist not only synchronously—that is, in the simultaneous events of the present, the cross-section—but also in diachronic systems such as the pendular movements of history mentioned above: love turns into hate, helplessness into a craving for power, masochism into sadism, and vice versa. This idea suggests interesting links to the phenomenon of fluctuation, which consists in rapid shifts between two opposite states of mind and which may be involved when normal affective-logical systems of reference become pathological. Fluctuation and its analogies to the formation of what Prigogine has called "dissipative structures" will be discussed in detail in Chapter 6. We can observe similar processes at work in the psychosocial field, such as the manifold interaction of extreme positions in politics. This observation again makes it clear that these phenomena can be properly understood only through a synthesis of psychoanalytic theory and systems theory.

I can describe here only in outline the way in which the original polarities form more complex structures. Basically they arise from a combination of many different bipolarities. It should be noted further that two opposites necessarily lead to a third phenomenon, namely a *middle*, an *in-between*. Bateson must have had something similar in mind when he remarked, in connection with binocular vision, that *"relationship is always the product of a double description."* [22]

This middle already contains the seeds of further development, however, as we can again see with particular clarity in the psychosocial field. The position of political moderates cannot be defined at all without the existence of the extremes; this fact may thus cause one moderate position to appear slightly more "radical" than another, making the formation of a more truly "moderate" middle group necessary, which in turn may set in motion yet another process of differentiation. Thus in a sense the middle "needs" the extremes. This fact places all kinds of marginality—including that of psychiatric patients—in a new light.

The same applies to many (perhaps all?) other psychosocial structures. The fact that two opposites necessarily create a third component, namely a relation and thus a *relativization,* was discussed in Chapter 1 in connection with the various constellations possible in the familiar triad of mother, father, and child: the child cannot truly perceive the third component, the father, until the child has achieved separation from the mother, until he has dissolved the original, narcissistic union and they have become two distinct poles or entities. Similarly, the child cannot acquire his own real identity until he becomes fully aware of the difference between his mother and father (in the oedipal phase). And finally he achieves genuine autonomy and psychological maturity (usually late in life, if ever) only when he has succeeded in integrating both with all their contradictions. This means in part the ability to accept their good *and* bad sides—which are always experienced intrapsychically as extremes—without negating the one or the other.

In summary, we may draw the conclusion from such obviously ubiquitous patterns that *absolutely nothing can exist without its corresponding counterpart.* The nature of the physical universe, which consists of positive and negative electrical charges, matter and antimatter, matter and energy, and so on, supports this view. It is most likely that all these convergences are connected with the absolutely central element of equilibrium. Equilibrium is also an essential part of systems theory, as the preceding chapter made clear. For this reason I have arrived at the conclusion that this theory must imply a basically polar structure of all differentiations or systems: the universe as a whole with its endless number of subsystems can be regarded as one gigantic process of equilibration. It is based on sets of equilibria or "equations" between the most various components; that is, in the last analysis it is based on parts and their counterparts.

These general considerations seem to lead straight to those comprehensive doctrines of dualism of which there has been no lack in both Eastern and Western philosophy, from Heraclitus to Hegel, and from *yin* and *yang* to Zen Buddhism. We have clearly hit upon fascinating questions for both philosophy and science, which our specific subject matter will not permit us to investigate in further detail. I would therefore like to stop here and summarize the most important results of this chapter.

The preceding discussion has shown that differences lead to differentiations, and differentiations to structures. It has shown further that structures and systems are virtually identical and can be generally defined as the product of an invariance and a variance. We may regard equilibrated affective-cognitive schemata as typical structures or systems in this sense; at the same time they represent affective-logical systems of reference, which on the one hand result from our interaction with the reality we encounter, and which on the other hand condition this interaction. The human mind obviously consists of a hierarchy of such systems of reference. Much evidence exists to suggest that the mind has a fundamentally polar or binary character.

4   On Language and Consciousness

Ideas form a complete system within us, comparable to one of the
natural kingdoms, a sort of bloom whose iconography will be traced
by a man of genius who will pass perhaps as mad.

—Honoré de Balzac, *Louis Lambert*

This chapter is devoted to the mysterious phenomenon of human
consciousness and its connections with language. We shall be concerned here not only with the "nature" of consciousness (its genesis,
structure, and function) but also with the role that certain phenomena
play in its formation: the differentiation of systems of reference and
the "extraction of invariance," that is, a condensation or abstraction
of information. As the example of the table concept has already
shown, language itself represents a typical condensation (*Verdich-
tung*) of a large number of concrete manifestations; it is only a small
step to the conclusion that consciousness and language are closely
related and may even be identical. We are certainly aware of what we
are able to express in words; in the same way the term *inexpressible*
is virtually a synonym for *unconscious*. The recent discovery of an
asymmetry in certain regions of the human brain that are associated
with conscious use of language and are lacking in animals appears to
support this hypothesis. Thus a closer look at the connections between consciousness and language may help to bring us closer to our
goal, which is to understand the psyche and also "insanity" as a peculiarly altered state of consciousness.

Consciousness and language, both very important fields for psychology and psychiatry, are extremely complex phenomena. Attempts
in the literature to deal with both together or their relationship to
each other are exceedingly rare. Clearly, the problem belongs to no
single discipline; various aspects are claimed by linguistics, psychol-

ogy, and philosophy (that is, the humanities), whereas others belong to natural sciences such as biology, neurophysiology, and medicine. As a result, most authors have concerned themselves with either language or consciousness, and almost no one has tried to integrate the two. Thus Chomsky's *Language and Mind* presents a comprehensive survey of linguistics but makes few references to the problem of consciousness; the same is true of Bierwisch's summary.[1] Piaget's work contains many interesting ideas on the importance of language in cognitive development—to which we shall return shortly—but as far as I know he did not explicitly address the problem of consciousness in this connection.

Similarly, authors who have investigated the phenomenon of consciousness usually mention language only in passing. In the last century, when Wundt, Wernicke, and others carried on the tradition begun by Leibniz in their studies of the nature of consciousness, the science of linguistics as we know it today was still in its infancy. Later, interest in the question of consciousness shifted away from psychology into the fields of neurophysiology and psychiatry. In recent times the French psychiatrist Henri Ey used the older work of Jackson and newer research on brain structure and functions to develop a differentiated theory of consciousness; his findings suggest a complex structure corresponding in large measure to the hierarchical organization of the regions of the brain involved (such as the cortex, reticular formation, centrencephalic projection system, and rhinencephalon). Even in this impressive synthesis, however, Ey does not go into the phenomenon of language at any length.[2]

One interesting study of language and consciousness has been undertaken by the Nobel laureate Sir John Eccles in conjunction with the philosopher Karl Popper. In their fascinating book *The Self and Its Brain* Eccles discusses the findings on split-brain patients (whose two brain hemispheres have been separated by surgery) and offers the hypothesis that a close connection exists between consciousness and the language centers of the left cerebral cortex. However, Eccles does not take any of the findings of modern linguistics into consideration, and—rather surprisingly for a neurophysiologist—he treats consciousness ("the self-conscious mind") as a wholly immaterial entity. He represents it as somehow located above the left hemisphere, connected with the brain only by a number of hypothetical open or closed "modules" in an equally hypothetical "liaison area" of the left cerebral cortex.[3] Apparently this "self-conscious mind" is supposed to be able to make choices, learn, and even feel wishes and desires quite independently of physiological processes in the brain, although these wishes and desires exert an active influence on the "neuronal" apparatus. Eccles writes, for example:

> the hypothesis is that the self-conscious mind is an independent entity . . . that is actively engaged in reading out from the multitude of active centres in the modules of the liaison areas of the dominant cerebral hemisphere. The self-conscious mind selects from these centres in accord with its attention and its interests and integrates its selection to give the unity of conscious experience from moment to moment. It also acts back on the neural centres.[4]

In other words, Eccles' theory of the self-conscious mind suggests a little organism like a homunculus that has no actual connection with processes in the brain. This strikes me as more of a philosophical than a scientific view, however, and it does not lead us much further, since the problem of the relationship between the brain and consciousness is not thereby solved, but merely displaced a step upwards or outward in the unexplained quantum leap from the "open modules" of the "liaison brain" of the left cerebral cortex to "the mind." In addition Eccles is concerned primarily with only one particular aspect of consciousness, namely self-awareness or the self-conscious mind. Both psychoanalysis and the work of Henri Ey indicate clearly, however, that this represents only an especially differentiated late form of an extraordinarily complex phenomenon.

For our purposes we might do best by attempting to grasp the phenomenon of consciousness as a whole. Only then will we have a broad enough basis on which to proceed and to relate the idea of consciousness to that of language with any success. We must also avoid thinking of the latter exclusively in terms of the sophisticated tool of present-day adults, which is the form in which we most often encounter language. Instead we should recognize that language represents a special case and the end result (so far) of an immensely long process of development, whose far-reaching ramifications have been explored by both genetic epistemologists and structural linguists.

The Concept of Consciousness

The literature presents consciousness as a complex and elusive phenomenon. Many authors do not even believe that it can be defined, since every definition would mean a limitation, a choice of some aspects to the exclusion of others.[5] Leibniz understood consciousness to mean "the total content of our experience of self"; Jahrreis saw it as "a peculiar degree of clarity, fullness, mobility, tempo, and hierarchical order of inner experience and the psychic functions." Karl Jaspers defined consciousness as "every manner of inner experience," distinguishing three aspects:

> It firstly implies *awareness of experience* and as such is distinct from loss of consciousness and what is extra-conscious; secondly, it implies *awareness of an object,* knowing something, and as such is distinct from unconscious subjective experience, in which "I" and "object" are as yet undifferentiated; thirdly, it implies *self-reflection,* awareness of one's self, and as such is distinct from the unconscious experience where I experience the self and the object as separate entities but am not explicitly aware of this differentiation.[6]

At the same time, however, Jaspers emphasized that the life of the mind cannot be understood merely as consciousness and from consciousness alone. An "unconscious foundation" must be assumed to exist as well, even though its existence can never be directly proved. "The life of the mind which is immediately accessible and which we actually experience is like foam floating above the depths of an ocean." What is outside our consciousness takes the form of everything "which we do not notice or pay attention to but nonetheless experience, which we do not intend to do but nonetheless do, which we forget and do not remember," and—most important for our subject—everything "which does not become concrete, which is not grasped in words." Ludwig Pongratz assumes the same relationship between what is unconscious and wordless, on the one hand, and between language and consciousness on the other, when he describes as "conscious" "everything which is communicated in words or at least communicable." His formulation is also notable in that consciousness represents a "cognitive presence of something: This means that consciousness always involves a more of less clear knowledge of something here and now."[7]

Also of interest in our context is Henri Ey's emphasis on the concept of the *field of consciousness* as the "scene of current experience in time and space," which is constantly changing, purposefully directed, and closely tied to the actions of the subject. According to Ey, the various aspects of this field form a "vertical structure and vertical dynamic" of consciousness, which are connected to processes of activation and deactivation between cortex and brain stem, and thus also connected to various stages of attention and vigilance, the rhythms of sleeping and waking, and so on.[8] Thus, in this view as well, consciousness is by no means a single phenomenon, but a multifaceted one that is constantly in flux; its hierarchically ordered levels range from the faintest traces of awareness to an intense clarity and full presence of mind that includes a sense of self and of the world around this self.

It should be growing clear that this view of consciousness cannot simply be equated with a particular waking condition of the brain such as might be registered by an electroencephalogram. It is something far more complex, something intimately related to *knowledge,* either of oneself or of the world around one. "Consciousness is always knowledge of something, always related to something," says Christian Scharfetter.[9]

I follow Pongratz in taking the view that the many diverse forms in which consciousness manifests itself can best be grouped for our purposes under the following extremely simple definition: *Consciousness is that which is known in general as well as at every single moment.*

This definition takes into account that consciousness is subject to the constant changes mentioned above; that it contracts and expands; that it directs its beam on certain areas like a moving searchlight, allowing other areas to lapse into darkness; it takes into account that consciousness can be either bright and clear or murky and confused, depending on our vigilance and the state of brain functions such as sleeping, waking, and dreaming. Most important, this definition makes it clear that consciousness has a genesis and undergoes development, which has its ontogenetic origins somewhere in the first months of life and its phylogenetic origins in the evolution of complex organisms. At the same time many levels of consciousness exist: I may "know about something," as when I put together a piece of equipment in the laboratory, concentrating totally on the task at hand and not thinking about myself. While I am thus occupied, I resemble—perhaps more closely than we usually think—an animal that has actualized certain internal schemata to build a nest. On the next level, I may "know that I know something," if I observe myself putting the equipment together; or I may even "know that I know that I know something," as I observe myself observing; and so on. We float back and forth between such levels of consciousness or abstraction; the example above is intended to give only a rough indication of how this occurs. It seems obvious that the higher levels are accessible only to human beings. This kind of consciousness changes in the course of a human life and in the course of history, and its individual and social aspects affect one another profoundly. Many pieces of conscious knowledge are transmitted to individuals by society, so that they share an awareness, a certain "spirit of the times." Both individual and supraindividual consciousness fluctuate from moment to moment, but both are also subject to a continuous process of change and extension over longer periods. As human knowledge constantly expands, we realize that this process has reached its highest level of sophistication (so far) in the thinking, speaking, writing, calculating, knowing, cultured, and self-aware adult of the present era.[10]

This point of view emphasizes the definition of consciousness as identical with knowledge. By this I do not mean a purely cognitive store of knowledge, however, but rather an actualization of knowledge that changes from moment to moment and is actively experienced. This process of actualization has a cognitive *and* an affective structure, that is, a typically affective-logical structure, rising from an unconscious foundation like a mountain peak above a sea of clouds into the light of a more or less clear awareness. Scharfetter makes this point very well: "People in a state of waking do not have consciousness, but exist consciously, are themselves consciousness in various states of waking, sensation, experience, feeling, mood, rational knowledge, and activity."[11]

This kind of consciousness implies an element of feeling that is explicitly physical. Momentary physical sensations and sensory impressions[12] (or our processing of them; see the section below, "Language, Consciousness, and the Brain"), together with the memory traces they evoke, constitute our consciousness and constantly "feed" it. The information it is continually receiving, and particularly the affective (or motivational) component of this information, can be regarded as a source of energy, which functions like a generator, providing the necessary "power" to keep the flickering light of consciousness burning. As we shall see in more detail in Chapter 6, experiments have shown that total sensory deprivation leads rapidly to a profound disintegration of consciousness into psychosis.

The question then arises whether animals, small children, or undeveloped adults in so-called primitive cultures have a consciousness— or rather, what kind of consciousness they have, since it is clear that definite boundaries or gaps between levels of consciousness cannot and do not exist. As everywhere else in nature, there exist only continuous and gradual processes of development. Sensations, vigilance, attention, and obvious "knowledge of something" occur in animals far down the evolutionary scale, and of course in infants and "primitive" humans as well. To a certain degree even insects and small mammals such as mice and rats display constantly changing levels of vigilance and are capable of directing their attention to one thing or another in different situations; this is obviously true of cats, dogs, or apes to an even greater degree. They are able to learn, and after some time clearly "know," certain things about their territory, sources of food or danger, and so on. This knowledge—or consciousness—is quite differentiated, related to space and time, and emotionally colored—that is, structured in a typically affective-logical manner. They bring a particular inner *order* to their external environment; they "know" about love and danger; they follow, anticipate, and "know" a number of basic rules and rhythms. Of course this has little or nothing to do with reflection or self-awareness in the human sense. However, the human infant in the first months of life has a form of consciousness barely distinguishable from that of higher animals, and we may assume that the same holds true for "primitive" man in the earliest stages of his evolutionary development. Both higher mammals and human infants form sensorimotor schemata that are in principle quite similar, as Piaget observed. These lay the foundations for later, much more highly developed cognitive or cognitive-affective schemata. For a few months the higher mammals clearly outstrip human infants in this respect. Thus human and animal "consciousness" must possess a very similar structure for a period of time. But then this development progresses much further in human beings: from a certain point on, human consciousness grows in a peculiar manner, until it finally becomes sharp and clear. We might compare it to a film projector, whose blurred image can be improved by adjustment of its mechanisms.

I have already suggested that this phenomenon of "getting a sharper picture" is decisively influenced by language. The emergence of a clearer consciousness in a small child goes hand in hand with its acquisition of language, from quite an early stage. What we say and can "put into words" is obviously conscious, whereas what is unsaid and unsayable appears to be largely inaccessible to our conscious minds.

Before we pursue this hypothesis further, however, we must first clarify what is actually meant by "language."

The Concept of Language

Since the time of Ferdinand de Saussure linguists have ceased to regard language(s) as merely the sum of words and sentences that can be constructed according to certain historically determined phonetic and syntactical rules, in German, French, English, and so on. They have come instead to see language as something far more general, namely as *a structural, synchronic system of conventional signs* ("signifiers") between which definite relationships exist and which function as a code for something to be described ("signified"). In a similar manner the abstract signs of the alphabet stand for particular sounds, and abstract algebraic symbols represent particular relationships or events in the physical world.

The findings of linguistics on the inner structure of language(s) are far from complete. Much research is still being devoted not only to minor, individual problems but also to central questions: How did these systems of signs originate? How are the simplest basic elements ("linguistic universals") combined? (This combination is thought to occur according to a set of rules which are probably largely unconscious and which are usually referred to as "generative grammar.") And, in this context, to what extent is language development innate and to what extent acquired? Despite the fact that such important questions remain unresolved, the fundamental approach of modern linguistics can contribute a great deal to a better understanding of how human consciousness is structured. In particular, de Saussure's distinction between a "signifier" and a "signified," which is at the core of all modern structuralist thinking, proves to be central to our line of questioning. The possibility that our conscious utterances have an "unconscious foundation" is a question that linguists have been debating for a long time and one that represents an important aspect of the problem. And finally—following the line of discussion in Chapter 3—we must concern ourselves with the wealth of evidence suggesting that language has a dual structure.

But before discussing the significance of de Saussure's approach, I must introduce the concept of the semiotic function. The study of *the unconscious foundations of language* began in the 1930s, influenced by the development of psychoanalysis, with Troubetzkoi's four-point program (which was originally limited to phonology) for studying not conscious linguistic phenomena but their unconscious foundations; not the single elements of language but the system of relationships between them; not their classification into systems but the actual systems themselves; and not special elements of language but those elements having a general and absolute character.[13] Later Chomsky introduced the fundamental distinction between the (immediately recognizable and conscious) "surface structure" of a language and its (only indirectly evident and partially unconscious) "deep structure." Chomsky regards as unconscious those underlying rules that determine linguistic behavior and enable even a small child to construct a virtually unlimited number of correct sentences, many of which it can never have heard before. Modern linguists know (or "are conscious of") only some of these rules, which form the basis of an implicit "language competence" and, in their totality, a "generative grammar" (Chomsky) of whose structure the speaker is in fact completely unaware.

If psychoanalysis has had an influence on developments in linguistics, clearly the reverse is also true: the findings of modern linguistics are important for the debate of the *structure of the unconscious,* which—despite the fact that psychoanalysis has been around for more than seventy-five years—is still going on. We seem to be able to get a clearer idea of this structure here than just about anywhere else. What becomes evident is the fact that in most cases we are as unaware of the rules governing our speech as we are of the rules governing our feelings and behavior! In other words, *the unconscious consists primarily of a set of rules.* When it is a case of rules for cognitive behavior (including language), we may speak with Piaget of a "cognitive unconscious"; when it is a case of behavior in the area of emotions, we may follow Freud and speak of an "affective unconscious." However, this view does not compel us to make any sharp distinction between the two. On the contrary, their correlation emerges once again: not only do affect and intellect join together—in both the unconscious and the conscious mind—to form the inseparable whole of affect-logic, but the cognitive and the affective unconscious must possess quite similar characteristics of form and structure. In principle a set of rules must be structured like a language or—to put it abstractly—like a system of dynamic relationships between more stable single elements. This is precisely the type of system apparent in the surface structure of language, where predicates, conjunctions, and so on indicate dynamic relationships between substantives. Lacan's famous remark that the unconscious is structured like a language takes on a new and more profound significance in this context. In addition we begin to suspect that what the system of language expresses and gives concrete form to is characterized by logical necessity and general validity, namely the organization of a system or structure as such, as a "totality with relations (= transformations) existing between individual elements." All the immensely subtle possibilities of language—including the possible combinations, connections and separations, inclusions and exclusions, but also all the semantic shades of meaning of single words—would thus represent the (almost) complete range of logical operations (or "manipulations") that can be performed with the elements of a given system. The performance of these operations would be preprogrammed in the unconscious, however, in something like programmed microprocessors. They would correspond exactly to the "linguistic universals" mentioned above. Remaining largely unconscious, they would then have to form the basis of the generative grammar whose patterns are accessible to the rational mind only with great difficulty, if at all. We shall see later on that Piaget, in contrast to Chomsky, has put forward a plausible hypothesis for the origin of these "microprocessors."

In general it appears that language offers us a kind of "window" on the mind, through which we can catch of glimpse of its structure. From the simplest sensorimotor schemata to the highest levels of mental activity, this structure is both necessary and similar; it has an affective-logical character throughout. Only a small part of this uniform structure rises into the light of consciousness, however; the much larger and more significant portion remains hidden in a broad and dark unconscious foundation.

But what distinguishes these two components and causes the shift or condensation from unconscious to conscious in a particular zone? This question seems more profoundly mysterious, more amazing than ever. Some additional findings of modern linguistics on the structure of language may be of interest as we pursue an answer.

According to Piaget all cognitive differentiation has its origins in basic and dual biological rhythms, consisting in departure from and return to a particular physical state. This can already be observed in the earliest, largely inborn processes connected with sucking and grasping reflexes. I argued in Chapter 3 that such dual rhythms can and must be regarded as absolutely fundamental, since the basic dynamics of every homeostatic system consist of a dialectical process, the disruption and reestablishment of a state of equilibrium. It also emerged that, as such a process is repeated and establishes physiological pathways in the brain, a structure must arise of necessity. This structure is the product of an invariance (the original state, which always remains the same) and a variance (the possible deviations from this state). It became evident further that a dual or binary structure represents the simplest and thus the most probable form of every differentiation. It is thus worthy of note that a number of linguists have found evidence pointing to such a binary structure of language. Bierwisch, for instance, has mentioned that as long ago as the 1930s Hjelmslev's Copenhagen school of linguistics developed a hypothesis of duality; following de Saussure's taxonomy, they postulated a combinatory algebraic structure of language, characterized by a series of logical binary divisions.[14]

According to Hjelmslev, the first fundamental distinction between meaning and expression (signified and signifier) is followed by the distinction between "form" (the relation between pure values in de Saussure's sense) and "substance" (the nonlinguistic correlation in which the form manifests itself). This leads to a combination of possibilities resembling the decision tree, namely four constellations or "streets," ordered in pairs. Many more polarities occur further down the tree, such as the difference between nouns and verbs, verbs and adjectives, and singular and plural.

We can view language as a whole, therefore, from the simplest phonological elements to the most complicated semantic shades of meaning, as a chain of binary components existing in a purely logical and essentially mathematical relationship to each other. Together they form a system of "figures" or "combinations of figures" that, far more than phonetic signs, represents the essence of language. The modern American school of linguistics, with its most prominent representative Noam Chomsky, has repeatedly attempted to illustrate both the surface structure and the deep structure of language with just such a branching system of elements, usually ordered in a binary fashion. Chomsky also makes frequent mention of "cyclical operations," inborn principles of organization that determine the structure of universal grammar. He writes in this connection that certain "abstract and partially universal principles must be postulated which govern human mental abilities."[15] Chomsky does not take the next step, as Hjelmslev did, and postulate a universal binary structure of language, nor does he refer explicitly to the related work of Piaget; nonetheless we cannot fail to recognize a number of similarities between their ideas.

Considerable differences of opinion exist between Chomsky and Piaget, however, on the subject of language development and the degree to which it is acquired or inborn, even though linguists have not studied this phenomenon directly in children to the same extent as genetic epistemologists.[16] Chomsky maintains that the basis of "generative grammar" consists in a "general language competence" that is essentially inborn. Piaget, on the other hand, points to the importance of the differentiation process through which basic sensorimotor schemata are formed in the first year of life by means of assimilation and accommodation; these schemata precede the acquisition of language and represent its natural foundation. According to Piaget, language develops toward the end of the first year of life as part of the gradual development of the *semiotic function,* the ability to grasp concrete facts increasingly by means of signals, symbols, and signs in de Saussure's sense.[17] Thus for Piaget language is far from representing something new; instead *it begins by attaching signs to behavior schemata (or their "abstractions") already established in the sensorimotor area.* This assignment of (phonetic) signs occurs in a constant process of development, in which to begin with specific sounds or sound combinations are attached to a few very general "concepts," such as particular, emotionally significant actions, objects, or situations. Later these early assignments of certain sound combinations to elemental experience take on increasing differentiation, as either the area of experience (the signified) or the sequence of sounds itself (the signifier) is expanded and determined more precisely.

In her two excellent surveys of the contributions of genetic epistemology to linguistics Hermine Sinclair offers several examples of very early language elements: they are "holophrastic," meaning that they consist of a single "word" having the equivalent value of a whole sentence.[18] It is most interesting that at the start they almost always signal the disappearance of something or someone, for example in French *aplu* and *allé allé* (for *il n'y a plus,* "there is nothing more," and *allé,* "gone away") and in English "all gone." Obviously this characteristic feature is connected with the child's most difficult intellectual task at this stage, that is, acquiring a sense of object permanence and grasping the fact that objects such as its mother can disappear and reappear in the same form.

Freud illustrated the affective side of this crucial step in cognitive maturation with the well-known little anecdote of the spool of thread. An eighteen-month-old child would play for hours with a wooden spool attached to a string; it would throw the spool over the edge of its crib over and over again, at the same time making the sound "o-o-o-o!" which to it meant "gone." Then it would pull the spool back with a joyous shout of "There!" It transpired that the child's untiring interest in this game was connected with its efforts to deal emotionally with repeated periods of its mother's absence.[19]

A little later such one-word sentences expand to two words ("Papa part" = "Papa's gone"; or "Sock dirty") and then to longer utterances of three words and more, whereby it is clear that the child is forming and integrating rules which are certainly unconscious and which may be regarded as the rudiments of Chomsky's "generative grammar." One interesting aspect of these first one- and two-word sentences is that, according to Sinclair, the subject and predicate are still fused; only later are they separated into two distinct components. This observation fits very well with the hypothesis that language development consists of a continuous process of creating two elements out of what was previously one. I see more evidence for the idea that this process of differentiation is fundamentally a binary one in Sinclair's remark that "linguistic universals" must in fact exist; however, these would not be based on the inborn "language competence" of Chomsky's theories, but rather on basic characteristics of the human intellect the biological roots of which extend down even to the level of neurological coordinations. For it is very likely that these, like many other biological processes, may be viewed as equilibration processes in homeostatic systems, which in the last analysis have a clearly binary character (that is, deviation from and return to an original state).

Finally, there is a wealth of material suggesting that not only language but all thought in general must have a binary structure; this idea pervades the work of Claude Lévi-Strauss, particularly his fascinating book *The Savage Mind*. Again and again Lévi-Strauss discerns polar structures behind the various and complex classification systems (taxonomies), kinship structures, marriage and eating customs, and the like among the ethnic groups he studied, mainly South American Indians and Polynesian tribes. At one point he summarizes his observations as follows:

> All that I claim to have shown so far is, therefore, that the dialectic of superstructures, like that of language, consists in setting up *constitutive units* (which, for this purpose, have to be defined unequivocally, that is, *by contrasting them in pairs*) so as to be able by means of them to elaborate a system which plays the part of a synthesizing operator between ideas and facts, thereby turning the latter into *signs*. The mind thus passes from empirical diversity to conceptual simplicity and then from conceptual simplicity to meaningful synthesis [emphasis added].[20]

And elsewhere:

> Apart from the fact that systems of classification, like languages, may differ with respect to arbitrariness and motivation without the latter ceasing to be operative, the dichotomizing character which we have found in them explains how the arbitrary aspects ... come to be grafted on to the rational aspects without altering their nature. I have represented systems of classification as "trees"; and the growth of a tree is a good illustration of the transformation just mentioned ...
>
> Starting from a binary opposition, which affords the simplest possible example of a system, this construction proceeds by the aggregation, at each of the two poles, of new terms, chosen because they stand in relations of opposition, correlation, or analogy to it.[21]

As examples of pairs of opposites structuring thinking, language, and social organization, Lévi-Strauss cites the polarities of left and right, horizontal and vertical, north and south, abstract and concrete, male and female; more global categories structured in a polar manner include synchrony and diachrony, universality and individuality, order and disorder, aggression and reconciliation, and war and peace.

Although ternary, quaternary, and other complex taxonomies can certainly be found,[22] they may be derivatives of binary systems, and we can see that anthropology offers a great deal of support for the notion that polar structures are the root and origin of all psychic differentiation. If this is indeed the case, then this approach would point, like so many others that we have already encountered, to a surprisingly simple conclusion: From the most primitive sensorimotor schemata occurring in animals to the most complex achievements of human thought, emotions, and language, the structural principles in effect appear to be of fundamentally the same kind. We can begin to get a glimpse of an overall picture—and a developmental process—with a magnificent continuity and consistency.

Nonetheless an immense gulf seems to exist, a decisive qualitative leap separating man from animals; this gulf must be connected with the nature and structure of human *consciousness*. We may draw this conclusion in the light of all the information cited thus far, even if we have encountered mainly instances of our similarity to animals. But what is this difference, or, better, what "makes" or "brings out" this difference between human and animal "consciousness"?

However we look at it, the most important difference comes down to human use of *language*, which thus appears to be at the bottom of human consciousness. It appears clear that the process of attaching abstract acoustic signs to sensorimotor schemata—which constitutes the essence of language, as we have seen—must have something to do with the growing clarity of consciousness, as well as with the polarization of the human psyche into feeling and thinking, body and mind. Language and consciousness are obviously very closely related, but now we must ask whether they are not in fact identical. Is it essentially a case of one single phenomenon to which only our lack of insight has led us to give two names?

Are Language and Consciousness Identical?
The Semiotic Function

A great deal does indeed suggest that the specific consciousness of human beings and our ability to use language are more than just closely related; the one conditions and "brings about" the other, so that we must in fact regard them as a single phenomenon: I do not become truly aware of what I experience until I am able to put it into words. Before this, in a preverbal stage, knowledge and consciousness are much closer to a diffuse feeling. They possess nothing like the clarity of what we can express in words and of what, through the use of language (perhaps even including the language of mathematics, a formalized "metalanguage" with a maximum degree of precision), can be connected and related to other things, which then also enter our consciousness and language.

We must also consider, however, that in addition to language we possess many other forms of expression—music, drawing, and gesture, for example—that are also connected with consciousness. I am tempted to say that they *create* consciousness, but is this really so, or do they merely *condition* consciousness, presupposing or indicating its existence?

This is obviously the crucial question: Does language, or do other sign systems, *create* "consciousness" (knowledge and understanding, and in the end knowledge of oneself), or is it merely an indication of the existence of consciousness? Does consciousness exist *before* these signs? Do these signs—in this case it does not matter *which* signs— merely express preexisting cognitive-affective knowledge?

Piaget and his school, who as far as I know are the only ones to have studied this question in detail, have a definite answer: the latter is the case. A preverbal "logic of action" exists long before it can be expressed in any language of signs. Before such logic takes the form of words and thus becomes in a certain sense (which I attempted to define in Chapter 2) "mind," it is "nothing but" sensorimotor-affective activity, or "body"—concrete, mainly physical actions and a form of experience that is without doubt closer to immediate feeling than to mediated thinking. But this largely "external" feeling is internalized to an ever greater extent as times goes by, and coordinated in increasingly meaningful and complex sequences. Toward the end of the first year of a child's life, but above all in the second year, something new and decisive happens that has immense consequences for all further development. Interestingly enough this is connected with acquiring object permanence, a first, clearly internalized, cognitive and affective invariance in a world that previously consisted almost entirely of variances and therefore had very little structure.[23] This decisive step is the development of the *semiotic function*, and it means that the child gradually becomes capable of symbolic play, of imitative behavior deferred in time (indicating an ability to retain mental images), and finally of attaching certain phonetic sounds to certain experiences. In sum, the child becomes capable of *reproducing reality by means of signs that are obviously different from what they refer to.*

This ability to separate into two components a previously undifferentiated mode of experiencing the world, namely a signifier and a signified (an ability that the higher mammals possess to only a rudimentary degree at best), constitutes the essence of the semiotic function. Language is only one particularly important and privileged manifestation of this ability. Some of the others are the above-mentioned symbolic play, deferred imitation, drawing, gesture, and the capacity to draw upon mental images from memory. In children who can form adequate early sensorimotor schemata, the semiotic function apart from language will develop in an almost normal manner despite handicaps: deaf and dumb children present almost no evidence of disturbances in this respect, whereas blind children, because of their much more deficient sensorimotor schemata, have considerable difficulties. Language is therefore only a symptom, in fact, and not the driving force behind cognitive development. "Language is not the source of logic, but is on the contrary structured by logic."[24]

It is even the case, as Sinclair reports, that logic goes beyond language to some extent, since some logical operations and possible combinations cannot be expressed in words. In this sense language resembles thought, in that both represent merely a (partially inadequate) translation and formalization of physical experience (action).

At the same time it is the highest medium in which human knowledge—and thus also consciousness—can be expressed, conveyed, and, as Piaget emphasizes, socialized. But Piaget's findings teach us that language clearly does not create or "bring about" consciousness; consciousness exists before and separately from language, and language is to a certain degree only an indicator of its existence and structure. Even if we consider the semiotic function in its entirety, the conclusion remains the same: mental images, memory, deferred imitation, significant motor activity and gestures, drawing, music, and so on are just like language, in that they express and transmit evidence of human consciousness rather than creating it. Its origins thus remain a mystery.

A closer look reveals, however, that even genetic epistemologists are not entirely certain about how matters stand. Bärbel Inhelder, Piaget's associate and an expert in the field, writes in her survey on the state of research:

> We still do not know enough about the links between sensorimotor and symbolic (or semiotic) behavior. Symbolic behavior is sometimes considered to have different origins from sensorimotor behavior—the two slowly converging; other psychologists consider that a continual process of interiorization takes place. While we favor this second working hypothesis, it is a rather weak one since it tells us no more than that processes similar to sensorimotor development take place without any external manifestations.[25]

A little later Inhelder presents a highly instructive illustration of motor symbolism as one aspect of the semiotic function that Piaget and his disciples are fond of citing; it suggests strongly that semiotics or the use of signs not only reflects and expresses consciousness but also can actively contribute to its development in a dialectical process, at least during the early years of life:

> At 1;4, Lucienne tries to grasp a watch chain which she has seen being put into a match box which she does not know how to open. The opening is reduced to 3mm. As a result of her previous experiences she possesses only two schemes: turning the box over in order to empty it of its contents and sliding her finger into the slit to make the chain come out. She immediately tries these two processes, which fail. A pause follows during which Lucienne manifests a very curious reaction, bearing witness not only to the fact that she tries to think out the situation and to represent to herself through mental combination the operations to

be performed, but also to the role played by imitation in the development of representations: she mimics the widening of the slit. She looks very carefully at it, then several times in succession, she opens and shuts her mouth, at first slightly, then wider and wider. She wants to enlarge the slit. The attempt at representation which she thus furnishes is expressed plastically, that is to say, due to inability to think out the situation in words or clear visual images she uses a simple motor representation as signifier or symbol.

Immediately after this phase of plastic reflection, Lucienne unhesitatingly puts her finger in the slit, pulls so as to enlarge the opening and grasps the chain.[26]

It seems quite clear that imitative, symbolic representation of a concrete sensorimotor process (Lucienne's repeated opening of her mouth *instead* of the matchbox) in this case runs parallel to or even *precedes* the formation of the corresponding sensorimotor schema, rather than vice versa. It thus appears reasonable to suppose that it is precisely this formation of signs that sharpens understanding and consciousness, or at least that these two processes are intimately related: in this very early stage the formation of signs and the growth of consciousness appear to represent the same phenomenon, just as we originally assumed in the case of language; it is possible that one cannot occur without the other. Only later, when a sign has been formed (and *thereby*, I am tempted to say, a firm pathway for a new element of consciousness has been established), only then does it appear as if this kind of *condensed* knowledge (to use a term that I will discuss later) could exist separately from the sign for it—in other words, as if the signs were mere "passive" expressions of a previous knowledge and understanding. In fact, however, and despite all appearances to the contrary, I believe that this separation is not legitimate, not even in the case of adults. Logic and consciousness can probably never exist independently of their corresponding system of signs, which gives them order and structure. These systems are merely internalized in adults to a large degree: we think in words, images, gestures, in ideas related to space and time, and perhaps—if we have developed such systems—also in tones, colors, and algebraic or other formulas, even if some of them do not reach the stage of expression. On the other hand, expression itself in a system of signs (of any sort) clearly contributes a great deal to the growth of consciousness; expressions such as "If I could only get it down on paper" or "If I could just find the word for it"—or perhaps even "the music for it"—

indicate how we try to increase our conscious awareness of things. The German poet Heinrich von Kleist had much the same thing in mind when he altered the familiar French phrase "L'appétit vient en mangeant" ("Appetite comes as we are eating") to "L'idée vient en parlant" ("Ideas come as we are speaking").[27]

Our internal *mental images* are particularly interesting in this connection, and also in a therapeutic connection, as we shall see later. They are thought to be associated primarily with the *right* hemisphere of the brain, and thus with the global, intuitive, and emotional mode of experience. Much evidence suggests that a concentration or condensation of images plays a central role in the emergence of a clearer consciousness, namely the role of mediator between concrete actions and abstract ideas. Indeed in our mental images extensive diachronic sequences are first joined together in synchronic or simultaneous wholes. One indication of this mediating function is the extreme specialization of cells concerned with vision in the human brain. One could even imagine that the optic subsystem acts as a kind of "pacemaker" (or "crystallization seed") within the whole sensory system, as a denser "ordering of experience" (both cerebral and psychic) is formed on a higher level of abstraction. Scientists, inventors, and creative thinkers of all kinds often report that in their search for answers to complex questions the "illumination" came to them in pictorial form, sometimes even in a dream. Two famous examples are the discovery of the closed-loop structure of benzene by Kekulé von Stradonitz (who had a dream about a snake biting its tail and at once "saw" the ring as the long-sought solution to his problem)[28] and Crick and Watson's discovery of the double-helix structure of DNA. Large areas of higher mathematics are accessible only through visual representations such as curves and parabolas. Graphic representations (including cave paintings), dance, and gesture, which reveal with particular clarity the transition from sensorimotor activity to symbolic imagery, must certainly have played a significant part in the origin of human consciousness. The extravagant gestures of orators or orchestra conductors also reveal the existence of a complex but only dimly realized world of inner spatial and visual representations, which provides a framework for our thoughts and acts as a nucleus or seed around which consciousness at times may "crystallize." Metaphorical, "analogical" thinking is far closer to the affective pole than is the "digital" thinking of language; it is also more informative and contains more levels of meaning. This probably explains the immense force of metaphorical descriptions in the development of consciousness. Some of them, such as the parables of Jesus in the New Testament, have maintained their power to move people for millennia. Modern advertising techniques make use of the same effect, as does Milton Erickson's brilliant (and typically "right-brained") picture language or Leuner's catathymic picture experience (see Chapter 7).

The evidence leads us to the conclusion that the relation between semiotics and the development of consciousness must be *circular* rather than linear: On the one hand, a sign expresses some kind of mental condensation, but on the other hand it also furthers and strengthens such condensation. However, even if we consider the semiotic function as a whole and not merely language, we have not explained the riddle of how consciousness arises, although we have certainly come a step closer. Perhaps we will be able to make more progress on this point if we can reach a better understanding of the key idea of mental condensation.

Abstraction and "Translation": Processes in the Creation of Consciousness

The previous chapter attempted to show that the affective-logical systems of reference that determine our knowledge—and thus our consciousness—of ourselves and the world around us are formed in a step-by-step process as a child grasps the existence of invariances, that is, similarities or regularities in the chaos of sensory impressions with which he is first confronted.

This process has the typical features of an *abstraction,* a grouping of heterogeneous elements under a common heading, whereby the heading itself is made possible by the discovery of an underlying shared feature in what had previously seemed to be a variety of occurrences without any order to them. In other words, when this variety is grasped as a totality, it is consolidated into a structure consisting of an invariance and its corresponding variance. Examples of this in a child's early life are the fusion into a whole of different sensory aspects of a physical object (such as a toy), a repeated experience (being rocked, fed, or bathed), or a person (the mother) who goes away and comes back. The brain is apparently capable of grasping an invariance from frequent repetition of identical sensory stimuli. There is no reason to assume that the vastly more complex abstractions of later stages, up to and including the highest levels of logic and mathematics, represent anything fundamentally different. In the language of mathematical group theory, what we have is a case of creating relations or "morphisms" (either simple or complex) between elements of two wholes (or systems, or structures; see the drawing) that were originally separate. The result is a system of a higher order, which includes the former two systems by condensing them into one. What occurs is clearly a kind of "translation": *Systems (or reference) of a lower order are "translated" into something different, new, and more abstract.* Years ago Arthur Koestler demonstrated through a number of convincing examples that this fusion of previously unconnected systems of reference into a higher-order system constitutes the decisive creative act in every scientific or artistic discovery, as well as the basis of humor.[29] There is interesting evidence for the hypothesis that we can extract common information from various sensory areas thanks to very complex "crossmodal connections" in the brain; this process may play a key part in the growth of human consciousness.

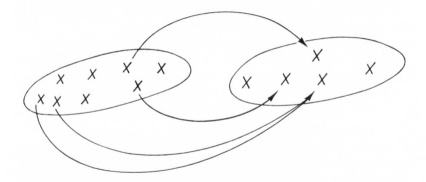

In addition, an important link exists to the Piagetian concept of *reversibility*, the creation of a reciprocal relationship between two related processes, which together form a kind of part and counterpart. This was illustrated in Piaget's experiment with beads, which were placed in glasses with different diameters and heights (see Chapter 2). But, as we are now in a position to recognize, this process is equivalent to extracting an invariance; in the experiment with the beads, the child suddenly realizes that the glasses always contain the same number of beads, whether the glasses are short and fat or tall and thin. Piaget illustrated the same developmental step in many other brilliantly simple experiments, including a roll of modeling clay pulled into different shapes and a string pulled in a right angle around a nail. (The length of the two portions of string varies reciprocally; naturally the total length remains constant, a fact that the child can grasp only at a certain stage of development.) The decisive creative step in the recognition of such reversibility (a step that also creates, expands, or consolidates consciousness) consists once again in establishing relations between two previously isolated groups of phenomena, that is, between two systems of reference.

This same process, which we may legitimately regard as one of *increasing the order of harmony* in systems of reference on the basis of invariances, is also without doubt in the interests of *economy*. It reduces the heterogeneity or "tension" between previously unconnected systems, thereby also reducing the total amount of energy needed to keep them all in balance despite all deviations (that is, despite all variance). Psychologically the harmonization of two or more systems of reference that are actually concerned with the same thing involves a resolution of disturbing contradictions (discussed in the next chapter). As we have seen, such a resolution of contradictions— a reduction of complexity—is a pleasurable experience, or an avoidance of unpleasure, and it offers an excellent illustration of how fruitful a combination of psychoanalysis and systems theory can be.

One appealing (but as yet unverifiable) theory holds that these processes, functional systems, and degrees of tension may occur not solely on psychological (sensorimotor-affective) and abstract mathematical levels but also on analogous electrochemical levels within the brain. We could imagine, for example, the spatial and temporal harmonization of rhythmic impulses, patterns of excitation, and electric potentials between previously independent neuronal networks (which represent systems of reference at the same time); this would lead in turn to the creation of new and higher networks. Both Changeux and Schneider have something similar in mind: "The formation of more abstract operations is connected by Changeux on a neurobiological level with the elaboration of the circuits involved in processing of neuronal data."[30]

These concepts are fully consistent with the ideas of genetic epistemology, in particular with Piaget's central concepts of "reflective abstraction" and "optimizing equilibration," the basic process of all cognitive differentiation. They are also consistent with the idea of affect-logic developed here from a basis of psychoanalytical thinking. The increasing condensation and integration of affective-logical schemata is equivalent to the (pleasurable, tension-reducing) harmonization of heterogeneous elements or "disturbances" in the formation of higher-order systems. Such integration is clearly governed in all respects by the same laws of economy and equilibrium that play a fundamental role elsewhere in nature.

From a theoretical point of view it is also noteworthy that the process of abstraction, or of extracting an invariance from an ever-widening range of variances, represents the exact opposite of the process by which a natural differentiation is created: a differentiation or structure arises by the addition of more variance or information to an invariance. The invariant table principle of our example was differentiated by varying the material, shape of the tabletop, shape and height of the legs, and so on. Conversely, the extraction of an invariable from a large variety of objects leads to our recognizing a more and more inclusive (or more abstract) whole. As we encounter all sorts of tables—high, low, square, round, made of wood and of stone—we finally come to grasp the abstract table principle as such; only after this has occurred can we attach to it a specific sign, the phonetic sequence "table," that encompasses all this variety.

We may think of the whole framework of sensorimotor-affective schemata constituting the "mind"—and, as we shall see later, consciousness as well—as a kind of cerebral data-processing apparatus. During the processes of recognizing reality, this "apparatus" runs, so to speak, through the development of the world as it was illustrated by the decision tree, but in the opposite direction: at the outset it is confronted with an immense number of heterogeneous single elements; its task is to group them into larger and more inclusive wholes, through a step-by-step recognition of the invariances that these elements contain (see Figure 4). The cerebral apparatus thus proceeds from the specific to the general, as Lévi-Strauss has emphasized. We might compare the way the mind is "thrown" into the world to the way in which a space probe is fired at Venus, but one marvelous difference is that the human psyche, unlike a manmade apparatus, is

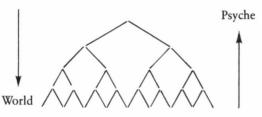

Figure 4.   Recognizing invariance.

able to learn from the environment it encounters and constantly develop and improve itself. The environment into which the psyche is thrown and which it must decipher, however, has obviously developed in a contrary manner, that is, from the general to the specific. It has grown from the original form of a molecule, a plant or animal species, into the multitude of existing phenomena. Thus both psychoanalysts and genetic epistemologists agree that an infant's cognitive grasp of its environment can extend at first only to heterogeneous fragments; even its mother cannot appear as more than a partial object—a breast, face, warm and comforting "something," which appears and disappears without the infant's definite recognition that she is separate from itself. This state of affairs can change only after a long, intensive process of affective and cognitive condensation, when the infant acquires a sense of object permanence and is able, during the second half of its first year, to join all the elements of the mother together in a distinct and constant affective-logical unit. As is well known, this developmental step is of the greatest importance in the ability to establish the boundaries of one's self.

The example of differentiating tables also made it clear that it is possible to regard all technological developments in the same terms: all inventions and discoveries, from the most primitive tool to the most complicated new machine, are based on extractions of an invariance, a process that is always structured in the same way. The following example necessarily simplifies a complex circular process.

Once an immense number of individual actions of, say, hitting something or cutting something into parts (or the operative sensorimotor-affective schemata underlying them) have been mentally condensed into a whole; once the essentially abstract principle behind them has been grasped intuitively, then the step to actualizing this principle in the general form of a hammer or knife (which can then undergo all possible transformations) is only a small one. Perhaps the most ingenious condensation of such sensorimotor action sequences (or schemata) was the invention of the wheel, since it represented such a leap, but modern inventions such as knitting and weaving machines and the gasoline engine are also based on the discovery and application of a general principle or abstraction behind the most varied kinds of concrete single operations. It becomes apparent that in instance after instance condensation and extension of information occur simultaneously. Abstraction and generalization are obviously reciprocal phenomena, that is, reversible operations in the sense of genetic epistemology. They belong together in exactly the same way that the (external) world and the (internalized) mind do in their reciprocal development: Something invariable (a whole, an essence, a principle, a structure) must be recognized in a large number of different phenomena before a generalization becomes possible; once this principle has been "extracted" or "abstracted," it can be modified to produce new variations of it.

The continuity of all development in nature—in which we must include the human mind and all its products—is truly astounding from this perspective: in all its achievements, including technology and culture (philosophies, religions, science, forms of social organization, and so on), the mind uses the same general principles of ordering and organization in all stages of its development. These principles consist, in their turn, of a direct, consistent sequence of fundamental equilibrating processes of differentiation rooted in biological, physical, and—in the last analysis—mathematical laws.

The gradual emergence of consciousness now appears as one aspect (though certainly a central and highly unusual one) of a continuous process of condensation, as more and more information is grouped under common and hierarchically ordered headings. Cognitive-affective schemata of a lower and simpler order are continually and successively translated into schemata of a higher order. Even the semiotic function no longer appears as something entirely new; instead it proceeds from signals, which may still be very concrete, through the intermediate stage of symbols, to the completely abstract level of arbitrary signs. (The sum total of human civilization and technology may even be regarded as a set of extremely complex signs standing for the abstract, intellectual processes of condensation and differentiation that they represent.) What we are confronted with is thus not something completely new, but a series of (certainly immensely significant) phenomena in a continuous process of development leading to an ever more comprehensive rationalization, equilibration, harmonization, and, at the same time, differentiation of the psychic and cerebral structures involved.

Even the first sensorimotor-affective schemata formed by animals and human infants on a foundation that is in part inborn and in part acquired represent condensations or abstractions, in a manner of speaking: they are already the result of a process of internalization, a condensation of the most varied specific events. They equilibrate and *condense* everything that has hitherto been encountered into a single, compact, gestaltlike schema, which sums up this experience. Without doubt this is accomplished by the typical process of extracting an invariance—a process accompanied by a simultaneous recognition of the range of possible variance—at the cost of some loss of information. In short, the most important aspect of this process in general terms is that it condenses an extensive set of diachronic events into a timeless, synchronic schema. Our spatial and temporal conceptions of the earth or the cosmos are influenced by this process to such an extent that the specific experiences, thoughts, and observations of countless generations fuse into a single overall schema that determines our view of the world. *As such abstractions develop, there also develops to a precisely corresponding degree a kind of internalized "knowledge" or consciousness, which grows clearer with each step of the condensation process described.*

Seen from this point of view, worms, migratory birds, and of course the higher mammals and primates possess traces of an "intellectual" or "abstract" knowledge or consciousness, gained from encounters with and adaptation to the environment, and partly implanted by heredity through the process of natural selection. Consciousness in this sense appears as a function of the brain's capacity to process data; the extraordinary capacity of the human brain permits us to process *more* information and to condense and store more of the information received than any animal can. This also means that human beings will possess information about themselves and their environment organized into systems of reference of a far higher order than ever become available to animals. The development of more and more condensed knowledge of themselves (in a process that has by no means come to an end yet) goes hand in hand with new levels of reflective abstraction and the possibility for human beings to "know that they know," to "know that they know that they know," and so on.

One key point takes us a good deal further toward solving the puzzle of what human consciousness is: The enormous *qualitative* leap to the development of consciousness is made possible by what is at first merely a *quantitative* difference, namely the much greater condensation of information in the brain. Human beings possess a highly differentiated apparatus for processing data, which can integrate the different sensory impressions reaching it via a large network of cross-modal connections in sophisticated ways. The efficiency of this apparatus is also greatly increased by highly developed forms of social interaction and by information handed down from generation to generation. Human and animal brains can be compared, respectively, to captains of modern oceangoing ships equipped with sonar, satellite television, radio, and telegraph, and the sailors of previous centuries. The former will have a much richer, clearer, and denser world view (that is, knowledge and awareness of the environment, themselves, and their own place in it) at their disposal at all times than their less well-equipped predecessors. Furthermore, this interpretation seems to provide a key to a better understanding of *language* and the semiotic function: From a certain point on, the feeling and knowing that have been more or less dreamlike and unconscious reach such a—previously unknown—degree of density, focus, and clarity that consciousness finally "dawns on us." It is precisely this cerebral and psychic condensation that, we may assume, provides a basis for the emerging signs of the semiotic function. (These may be a deferred imitative gesture, a mental image, an idea, or a sound.) The dawn of human consciousness, the use of signs and a progressive ability to abstract (to condense information) would then be actually a *single* phenomenon, a process with somatic and material aspects as well as psychic and immaterial aspects. Whichever of these aspects manifested itself, either the concrete or the abstract ones, the same one process would still be involved, just as a fire is simultaneously a gleam of light, a chemical process, and an abstract event with an abstract relation to other events. The semiotic function makes its appearance when, and only when, the condensation of information about diachronic events (actions, experiences) in space and time has attained such a high degree of compactness that it can be *compressed* into a single idea and hence into a sign. In other words, the semiotic function indicates the level of consolidation that has been reached, while at the same time helping to stabilize and organize it. It thus appears as a "milestone" or edifice to which one element after another of the new system of reference being constructed is added. Each of these elements is cemented by the semiotic function and given a form, which allows it to be recognized again later with growing ease and brought into connection with other, similar elements. According to René Spitz, one particularly important milestone of this kind is the word *no;* when children acquire the ability, around the age of eighteen months, to refuse or negate something, this word reflects a first and fundamental separation of the self from the world around it.[31] A similar but even larger step is taken some time later, when children learn to use the pronoun "I."

Language, much more than any other medium of expression, is a precise, subtle, and convenient system of signs. It offers the user a wealth of "prefabricated" operational elements or, in computer terminology, "microprocessors." There can be no doubt that their use leads rapidly to an immense burst of progress in organizing consciousness.

The relationships revealed to consciousness by the use of language grow increasingly well organized, codified, and also *socialized* as the speaker learns to use the new signs (and their corresponding dynamisms) according to established rules and *conventions*. This means in turn that the single operations and relationships contained in these microprocessors grow more and more automatic. Once they have been constructed "in a state of full awareness," they tend to sink back into unconsciousness. This is a highly interesting function of consciousness, which I shall discuss in more detail in a few pages.

Language, Consciousness, and the Brain

The preceding discussion suggests a hypothesis that we can now summarize as follows:

> *Consciousness results from a process of progressive abstraction and condensation of affective-cognitive systems of reference. Abstraction means the extraction of an invariance, that is, economical translation into a system of reference of a higher order. This is marked, stabilized, and organized by the semiotic function, and by language in particular, whereby the foundation is laid for further abstractions on even higher levels.*

A number of findings concerning the structure and functions of the human brain lend support to this hypothesis. The most important of these are the following.

1. The brain is an immensely complex structure; as Eccles stresses repeatedly, no other known material shows such a highly complex organization (interestingly, it also consumes a maximum of energy, relative to the rest of the organism). The brain is designed primarily to assemble and process information, in the broadest sense of the word. It consists of an almost unimaginably intricate network or set

of circuits, in which virtually every part is potentially capable of communicating with every other part. Seen as a whole, the brain forms a typical open system as defined by systems theory. It is connected via the sensory organs with the environment and is also, as we saw, connected with the "system" of the body, together forming a system of a higher order. The brain is divided into a huge number of functional subsystems with a hierarchical order. Every one of the approximately 10 billion nerve cells of the neocortex, each with hundreds or thousands of synaptic connections, forms in itself an immensely complex subsystem. Other functional units that have been clearly identified are the 1 to 2 million vertical columns, or "modules," in the cortex, each about 3 mm long and ½ mm thick. Every column consists of up to 10,000 nerve cells linked to each other in a great variety of ways; such a column thus represents a kind of "microcircuit" of almost inconceivable intricacy. These modules can in turn be regarded as an enormously complex interconnected set of "power units"; they maintain a balance between themselves and at the same time function as elements of countless larger systems.[32]

2. The brain (and with it the entire nervous system) can be viewed as an organ whose specialization is *condensing* information. Optical pathways from the eye to the visual area of the cortex represent one particularly well-researched area that illustrates this point. These pathways are organized in such a way that chains of neuronal systems relay information according to the all-or-none law: they fire—pass their information along to the next relay station in the chain—only when the activity of several neurons ahead of them in the circuit has reached a certain level. Eccles writes in this connection: "Already in the nervous system of the retina there has begun the abstraction from the richly patterned mosaic of responses by the retinal receptor units into elements of pattern, which we may call features, and this abstraction continues in the many successive stages that have now been recognized in the visual centres of the brain.[33] As I mentioned before, it is now also known that particular cell clusters recognize only one certain kind of optical element (with a horizontal, vertical, or diagonal orientation). In other words, they extract this kind of invariance from what may otherwise be quite heterogeneous information. All information circulates in the brain in the form of electrical impulses, which can undergo extremely complex modulations. Thanks to a variety of ingenious structures in the sensory organs, all events can be "encoded" in these impulses, which is to say that in a certain sense

they are once again "condensed." Another aspect of the condensation process is the interplay of inhibiting and activating signals that repeatedly connect and disconnect subsystems; this is a dynamic process of almost inconceivable subtlety, resembling the continuous opening and closing of valves and locks in an intricate canal system.

3. This network of connections in the brain is in part inborn, but it is expanded and actualized through use. Eccles writes: "the more a particular spatiotemporal pattern of impulses is replayed in the cortex, the more effective become its synapses relative to others. And by virtue of this synaptic efficacy, later similar sensory inputs will tend to traverse these same neuronal pathways and so evoke the same responses, both overt and psychic, as the original input."[34] New research very relevant to our discussion here has shown that the fine neuronal structure of the brain does not form completely until after birth. Most of this structural growth occurs in early childhood, but some of it continues even into old age: information (both action and experience) reaches the brain and influences the growth of dendrites (extensions branching out from nerve cells). This results in a large number of new connections between neurons and neuronal systems. Experiments of newborn cats have shown that if they are prevented from performing certain actions at a critical point in their development—if, for example, they are blindfolded and not allowed to use their eyes—then these neuronal connections fail to grow. Today brain researchers speak of an activity hypertrophy or an inactivity atrophy of brain regions, as in the case of muscle tissue. Thus we can compare the growth of brain structure in the course of a human life to the construction of a road system in trackless territory, just as the words of Antonio Machado at the beginning of this book suggest. Whether these connections remain narrow pathways or become large highways depends on how much they are used. In the brain this "territory" is so plastic, or adaptive, that almost every point can be connected with every other.[35]

4. The human brain is more complex, and equipped with more and better crossmodal connections (between the regions of the brain associated with the various sensory organs), than are the brains of all other animals, including primates. It has a greater capacity and can thus connect more information and consolidate it into wholes of a higher order than any animal brain.

5. The human brain is unique in possessing a functional anatomical asymmetry in its right and left hemispheres. This fact has grown in-

creasingly clear in the wake of Sperry's work on split-brain patients (for which he received the Nobel Prize). In the right hemisphere there tend to be concentrated the synthetic, pictorial, musical, and unconscious functions, while analytic, deductive, language, and conscious functions are more associated with the left hemisphere. The right hemisphere is thus more closely connected with the analogical thinking of early developmental stages, that is, with primary processes; it is the area associated with our dreamlike, intuitive, creative thinking and directed toward grasping wholes. The left hemisphere is more related to the digital, rational type of thought and connected with secondary processes, language, logic, and the grasping of details. Both regions normally interact, of course, but they do so in a highly sophisticated manner that we do not yet fully understand. Fascinating parallels suggest themselves, including the notion that the functions of invariance and variance, whose interplay permits us to recognize structures, might be associated with the two hemispheres of the brain, invariance in the right and variance in the left. Other fundamental bipolarities such as synchrony and diachrony or feeling and thinking could conceivably function in an analogous manner.[36]

These few basic facts of brain anatomy and physiology clearly lend support to the hypotheses about the structure and function of the psyche developed above. We find striking parallels between the specifically human phenomena described, between the cerebral and the psychic: a high degree of differentiation in the intellectual sphere corresponds to a high degree of differentiation in the material of the brain; in all probability equilibrated affective-cognitive schemata correspond to analogous neuronal networks and patterns of excitation, and the continued growth of these networks as a result of action probably corresponds, on the cerebral level, to the simultaneous effect of experience on the psychic level. It seems equally clear that connections exist between the process of mental condensation (or abstraction) and the structure and function of the central nervous system, which is constructed so as to provide the best possible condensation of information. Furthermore, the contrast between the analytic capacity to use language and the semiotic function, on the one hand, and a more intuitive, emotional grasp of wholes on the other corresponds to the asymmetry or *polarization* of the psychic apparatus. Many other parallels between psychology and brain physiology will no doubt be discovered in the future. On the basis of specific manifestations on a concrete level we may draw a more abstract conclusion, namely that both psychic and cerebral phenomena are characterized by *a process of increasing differentiation and also by a process of progressive ordering or harmonization of an (open) system of relations between single elements.* This takes us right to the heart of the mind-matter problem that Popper and Eccles discuss in detail.[37] It would lead us too far afield to go into this subject here, but I would like to emphasize once more the key role played by the *condensing* of information. The internalized schemata that we have come to recognize as the constituent elements of the psyche represent a tremendous consolidation of an almost infinite variety of specific actions and events; at the same time they give these events a certain order: a concrete, material, diachronic sequence of events becomes a synchronic or timeless "concentrate." Even the order that we can observe in human brain matter can be regarded as a reflection of such events, given the plasticity of the brain that we know exists. In a broader sense the same holds true for hereditary cerebral structures (which have been selected for their efficiency), and perhaps it holds true for all matter as such. Mind and matter, body and spirit, appear as two aspects of one whole from this perspective, polar opposites on the one hand, but identical in their abstract structure on the other. Both are, in a manner of speaking, equally necessary, important, and "noble"; the essence of the whole that together they constitute appears to consist of an *increasing order between relations.*

The Function of Consciousness

It now remains to try to get a clearer sense of the function of consciousness within the psyche as a whole. I mentioned at the beginning of this chapter the fact that consciousness fluctuates greatly in clarity, quality, and focus—a phenomenon that is usually referred to as "attention" or "concentration." It is obvious that one major purpose served by attention is coping with daily life; directing our awareness toward things that might mean danger, difficulties, or change is a deeply rooted biological reflex. But it is just as obvious that this shifting focus of consciousness can illuminate only a tiny sector of what we encounter and must deal with. The great majority of our sensorimotor-affective reactions occur automatically, outside the sphere of awareness. We have seen that the unconscious can be understood as a system of rules, consisting of operational schemata and systems of reference with a typical affective-logical structure.

It is now most important to recall an aspect of this question that has already been touched upon: These unconscious behavioral schemata (at least those that are not inborn)[38] *did* have attention focused on them for a period of time. They were "illuminated" by consciousness at the time when they were being acquired and formed. Nothing illustrates the acquisition of a new affective-logical schema better than the typical process of learning a new skill:

> I am playing the flute and keep stumbling over an apparently simple trill. Now I direct my attention—the focus of my consciousness—entirely toward this trill. Playing very slowly, I discover that the difficulty lies in a slight, involuntary movement of my ring finger when I move my little finger. I practice moving these fingers in opposite directions for a long time, very consciously, slowly at first and then faster and faster, until the difficulty disappears. As I go on, I succeed in playing the trill more and more automatically, until finally I am no longer conscious of the problem I had to overcome.

This example may seem banal, but it deserves some closer analysis. First of all, we should realize that playing the flute, like every other learned activity and skill (and all behavior in general), consists of nothing but an increasingly well coordinated set of sensorimotor-affective schemata, which at first must be laboriously constructed and joined together like the links in a chain, in the full light of awareness. As they become more automatic (and simultaneously become fused into wholes of a higher order), they also tend to sink back into the dark regions of the unconscious. Constructing such a schema is a highly complex business, although it might not at first seem so. In this example, finger movements are far from being the only factor; there are also optical ones (connected with reading the music), acoustic ones, complicated movements of the mouth and tongue, and controlled breathing; on other levels there are also affective, intellectual, and abstract components. All of these must be coordinated with one another, something that certainly can happen only with the aid of complex crossmodal connections. Many different monitoring and feedback mechanisms are necessary for the schema to reach a harmonious state of balance. And finally, it is interesting to note that one sensorimotor schema involved in this example is the involuntary synergic movement of two fingers, which is certainly inborn. Although this schema is normally advantageous, because it makes grasping objects easier, here it had to be modified and further differentiated. This appears to be possible only when attention is sharply focused—that is, in the realm of consciousness.

We have already come to see consciousness as a particularly concentrated form of mental activity, and one that consumes a great deal of energy; using this perspective, we might compare it to a brightly lit workshop where bits of information are assembled into new microchips. In this workshop they are fitted into existing cognitive-affective schemata, with the presumable result that these schemata gain considerably in precision, flexibility, and solidity. Once assembled, these now modified schemata are "broken in" and "polished," that is, coordinated with other schemata. As soon as the new situations have been processed, encoded, and become automatic, however, the energy-consuming luxury of conscious awareness becomes superfluous or even a hindrance. An easy example is trying to walk or talk and be aware of every involved movement at the same time. Many mechanisms, once established, function much better unconsciously than consciously, and it takes a great deal of effort to become consciously aware of their details.[39]

This is equally true, however, for "defective constructions" resulting from traumatic experiences and negative environmental influences—or possibly, as Freud thought, from constitutional deficiencies in the ability to respond to such influences; it is such defective constructions that appear to underlie neuroses and other forms of disturbed behavior.

All the evidence—particularly the recently developed psychoanalytic understanding of the nature and formation of internalized object representations, which will occupy us in the next chapter—does in fact suggest that the typical affective-logical representations of important people in a small child's life (mother, father, siblings, and so on), of the self, and of their mutual relations are formed in exactly the same manner: they are a condensation or abstraction of specific experiences of which the child was certainly aware at a particular point in time. Very early and intense affective impressions must obviously leave an especially strong stamp. Such affective-logical schemata combine to form a comprehensive intrapsychic system that may be viewed as a schematic reflection of external, extrapsychic systems and transactions such as occur in a family. Depending on what happens in daily life, different parts of this schematic condensation of the past in which our knowledge and experience are stored become reactivated. We could compare this to using a flashlight to find our way through a network of intersecting paths created by frequent previous use. Our attention is like the beam in the darkness, enabling us to find the path. Directing the beam of the flashlight corresponds precisely to the shifting nature of human consciousness. Consciousness and attention are therefore inseparable: where our attention is, there our consciousness is also (on widely varying levels of abstraction). This statement may seem innocuous, but it has far-reaching implications. It means that a dream consciousness exists, and hypnotic, meditational, and psychotic consciousness; it means that the concept of consciousness includes more than we normally think of. There is considerable evidence that what has just been said about the role of consciousness in the process of adding new information to existing affective-cognitive systems of reference also applies to these other states of consciousness. We will see in the final chapter that this has interesting implications for therapy.

Before we take a closer look at the important concept of information in this connection, we must clarify the role of the semiotic function, and of language in particular, in the process of constructing and adding to systems of reference. It appears that from a certain point on, language acts like a mold or die for casting, shaping and forming the elements to be fitted into the construction and bringing them into line with customary usage. The latter contributes greatly, of course, to the efficiency of such systems. Language thus has a special function within the whole complicated process that occurs when human beings direct their attention to something new and unusual:[40] This function is *the further differentiation of the psyche under especially favorable conditions*—a revolutionary change that has made possible the differentiation of human behavior beyond the operational schemata of animals. For all their complexity, animal schemata are still much more elementary and to a much greater extent inborn.

This approach enables us to frame the tricky question of the difference between human and animal consciousness (or "knowledge of something") a little more precisely. We are "conscious" at any moment of what we have focused our attention on. Animals' awareness certainly resembles human consciousness most closely in this attention reaction. Otherwise, however, an animal's "knowledge of something" is much more unconscious than human knowledge—a way of stating it that only appears paradoxical. The behavioral schemata associated with the primary or secondary unconscious (that is either inborn or acquired with a temporary focus of attention) still contain a kind of knowledge that under certain circumstances may be quite differentiated. This knowledge represents the mental concentrate of physical experience. In the case of animals, not only is a much larger portion of this knowledge inborn, but also it is abstracted and concentrated to a much smaller degree. For this reason alone animal perceptions must be quite different from human ones: the lack of sophisticated crossmodal connections contributes to the fact that what animals are able to focus attention on is much more elementary and isolated than in human beings. A cat, for example, reacts quickly and accurately to certain noises and movements such as might be produced by a mouse, but it is not capable of placing them in a larger perspective. Both consciousness and the unconscious appear much more rudimentary, schematic, and fragmentary in animals than in human beings; their consciousness functions on the level of automatic reflex and is able to combine much less information into a whole of a higher order. What animals lack, above all, is the ability to condense information to the point where they could "know that they know" something and attain the stage of human self-awareness.

Returning to the problem of information and its integration into existing systems of reference in the light of consciousness, we are now in a position to define this central concept in terms of affect-logic. As I mentioned earlier, information—that is, a new element or "bit"—is often defined today as "a perceptible difference." According to Shannon and Weaver, a bit is the amount of information necessary to permit a choice between two equally probable alternatives.[41] This definition fits in very well with the ideas developed earlier on the nature of differentiation, but it takes only the cognitive, structural aspect of information into account. All our conclusions so far, however, have indicated that information is something double and bipolar, with an affective as well as a cognitive component. Everyday experience teaches us that purely cognitive messages do not truly become information: they will not draw out attention sufficiently. If they do not enter the focus of our consciousness, they will never be integrated into existing affective-logical structures and behavioral schemata by the processes of assimilation and accommodation. A mother can tell her child a hundred times to clean up his room or not slurp his soup, but her words will have no effect unless or until they are accompanied by emotions. These feelings—anger, rage, tension, or the prospect of a reward, pleasure, affectionate attention—will give her words enough emphasis that they finally make an "impression." Adults behave in just the same way in the face of commands and instructions, indications of possible dangers or sources of pleasure, and reports of disasters in distant countries. We hardly register them, and they have virtually no influence on our behavior unless they are simultaneously provided with some sort of affective stamp or "imprint." Modern advertising experts have grasped this only too well. The internalized schemata and structures governing our behavior necessarily possess a considerable degree of inertia. They are open systems, but ones that have been formed and equilibrated with strong homeostatic mechanisms on the basis of experience and a great deal of previously acquired information. In his important book on the equilibration of cognitive structures Piaget demonstrated how new information is acquired in three phases. In the first or α phase this information is simply dismissed and denied (repressed). In the following (β) phase it is placed next to the old information without any connection, in an unstable, flickering, back-and-forth state. Not until the third (γ) phase is it integrated into a new and expanded (optimized) schema. (It again seems odd that Piaget could neglect the affective components of this process to the extent he did, given the way he himself emphasized the annoying disturbance that everything new entails for familiar ways of looking at things.)

> In an experiment children were asked to predict the direction of water level in a decanter that was presented first vertical, then lying down, then turned upside down, and finally inclined at 45°. Children between the ages of 5 and 7 will draw the water level of a decanter tipped at an angle of 45° either placed against the side of the decanter or parallel to the inclined base. The intermediate phase showed a series of characteristic compromises such as drawings in which the water level was shown as curved. Finally, at about the age of 9, the children were able to "optimize" their perception of the properties of water and to realize that the water level always remains horizontal, no matter how the container is inclined.[42]

It is hard even to imagine information consisting solely of affect, such as pure fear, rage, or pleasure. Even the strongest emotions connected with extreme situations such as catastrophes or war remain connected with some kind of situational or other cognitive elements. At the very least they are linked with certain structures of time and space, which are stored as information associated with the affect. Indeed we must assume that the affects of newborn infants, which appear almost pure, must in fact retain some rudimentary cognitive elements (perhaps temporal ones) in order to be registered at all and to become bits of new information in their forming sensorimotor schemata.

In sum, from the point of view of affect-logic, information—something that "informs" existing affective-cognitive structures—is always and must necessarily be *an affective as well as a cognitive difference*. It is clear that this view has many practical consequences, particularly for therapy.

Summary: A New View of Psychic Structure

The ideas presented above by no means represent a final "solution" to the complicated problem of language and consciousness. My main aim has been to approach the issue from the perspective of affect-logic while taking into account some of the latest research in different fields, especially brain physiology and Piagetian genetic epistemology. The result cannot be other than fragmentary. Nevertheless, even these incomplete results can prove helpful. We are able to conclude this investigation of normal psychic phenomena with a more rounded overall view of the psyche, a view that offers certain new aspects. The psyche now appears as a kind of "organ" connecting an organism and its environment; we might compare it to a net that, as it expands, creates denser and better links between the organism and the surroundings, thus enabling the organism better to master reality. A continuous process of exchange goes on between the organism and the environment via this net, which affects and transforms the nature of the net, or psyche, itself. The essence of psychic activity appears to be the *condensation* of information; this means that something diachronic (a specific event occurring in time: experience) is transformed into something synchronic or timeless, something abstract. What is it that is extracted and concentrated? Above all, it is *relations,* the essentially mathematical or abstract relations between the specific facts encountered. These relations will consist mainly of their points of similarity and/or difference. The psyche proceeds step by step to extract the invariances from a constantly growing range of registered variances, condensing experience (or action) and thereby acquiring a better grasp of the environment. As it does this, it runs through the reverse of the developmental process by which this environment came into being: the psyche proceeds by progressive condensation from the specific to the general, whereas the world grows by differentiating, proceeding from the general to an infinite variety of specific manifestations. At the same time, however, the psyche also knows this reciprocal process: ideas, cultures, and works of art proliferate like animal and plant species. Thus abstraction (the extraction of invariance from a multitude of varied phenomena) *and* generalization (the introduction of ever new variants in something invariable) prove to be the ubiquitous and polar principles behind all structures. They represent a particularly sweeping or fundamental instance of Piaget's "reversibility" of all intellectual operations.

Consciousness now appears as the product of an ongoing process of condensation, translation, *and* differentiation. The early stages of this process remained entirely unconscious for a long time. Consciousness is thus neither a sudden nor a specifically human phenomenon, but rather—like everything else in nature—something that develops slowly and gradually. As defined on its first level as "a knowledge of something," this sort of knowledge already occurs with the concentration of diachronic information into something synchronic in the lowest forms of animal life. In human beings, the increasing perfection of specific information-processing systems—that is, the progressive differentiation of neuronal material in particular tracts—brings with it higher levels of concentration, focus, and clarity. Finally the ability is acquired to distinguish between a signifier and a signified (in de Saussure's sense); these components can be manipulated intellectually and combined into wholes of a higher and higher order, until knowledge of knowledge (or knowledge of knowledge of knowledge) and an awareness of the self and its place in the whole become possible. This process is closely connected with the capacity to attach concise signs to information that has already been greatly compressed. These signs condense an immense amount of diachronic, specific material into a single, formulaic, and essentially abstract synchrony: the semiotic function appears first as an internal experience of images and then as *language,* which "expresses" the consolidated consciousness as well as stabilizing, structuring, organizing, and, above all, *socializing* it, by means of a system of firm rules and conventions. This represents, despite all structural continuity, a new organizing principle of revolutionary efficiency. It can vastly speed up abstraction and differentiation and can connect (virtually) all information-processing centers (the brains of individuals) into a single "pool." It also permits information to be transmitted economically from generation to generation, far more so than would be possible through selection and heredity alone. In this manner processes of concentration (and of ordering) are set in motion that have a range, flexibility, and speed hitherto unknown. Through ever new abstractions and abstractions of abstractions, human beings can arrive at a picture of themselves and the world that continues to grow more differentiated all the time. An immense number of "errors" occur, and detours arise, but these are only the extreme states of a self-regulating, equilibrating process that always seeks to achieve harmony and to reduce tension. The invention of computer technology has accelerated this process still further, but it is a small step compared with the acquisition of the semiotic function, even though they are structurally analogous phenomena.

The sensorimotor-affective schemata of Piagetian theory now appear as *the* key building blocks of the psyche, or as the threads of the psychic net of which I spoke earlier. In addition, despite its methodological problems Freudian psychoanalysis has offered substantial evidence that affective components must always be woven into these schemata. This means that there can be no pure logic, but only affect-logic: the life of the psyche goes on within a double system of combined thinking and feeling, body and mind, that seems to correspond in large measure to the polarity of concrete materiality and abstract relations. Not only thinking (and speaking) but also feeling appear as internalized and economical "trial actions" along what one is tempted to call the previously trodden pathways of affective-logical operational schemata. The striving for pleasure and avoidance of unpleasure, in which psychoanalysis sees the foundation of all human behavior, clearly represents only one aspect and expression, in the psychic realm, of a much broader principle, namely the striving for less tension, for balance and for more harmony within and between open but limited functional systems. The reasons for the existence of this striving can be seen as biological, and even physical and mathematical. It thus becomes the driving force behind all psychological and intellectual development, both individual and collective, in the sense of "optimizing equilibration." At the same time it supplies all operational schemata formed through action with a (biologically extremely useful) affective stamp. These schemata appear to be formed in the focus of consciousness or attention—a fact that offers a great advantage. Once they have been formed and have become largely automatic in their functioning, however, they are usually fused into wholes of a higher order and sink back into the darkness of the unconscious. The unconscious must therefore be regarded primarily as a well-organized set of rules or programs that determine by far the greatest portion of our behavior. The "luxury" of consciousness is obviously reserved for only a small proportion of our sensorimotor-affective activities. In our daily life, events may cause us to activate certain areas of these internalized schemata, to shine a light on them, so to speak, and direct our attention to them for a time. When we are confronted with especially difficult tasks (ones for which we have no automated schemata), we can use our conscious awareness for the purpose of *developing the psyche still further,* that is, for the purpose of integrating new information into existing affective-cognitive schemata.

These schemata represent typical *systems* (or structures) in the sense of modern systems theory. These systems function as systems of reference (or preexisting grids) and probably, in the last analysis, obey universal, mathematical laws of differentiation. Recalling this, we arrive at a picture of the psyche that possesses truly marvelous beauty. We might compare it to baroque music, or finely chased metalwork, or lace of immensely ingenious design. The "net" of the psyche has such an ingenious (and probably binary and symmetrical) design, which grows from a biological foundation and surrounds the most highly differentiated material known to exist, the human brain, like an invisible organ. Emotionally colored in all the infinite shades from pleasure to pain, and at the same time formed according to strict cognitive laws, the psyche in all its parts functions as a system of roads or channels, which are always created in concrete action, that is, in response to needs, and which are always designed to permit the best possible processing of reality.

Rising from dark depths, the psyche ascends through dreamlike intermediate stages; as the degree of condensation increases it achieves the highest clarity of a logic (or affect-logic) that has become fully conscious, decentered, reversible, and thus optimally mobile. There are convulsions and confused tangles along the way, to be sure, but seen from a higher perspective it advances in the end under the benevolent control of omnipresent laws of equilibration to a state of harmony with an equally harmonious and equilibrated environment into which the psyche is "thrown" (or perhaps rather "softly embedded"). If we also consider this marvelous construction that we call the psyche, the mind—or, to use a less scientific term for once, the soul—as being less static than these comparisons suggest, but instead as always in motion, like the surface of a lake ruffled by a pleasant breeze or sometimes tossed by storms, or like a fine, multidimensional net in a shifting wind, then we arrive at a total picture that we must contemplate with awe and amazement.

This gives us all the more reason now to inquire into the question of how this lovely structure can fall into all the "dis-order" that we are accustomed to call "mental illness," and "schizophrenic psychosis" in particular.

5 Contradictions, Paradoxes, and the Double Bind

A little boy complained to his mother, "Daddy hit me." His father came in and said, "Are you telling another of your lies? Do you want me to hit you again?"

—Johann Peter Hebel, in Gottfried Honnefelder, *Lieber Vater*

A Hypothesis about the Pathogenesis of Schizophrenia

In 1956 Gregory Bateson, the British ethnologist, anthropologist, and communications theorist, published an essay titled "Toward a Theory of Schizophrenia," coauthored by Jackson, Haley, and Weakland. The authors described in detail for the first time a mechanism which they believed was connected with the pathogenesis of schizophrenia, and which they called "the double bind."[1] What they had uncovered was the existence of highly confusing and paradoxical patterns of communication in the entire family constellation of of the individual who actually developed symptoms, the "identified patient." This article hit the world of schizophrenia research like a bombshell, breaking a dam of rigid views about this mysterious disorder and loosing a flood of publications (which continues to flow) on disturbances in schizophrenic communication. New techniques for treating whole families in therapy sprang up on all sides as a result and challenged the absolute dominance of psychoanalysis as the only form of therapy that could supposedly go deep enough to treat the "causes" of emotional disturbance. New "paradigms" of the familial and social environment of the identified patient were presented, though often in a one-sided, polemical manner, and began to gain ground on the older, purely intrapsychic theories as explanations of psychotic (and soon also neurotic) symptoms.

This countermovement, however, tended to neglect the interaction between social factors and individual, intrapsychic factors, a subject that represents perhaps the most interesting problem of all. As time went by it became evident that the disturbed forms of communication that had been identified, including the notorious double bind, were by no means specific to families of schizophrenics; they could be found in the families of other mental patients, too, and even in healthy families, albeit usually in a less extreme form. It proved virtually impossible to construct a valid, objective model of the complex phenomena involved in the double bind, and even the original proponents of the theory were unable to devise workable criteria by which the mechanisms could be diagnosed satisfactorily in individual cases.[2] The older school of conservative psychiatry, with its genetic and biochemical approach to the origins of mental illness (and corresponding emphasis on medication in treatment), responded by pointing to new research that once again confirmed the influence of hereditary factors in the pathogenesis of schizophrenia. With such evidence in hand this group tried to dismiss all double-bind theories—and with them much of psychodynamic, social, and communications research—as irrelevant, thus regaining a dominant position. As more time passed, the originators of the concept were in fact forced to lower their expectations of a major breakthrough in the understanding and treatment of schizophrenic psychoses. At a large conference in California attended by many prominent exponents of the double-bind theory twenty years after its inception (1977), Bateson's ideas still clearly held their fascination, but there was also clearly a sobering general sense of stagnation.[3] Jay Haley was particularly outspoken on this subject. Aside from a few new insights—namely that double-bind situations can have positive, creative, and therapeutic effects as well as negative ones; Singer and Wynne's interesting findings on disturbed patterns of communication between the parents of schizophrenics; and Scheflen's concept of a "single bind," that is, the persistence into early childhood of a symbiotic fusion with the mother as a precondition for the double bind—the conference produced little of value that was new.

Nevertheless a great deal of evidence suggests that Bateson and his colleagues were on the track of something important for the understanding of schizophrenia. The problem has been a lack of success in identifying the important phenomena precisely enough and in clarifying their position in the complex overall picture of psychotic disorders. Despite all efforts, particularly those of Bateson himself, to define double-bind phenomena within the framework of a larger epistemology,[4] we are still clearly lacking sufficient insight into the general context in which the processes described take place. In my own view the main task is to clarify the relations between affective, physical phenomena and cognitive, intellectual ones, and also the relations between interpersonal, social phenomena and individual, intrapsychic ones. Bateson's 1979 book contributes very little on the double bind beyond what he had to say in 1956, but the research by Singer and Wynne referred to above (which is distinguished by an excellent methodological approach) on the parents of schizophrenics shows that the track Bateson discovered has led to relevant findings. Although a number of objections have been raised,[5] this study leaves little doubt that the double bind is only one particularly malign form of a large number of ambiguous and confusing communication processes, many of which may be present simultaneously in the family environment of the patient. Approaches to the problem from an entirely different point of view have demonstrated in many families of psychotics the existence of similar phenomena, which are sometimes called "enmeshment" or "emotional overinvolvement."[6] The latter has been found to be connected to a significant degree with a greater frequency of acute psychotic relapses.[7] There is also a striking correlation between some of the observations made in the field of interpersonal communication, such as an inability to maintain a common focus of attention in a conversation, and many of the "thought disorders" that researchers have discovered in intrapsychic studies of schizophrenics over the past fifteen to twenty years.[8] It appears quite possible that underlying the two sets of observations are causes the same as or similar to those first described by Bateson in connection with the double bind. Furthermore, some creative researchers and family therapists have used Bateson's ideas to create more comprehensive and therapeutically useful concepts. Helm Stierlin, working in Heidelberg from a foundation of both psychoanalysis and family dynamics, developed the ideas of "delegation" and "the impossible mission," by means of which many parents of schizophrenics plunge their children into an insoluble existential dilemma.[9] Another extremely interesting approach was developed by Mara Selvini Palazzoli and her colleagues in Milan, using dramatic techniques to neutralize hidden paradoxes.[10] And finally, new psychoanalytic insights into the nature of pathological narcissism, particularly the views of Kernberg on the genesis and structure of internalized object relations,[11] can prove extremely valuable as we seek to understand the role that contradictions and double binds play in psychosis on both an intrapsychic and a familial level.

As is so often the case, we cannot expect to gain a better grasp of the phenomena described by Bateson and other communications researchers by studying them in isolation, no matter how sophisticated our techniques are. Such complex, seemingly insoluble problems will yield only to a combination of several approaches, some of which may appear antithetical. Because the ideas presented in the preceding chapters can make a contribution to such a synthesis, it will be useful first to summarize the most important points of this discussion and to add one more essential element.

Affective-Logical Systems of Reference: A Recapitulation

Though beginning from several different points of departure, our reflections on the nature of the psyche always converged on the central notion of an effective-logical system of reference. The phenomena studied with the intrapsychic approach of psychoanalysis and those observed in the family unit by systems and communications theorists show no fundamental contradictions over large stretches; on the contrary, there are many important areas of agreement. It is a clear case of complementary phenomena manifesting themselves in different ways on two levels. A comparison of psychoanalytic insights concerning affectivity and Piagetian theories of genetic epistemology, which deal with cognitive functions, opened a perspective from which to view the nature of affect-logic. This affect-logic, according to my central hypothesis, constitutes the actual overall character of the life of the mind. Accordingly I developed the concept of the bipolar, affective-cognitive schema as the most important element of the psyche, describing these elements, or building blocks, more precisely as typical open systems in the sense of systems theory. Over time these systems acquire a high degree of stability. The notion of a system proved to be virtually identical to the modern dynamic definition of a structure: we can define both in a general way as "the product of an invariance and a variance," a definition that also sheds some light on their origins. Furthermore it became clear that such intrapsychic structures or systems, which presumably correspond to analogous neuronal patterns in the brain, at the same time represent specific experiential systems of reference, that is, associative frameworks within which all our thoughts, feelings, and actions are located. Finally, from investigating the complex relationship between consciousness and language we arrived at a view of the psyche as an intricate network of such affective-logical systems of reference, divided into an infinite number of subsystems. By successive extractions of invariance from the variety of information encountered in the course of an individual's development, these systems of reference condense into an increasingly clear consciousness. This process is marked, structured, passed on from one generation to the next, and thus decisively accelerated by language and the semiotic function as a whole, in which internal mental images appear to play a crucial role.

We thus arrived at a view of the conscious and the (proportionally much larger) unconscious portions of the psyche as a complex network of affective-logical programs for behavior. Through the integration of new information (which must also be understood in terms of affect-logic) these rules undergo further differentiation, a process that appears to represent one of the main achievements of consciousness. To illustrate this I used the image of a beautiful lacy net spread out between the human organism and its environment, and also the image—perhaps less poetic, but more accurate—of a complex system of pathways, the appearance of which is determined by how much its various parts are used. The second image makes it very clear that psychic structures arise as a result of constant traffic back and forth between the inner and outer worlds, between centration and decentration, between subject and object, "I" and "thou," or, in Piagetian terms, as a result of an equilibrating, optimizing process of accommodation to and assimilation of the environment. Not only can the results of the latest neurophysiological research be fitted into such a description without difficulty, but so also can the recent insights of psychoanalysts such as R. R. Fairbairn, Edith Jacobson, Margaret Mahler, and Otto Kernberg on the formation and structure of internalized object relations.[12] To this we must now add the following points.

As I mentioned briefly in connection with the concept of invariance, Kernberg ascribes to affects the function of crucial "organizers" of developing psychic structures, especially in the early phases. Whatever is experienced in a particular emotional state becomes fused with the simultaneously occurring sensory (tactical, thermal, gustatory, optical, acoustic, proprioceptive) impressions and sensorimotor sequences into an affective-cognitive-sensorimotor conglomerate, which is at first very diffuse but soon becomes differentiated into clear polarities of pleasure and unpleasure. To begin with there also exist no clear distinctions between the self and the outside world, of course. We may postulate a matrix, wholly undifferentiated at the outset, from which the first internalized psychic "protostructures" presumably develop; these are fused "self-object representations," associated with pleasure on the one hand and unpleasure on the other. These constitute the most primitive, global affective-cognitive systems of reference; they are, as Kernberg observes, associated with intense feelings related to persons. Even at this early stage, as various events are grouped under one aspect (namely the same basic affect), a typical condensation, or extraction of invariance from a broad range of variance, is taking place. As Kernberg describes them, these early self-object representations are characterized by broad but diametrically opposed emotional categories, of the type "all good" or "all bad." As the cognitive functions mature, these categories undergo further differentiation into distinct representations of the self and objects, which for the time being, however, remain split into "all good" and "all bad" parts that lack any connection to one another. The realization that the pleasurable (= "good") and unpleasurable (= "bad") internal representations belong to the same entity—either to the self or to the first significant object, usually the mother—is achieved by means of a further and much more complex extraction of an invariance. According to Kernberg and all the other authors who have concerned themselves with this problem, the joining of both the good and bad aspects of both the self and objects represents an enormously significant step in development. These stages of affective-cognitive development can easily be illustrated by a diagram whose dichotomous form resembles the decision tree, which in Chapter 3 was postulated as providing the basis for every kind of differentiation (see Figure 5).[13] If conditions are unfavorable, this integration of the positive and negative aspects of the self and objects will be achieved to an insufficient degree or not at all. There is much evidence to support Kernberg's opinion that maintaining such a split into "good" and "bad" parts of the self and objects plays a major role in conditions not far removed from psychosis, mainly in "borderline personalities."

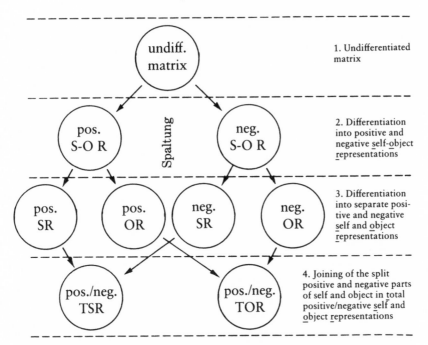

Figure 5.   Formation of self and object representations (courtesy of Dr. Dieter Signer, Bern, Switzerland).

These psychoanalytic insights can be combined with the ideas previously presented to provide an interesting approach to a more profound understanding of contradictory, paradoxical, and double-bind communications. Among other things, we shall see that internalized self and object representations are nothing other than the result of the interaction between the self and the object which actually occurred and which has become information in an affective-logical sense. They, too, represent a condensation or abstraction of reality, consolidated into an intellectual or cognitive-affective schema—in other words, a typical affective-cognitive system of reference that determines perception as well as feelings, thoughts, and behavior. Kernberg suggests that contradictory aspects of such schemata can be split off and isolated for purposes of defense—a notion that is confirmed by much clinical evidence. If we assume further that these fragments (such as a one-sided affective-logical representation of the self or a partner with an intense feeling of "all good" or "all bad" attached to it) can enter consciousness in isolation at certain times and are then able to determine feeling, thinking, and behavior, then we will indeed find many phenomena of the major "endogenous" psychoses and related conditions (mania, depression, schizophrenia, borderline conditions) more understandable. The inner confusion of such patients and the frequently contradictory forms of communication existing in their family environment can then be seen as closely related and interdependent: contradictory interaction between family members results in correspondingly contradictory internalized systems of reference, and vice versa. Accordingly, contradictions, paradoxes, and double binds can be understood as specific constellations in these systems of reference, similar in some respects but dissimilar in others.

In our discussion so far the "psychic system" has always figured as a double system, with one pole formed on the basis of affect and physical sensation, and the other on the basis of thought and intellectual processes, including language and the semiotic function. In a healthy organism these two aspects confirm and validate each other constantly; furthermore, such healthy individuals live in harmony with their environment, and especially with those closest to them, at least to the extent that clear and congruent affective-cognitive messages of one partner elicit unambiguous responses of both thinking and feeling in the other (although this by no means rules out all disagreement and conflict). It is obvious that such a style of communication in a family must lead to a much greater clarity in self and object representations (that is, to a clarity in the affective-cognitive systems of reference relevant to dealing with the self and others) than is the case if communication consists in an exchange of inconsistencies and ambiguities. This is true for all family members, but applies above all to growing children.

Contradictions

The preceding discussion leads us to the question: How should we now define a contradiction? According to the *Handbuch philosophischer Grundbegriffe* (Handbook of basic philosophical concepts) a contradiction exists when "two sentences consisting of a statement and a negation of that statement both claim to be true." The handbook goes on to say that the problem of logical contradictions has occupied philosophers and mathematicians since ancient times, and no one has yet come up with the full solution. Zeno, Plato, and Aristotle all built on the insight of Parmenides of Elea (504–450 B.C.) that "something cannot be and not be at the same time."[14] Philosophers up to and including Kant assumed that lack of contradiction was a formal prerequisite of every truth; Hegel was the first to envision the possibility that reality might contain internal contradictions. We must distinguish, however, between contradictions in formal logic and the kind of dialectical opposites with which Hegel was concerned. Today there is some evidence that everything that exists (or at least the way we are able to perceive what exists) has a dialectical, polar structure.

At the beginning of this century Bertrand Russell added an important new idea to this philosophical discussion with his doctrine of logical classes. The most important point he made for our concerns here is that a logical class cannot contain itself; it can be grasped only from a class of a higher order. Paul Watzlawick has explained this fundamental idea as follows:

> A class is the totality of all objects having a certain property. Thus, all cats, past, present, and future, [compose] the class of cats. [Once] this class [is established], the remainder of all other objects in the universe can be considered the class of noncats, for all these objects have one definite property in common: they are *not* cats. Now any statement purporting that an object belongs to both these classes would be a simple contradiction, for nothing can be a cat and not a cat at the same time.[15]

In other words, the class of cats as such cannot belong both to itself and to the class of noncats, but only also to a higher class such as that of mammals.

We shall see that according to Bateson an important part of the double bind consists in ignoring this principle of logic. But it is once again striking that until now only the logical, formal structure—the *cognitive* structure—of contradictions has been studied, while their *affective* side—including the tension, rage, fear, and perhaps joy they may arouse—has appeared to need no explanation. This approach applies to a large extent even to Bateson and other modern communications theorists. In my own view, however, these are precisely the key questions: When, how, and why do formal contradictions cause tension and rage, and sometimes even "insanity"? What contributes to the intensity of these feelings? How is this related to paradoxes and to the double bind? The concept of affective-logical systems of reference can help to answer these questions of crucial importance for practical therapy.

In formal terms we can define a contradiction as a localized *irreg-*

ularity in an otherwise equilibrated framework of relationships (that is, in a system of reference). We might compare it to a mistake in a piece of knitting or weaving or, perhaps more accurately, to a barrier in a system of otherwise passable roads. In affective terms such an irregularity means above all a *disharmony,* that is, the collision of one mood or frame of mind with another, contrary one. If I play cheerfully with a child for a long while, for example, and then suddenly shout at it angrily because it has made some tiny mistake, my behavior contains a contradiction that causes a state of emotional confusion at least momentarily. How serious this incident was and how consistent my further behavior is will now determine whether the disharmony recedes and is suppressed (although it may of course remain below the surface as an unpleasant memory and source of later disturbance), or whether it creates more and more tension, so that we break off our game and my partner must revise his picture of me. Simple contradictions have an analogous structure in all kinds of fields, from social interaction to the sciences and mathematics, and despite the infinite variations possible in different contexts, their affective-logical effect is always the same in principle: a dominant, coherent, and well-equilibrated system of thinking and feeling is disturbed. It is stirred up temporarily like the surface of a pool into which a stone has been thrown. After a while balance may be restored by a complete reabsorption or neutralization of the motion (in psychological terms by isolation or repression), or it may end in an alteration of the entire system, in a constructive, "optimizing" (or perhaps destructive and regressive) new adjustment. A simple contradiction—as distinct from paradox and the double bind, as we shall see—has the following essential aspects:

- There is a clear quantitative and/or qualitative disproportion between the dominant system of reference and the disturbance; the latter represents only a discordant "blip" in an otherwise homogeneous and concordant whole.
- The emotional tensions created by this heterogeneous element (as a rule some form of unpleasure such as uncertainty, anger, rage, or fear) remain relatively well defined and do not seriously threaten the functioning of the psychic system in the particular context.
- In the simplest cases the contradiction is readily apparent. It can thus be confronted directly in a verbal conflict, and, if both parties make the necessary adjustments, it may be resolved.

This definition does not require a contradiction on different levels of logic or communication. Unlike Bateson and several other authors who have recently concerned themselves with this subject, I do not consider contradiction on different levels as an absolutely essential element, but merely as a possible one. I hold this to be true even for paradoxes and double binds, which represent only special forms of contradictions. Thus in the example of my behavior with the child, the contradiction—the inappropriate angry reaction in the middle of happy play—can easily lie on the same level of logic as the predominantly friendly behavior. The two contradictory messages can also be expressed in a consistent manner, with friendly words, gestures, and body language at one time and angry ones at the other. Leaving aside for the moment all the implied levels of thought and communication, we can see that a contradiction is simply a statistic to begin with, namely the fact that *a rule is broken by an unusual occurrence.* It was necessary, we recall, for an emotional and/or cognitive regularity (invariance) to be grasped before we could form an internalized system of reference or complex of associated ideas. However, it lies in the nature of a contradiction that these associations of ideas prove to be no longer (or not always) concordant.

This represents the simplest and thus most easily recognizable instance of a situation in which all kinds of variations and complications are possible, leading to paradox and the double bind in a series of gradual transitions. In a verbal argument, for example, the focus may shift from a large and dominant system of reference to the particular, narrow area where the contradiction lies, with the result that two contradictory "truths" come to appear quantitatively of equal weight. This is the constellation of a typical paradox. The same thing can occur if the contradiction spreads out from an originally limited context—for example, if my behavior while playing with the child becomes so contradictory that a completely unpredictable situation arises. Furthermore, evident contradictions may become more and more veiled; logical levels may become confused; affective and cognitive messages may begin to contradict rather than confirm each other; and so on until a typical double-bind situation is reached. As the following example shows, the result must be increasing tension and confusion of both a cognitive and an affective kind.

A married couple comes to me for therapy because of a conflict that has been smoldering for years. They demand a psychotherapy session urgently just before Christmas. Both of them are tense, depressed, and aggressive. They report that they had experienced the last of several periods of reconciliation a few weeks before, including a feeling of closeness and sexual intimacy. Then they had begun to quarrel again over a misunderstanding of some arrangements, and the wife had deeply injured her husband by saying that she "didn't want to have anything to do with him anymore." Although she then completely "forgot" about this remark, her husband did not. On the other hand she complained bitterly that for weeks he had been refusing to participate in any of the family's Christmas preparations and had taken no notice of her conciliatory gestures.

In this marital conflict the confusion has arisen as a result of synchronic and diachronic contradictions, contradictory messages on different levels, misunderstandings, "memory lapses," and a constantly contracting and expanding focus of attention from areas of a higher order to those of a lower order. It appears possible that the spouses' treatment of each other is dominated alternately by first the positive and then the negative representations of object and self that Kernberg has described. In any event the systems of reference of ideal harmony, the Christmas spirit, and family unity alternate with those of bitter aggression and rejection. They determine all feeling, thinking, actions, and perceptions in alternating phases and thus represent quite consistent but contrary "worlds" or "truths" that can be pulled out—as if from a file—to be used for a while and then put back in a drawer out of sight. When we fall in love, have outbursts of rage or grief, or suffer illnesses such as depression or mania, we experience such displacements or "dis-orders" of an affective-logical focus in temporarily split-off contradictory areas of thinking and feeling. These phenomena can range from normal experiences of everyday life to the pathological.

If we apply these ideas about individual or family systems to larger contexts, they lead to a number of interesting general conclusions. There is no reason to assume, for example, that this kind of cognitive-affective shift of emphasis cannot occur in entire groups, communities, or even nations. The affective-logical world view of groups is determined by their present, past, and future "reality" (either anticipated or feared)—that is, by all concrete experience that has become cognitive *and* effective information in the sense described above. This world view must necessarily be different for every collective, despite considerable overlapping. This is one reason why—all propaganda aside—Germans and the British, Russians and Americans, Arabs and Israelis are capable of experiencing, in all good faith, very different and highly contradictory affective-logical "truths" in certain areas. The same can occur on other levels, between urban and rural populations in one country, or between management and labor, young and old, or men and women. When viewed from the perspective of affect-logic, so-called objective truths are nothing but consonances—internalized cognitive-affective systems that have been more or less harmonized and brought into balance by leaving out contradictory elements. This occurs so that these systems can deal as efficiently as possible with the reality that the person encounters. These consonances necessarily possess a high (but not absolute) degree of homeostatic resistance to change; otherwise they would not be able to function—a result that can in fact occur in certain pathological borderline conditions. In other words, these systems change only under the irresistible pressure of contradictions so severe that they cannot be isolated. The same phenomenon governs the development of scientific knowledge, as the modern philosophy of science has shown. The state of our knowledge at any given time, our truths, our philosophy—in short, the total of our systems of reference—appear from this perspective as an instrument for processing incoming information with the least possible tension. This instrument, which is well equilibrated, adaptable to events as they occur, and constantly undergoing slow transformation, can also be regarded as an organ designed to keep a balance between a human being and the total environment, including all the achievements of human civilization. Seen in this light, a human being and the environment together form a system of a higher order, certain elements of which (and also the *relations* between elements) come with time to be registered as invariances in the internalized and condensed cognitive-affective schemata, "instructions for acting," or "programs" that we call the mind or the psyche. This thought pervades contemporary thinking from the philosophy of science to ecology and structuralism. It has been most strikingly illustrated in Gregory Bateson's description of a man felling a tree with an ax, in which all three elements together—the man, the ax, and the tree—form a circular, constantly varying system without beginning or end. Within this system the man and his mind are only part of a more comprehensive whole.[16] Sartre described the circularity of the dominant philosophy of any epoch in a quite similar approach:

In certain circumstances a philosophy is formulated in order to express the general development of society; as long as this philosophy remains alive, it serves the people of its time as a cultural milieu . . . Sprung from social development, it is itself development and thus reaches into the future . . . Seen from this aspect philosophy has the character of a method of investigation and explanation . . . Thus philosophy remains effective as long as the usage which produced it, and by which it is constantly supported and illuminated, remains alive.[17]

Finally, it is especially interesting that contradictions do not always create only tension, are not always disturbing and destructive, but in some cases contain great creative potential: when the time is ripe, they can provide the impetus for an optimizing equilibration in Piaget's sense, leading to further abstraction and development of the entire cognitive-affective system in question. A famous example of this from the history of science is the orbit of the planets, which—in contrast to the movements of the sun and stars—cannot be understood from a geocentric perspective: their irregular wanderings in the night sky simply do not fit this idea, which was taken over from Plato and Aristotle and dominated all medieval thinking. This annoying contradiction certainly did not disturb most people, but it did lead astronomers throughout the centuries to invent the most extraordinary theories (for example, the theory that epicycles were tacked on to the original revolutions around the earth, comparable to the seats on a ferris wheel as they rotate on their own axis while revolving around the large circle). This contradiction also led to bitter disputes, which Arthur Koestler described many years ago in his fascinating book *The Sleepwalkers*. If we follow the development of astronomy from the earth-centered view of Ptolemy (second century A.D.) through Copernicus, Kepler, and Galileo to the heliocentric concept of Newton (1642–1717), we can easily recognize the stages α to γ that according to Piaget characterize all optimizing equilibrations. The strange mixture of old and new ideas in the theories of Copernicus is particularly instructive. As Koestler describes them:

At the beginning (Book I, Chapter 10), Copernicus had stated: "in the midst of all dwells the sun . . . Sitting on the royal throne, he rules the family of planets which turn around him . . . We thus find in this arrangement an admirable harmony of the world." But in Book III, when it comes to reconciling the doctrine with actual observation, the earth no longer turns around the sun, but round a point in space removed from the sun by a distance of about three times the sun's diameter. Nor do the planets revolve around the sun—as every schoolboy believes that Copernicus taught. The planets move on epicycles of epicycles, centred not on the sun, but on the centre of the *earth's orbit*. There are thus two "royal thrones": the sun, and that imaginary point in space around which the earth moves . . . In short, the earth appears equal in importance in governing the solar system to the sun itself, and in fact nearly as important as in the Aristotelian or Ptolemaic system.[18]

Astronomy is especially rich in examples of how contradictions to which little attention was paid at first (such as small irregularities in the courses of heavenly bodies) finally led to important new discoveries. Thus from discrepancies in the path of Neptune a student named Tombaugh was able in 1930 to deduce the existence of the planet Pluto.[19] Children's understanding of the world develops in principle in much the same way, as the example of Piaget's experiments with the surface of water in bottles shows. We should not be surprised, therefore, to see that even clinicians who used to see contradictory and paradoxical forms of communication as purely destructive and conducive to psychosis have begun to recognize their positive, creative aspects.

Paradoxes

According to definitions in most dictionaries, a paradox is more or less identical with a contradiction. Etymologically, *para-dox* means "a contradictory dogma," "an alternative truth." Some dictionaries emphasize, additionally, the surprising character of a paradox. *Webster's* defines *paradox* as "a statement that seems contradictory, unbelievable, or absurd, but that may actually be true in fact." In addition to Mara Selvini Palazzoli's book *Paradox and Counterparadox: A New Model in the Therapy of the Family in Schizophrenic Transaction,* the writings of Paul Watzlawick have done much to popularize the concept of paradox in psychiatry. He defines a paradox as "a contradiction that follows correct deduction from consistent premises."[20] The excellent article by Klaus Schäfer in the *Handbuch der philosophischen Grundbegriffe* takes the definition of paradox clearly beyond that of simple contradiction. Referring to Socrates, Jesus, Hegel, and Nietzsche, he stresses the creative aspect of paradox, which can expand awareness:

An event may be called a "paradox" when, and only when, the system D(oxa) affected by it becomes more complex, differentiated, substantial, flexible, open and richer through the appearance of this factor . . .

P(aradox) thus does not make D more predictable or convenient, but rather charges it with energy, adds conflict, gives it more risk and more appeal. Paradoxes raise the level and intensity of the relations and processes in a system and between the system and the environment . . .

Paradox offers the system the chance to criticize itself, to rejuvenate itself, and to expand its boundaries.[21]

These definitions will be of particular importance in clarifying the relationships between paradox and double bind in the next section. A little later Schäfer even says that "such a learning system might exist, for example, when two people talk to each other, when an interdisciplinary research team is planned and developed, when a movement or a group works for social change, indicates a path for others to follow, or experiments with possibilities for improvement."[22]

In Schäfer's view—which coincides with my own—a paradox is *more* than a simple contradiction as defined above. In terms of affect-logic we can define a paradox as follows:

A paradox results from the collision of two affective-logical systems, consistent in themselves but irreconcilable in combination, of the SAME *order.*

Thus, in contrast to simple contradiction, paradox does not consist in a limited inconsonance *within* a greater system of reference, but rather in a collision of two contradictory interpretations of reality, each having equal weight. (Metaphorically one could speak of two equally extensive and well-organized systems of pathways for mastering reality.) Paradoxically contrary truths must necessarily be both true and false at the same time. A well-known example from physics is the nature of light, which consists of waves and particles at the same time: both theories explain a number of observations, depending on the context and standpoint of the observer. These observations fit without contradiction in general theories about the qualities of waves and particles, but together they are completely irreconcilable, as long as no theory of a higher order exists that includes *both* sets of observations. In the field of psychology we can find something quite similar in Kernberg's "all good" and "all bad" representations of the self and objects, which are diametrically opposed but nonetheless refer to one and the same person. The fact that one can experience oneself or an important person such as one's mother or spouse as immeasurably good and loving and immeasurably bad and evil at the same time (or in rapid alternation) represents a genuine paradox. Such a radically contradictory state of affairs creates confusion; for this reason, as Kernberg explains, the two must be kept separate at first, split into two isolated, homogeneous affective-cognitive concepts.

Social, political, and ideological systems of reference such as the differing world views of Russians and Americans, Israelis and Arabs, and city and country dwellers, can also become paradoxes when they present the same claims to all-inclusive validity and collide with one another. *Within* each of these systems, on the other hand, observations and arguments from the "other side" remain mere contradictions, which can be endured or dismissed with relative ease. This difference, which is actually more quantitative than qualitative, explains the particular destructive force of the genuine paradox and also its creative affective (or affective-logical) force. It creates amazement, tension, confusion, and sometimes also irritation, aggression, and anxiety. The area in which the two systems of reference collide represents a zone of explosive instability and uncertainty; one could say that there is a war going on. This image helps to explain why both in society and within the individual psyche strong forces must continually be mobilized to eliminate such a trouble spot or at least to neutralize it.

Such a mobilization of psychic forces is connected in turn with a universally valid principle of affect-logic that becomes apparent only in situations of extreme conflict and seems to play a major role in mental disorder: *It is not possible to live in two different affective-logical systems of reference at the same time.* Every system represents a framework of internalized instructions for feeling, thinking, and behaving, which has grown organically out of concrete experiences in interaction with a particular environment and gradually established a subtle balance. At the same time, such a system is also a *system of values* motivating behavior. Contrary values can no more coexist than contrary moods, however. It is possible—and this is also highly significant—to conceive of different states of equilibrium for one and the same reality—or, one could say, different *Gestalten* or interpretations of reality. This ability provides a basis for the existence of paradoxes. In this sense, "truth" is multiple; every scientific theory, every world view, religion, political or other kind of ideology, and every personal philosophy represents a possible way of ordering the reality that is encountered and of establishing it in a more or less economical state of equilibrium. We are sometimes able to shift from one state of equilibrium to another, either for single, circumscribed concepts or for comprehensive "versions of the world" (two good examples from pathology are depression and mania, two paradoxically opposite interpretations of reality). But we do not appear to be able to change these affective-cognitive states of equilibrium at will. There are good reasons to assume that what we do above all is to regress and reactivate earlier affective-cognitive states that were established and equilibrated in early childhood. This is probably the case in certain kinds of depression, for example, which seem to affect only people who actually experienced during their first years extreme conditions of abandonment, anxiety, and hopelessness, which they consolidated into corresponding systems of behavior or reference. Later these systems are always available to fall back upon. New and progressive modes of thinking and feeling can be acquired only through the very slow and laborious achievement of new optimizing equilibrations—as not only all psychotherapists, but also teachers and members of the clergy know only too well. Certain fundamental ways of thinking and feeling with which we grasp the world (our basic relationships to other people and events, our self-image, and our ways of coping with "the way things are") may in fact be unalterable, having been established once and for all. This is suggested by such phenomena as "basic trust" or mistrust (Erik Erikson) and lifelong basic feelings of strength and success or weakness and failure, optimism versus pessimism, activity versus passivity, and so on.

In cybernetic terms these frameworks or systems of reference, formed through and validated by experience a thousand times over, through which we grasp reality, have as their primary purpose the reduction of tension—in principle something pleasurable—in an individual's dealings with the world. If, however, these frameworks are confronted with other, contradictory frameworks, this tension-reducing effect is lost at once, and a highly unpleasurable disorder results instead. Since ancient times people have pondered puzzles such as the paradoxical statement "'All Cretans are liars,' says a Cretan." Is he telling the truth or lying? This type of intellectual game can be both annoying and amusing, but in real life it is no accident that we avoid paradoxes whenever possible, for they produce a deep sense of uncertainty by placing in question our whole framework of values and relationships. Our essential psychic structures for surviving in the world are shaken to their foundations. If we realize this clearly enough, then we will be better able to understand the destructive effect of the double bind.

First, however, I would like to take a closer look at the *creative aspect* of paradoxes that Schäfer emphasized. Without doubt this springs from the same disorder previously described in negative and unpleasurable terms. Paradoxes are characterized by a zone of affective-cognitive instability and tension that virtually demands a restoration of order. One solution is to split the two components and to accept one and then the other in alternation; this is what Kernberg suggests happens with "all good" and "all bad" self and object representations. Other defense mechanisms include denial, repression, projection, and reaction formation. However, under certain mysterious but interesting circumstances something entirely different may occur: the two sides of the paradoxical contradiction are not negated, but affirmed. If this confrontation can be endured, a common aspect may finally come into view, previously not recognizable but now linking both components. This extraction of an invariance can now bring about the desired reduction of tension. Such an act of condensation creates an element of a higher order, which can be used to construct a new and higher system, that is, an optimized system. This is clearly what happens when a small child becomes capable of joining the good and bad sides of its mother (and itself) together into a new whole; every other solution of a paradox through optimizing equilibration is achieved in an analogous manner, in terms of both structure and the tension-reducing, pleasurable affective result. It is thus highly interesting to observe that intellectual development—and perhaps every other kind of development as well—follows Freud's pleasure principle in the last analysis. Generally speaking, however, the decisive creative step is probably always insight into the fundamental structure of the paradox—the realization that part and counterpart determine each other and are inextricably linked. A constantly recurring fusion of two radically opposite parts is necessary to create a true whole. This phenomenon certainly applies to the good and bad sides of both object and the self, but it may possibly apply in equal measure to such apparently independent and contrary value systems as capitalism and communism, right- and left-wing concepts, and police and criminals. To pursue this last point would take us too far afield, however.

There is good reason to assume that a developmental principle of great general importance lies hidden in the creative potential of contradictions and paradoxes. Something must be afoot when, as now, not only the humanities but also mathematics, physics, and even psychiatry all display a growing interest in paradoxes. This cannot be happening by accident, and I suspect the reason behind it is that paradoxes contain a basic developmental mechanism, one that can take two components and transform them into a third, new entity. We begin to see with growing clarity that this mechanism consists in *combining two systems to form a third as a result of "interference" in the border areas of overlap between the two systems.*

Let me use an image to make my meaning clearer.

As I write these lines I am sitting on the beach of a small bay in the south of France. The bay is surrounded by cliffs and protected from the strong wind, the mistral, which is blowing out to sea from the north. From time to time the wind stirs up the surface of the water with a gust; small showers create varied patterns of waves and then move on, leaving the surface smooth again. Farther out to sea, the wind blows up long retreating lines of spray.

Wind and water, which play the leading roles in this pleasing natural spectacle, each represent a large and dynamically equilibrated system: the wind blows southward in powerful gusts, following its own laws and creating a balance of pressure; the sea rests in its own horizontal and vertical equilibrium, and in its depths many dark, circulatory processes run their course, some rapidly and some more slowly. On its surface, however, that is, at the borders where the two systems touch, the two components interact to create phenomena of a new kind: the endless variety of wave structures—large and small, general and localized, permanent and momentary—are "translations," so to speak, of the constantly shifting wind structures into patterns that neither system could have produced on its own.

Something analogous must occur with the intellect and the emotions when in a paradoxical situation two cognitive-affective systems collide, each of which is equilibrated—and therefore stable—if taken by itself. This is true not only of mathematical formulas[23] but also of "equations" of an entirely different kind, such as all-good or all-bad images of oneself or others. The image above also demonstrates what must occur for two such systems to be able to "coexist" and create a new ordered structure: they must share some common element, an *invariance,* through which a constant *relation* can be established between them. In the case of wind and water, the common feature is clearly their characteristic flowing motion in waves. Unless such an invariance can become effective, the critical border area of the two systems will reflect only confusion (in psychological terms, tension and unpleasure). If a creative synthesis can be reached, however, relaxation and pleasure take their place. Interestingly enough, a similar phenomenon can be observed in animals: paradoxical contradictions can lead to disturbed behavior resembling psychosis in dogs. Pavlov demonstrated this early in the century with his famous experiments on conditioned reflexes, in which animals had to distinguish between a circle and an ellipse in order to get food. If the difference between the two figures was gradually reduced, until finally a distinction became impossible, the dogs' behavior would become unpredictable. They would become overexcited, lethargic, or even comatose, depending on their temperament. However, animals also demonstrate that overcoming paradoxical contradictions creatively is an achievement with a pleasurable side to it. Bateson reports one striking example.

In connection with his studies of logical classes Bateson was observing how dolphins were trained at the Oceanic Institute in Hawaii. A female dolphin had been trained in a first phase, A, to expect a reward of fish if she repeated a previous piece of behavior in the exhibition tank when the trainer blew his whistle. In a later phase, B, the dolphin received a reward only when she demonstrated a *new* and different piece of behavior, such as a new kind of jump. The "paradoxical" change in the usual rules at first led to a crisis. The dolphin did not understand it and became so disturbed that in order to preserve the relationship between her and her trainer, it was necessary to give many reinforcements to which the porpoise was not entitled (unearned fish). "In the time out between the fourteenth and fifteenth sessions, the dolphin appeared to be much excited, and when she came onstage for the fifteenth session, she put on an elaborate performance that included eight pieces of conspicuous behavior of which four were new and never before observed in this species of animal." From this moment on she had grasped the new rule; the tension disappeared; the synthesis between the two contradictory systems of reference (context A and context B) had been reached and thus also the leap to a higher logical class and level of abstraction.[24]

It seems reasonable to assume that analogous processes occur in every optimizing abstraction. One most interesting fact stressed by

Bateson is that in the critical phase before the resolution of the paradoxical contradiction the trainer continued to provide evidence of his
"affection" with extra rations of fish, despite the lack of success. We
shall see in the final chapter that this represents one crucial difference
between pathogenic and therapeutic paradoxes.[25] The unambiguously positive affective coloring of *both* contradictory contexts, A
and B, certainly is another important contrast to the malign form of
paradox.

The Double Bind

In their 1956 article Bateson and his colleagues did not offer a simple
definition of the double bind, but instead described six of its main
characteristics:

1. *Two or more persons* are involved. One, usually a child, is
   designated as the "victim"; the other, usually the mother, is
   seen as the inflictor of the double bind.
2. *Repeated experience* is assumed rather than a single traumatic
   event, so that the double-bind structure comes to be a habitual
   expectation.
3. A *primary negative injunction* ("Do not do thus and such") is
   established. Noncompliance is threatened with punishment,
   usually some form of withdrawal of love.
4. A *secondary negative injunction,* conflicting with the first on
   another level of logic, is also established, and compliance is
   again enforced by punishments that threaten survival.
5. A *tertiary negative injunction* prohibits the victim from escaping from the field.
6. *The complete set of ingredients* is no longer necessary when
   the victim has learned to perceive his universe in double-bind
   patterns.

The authors go on to particularize the situation with the following
points:

1. The individual is involved in an intense relationship in which
   he feels that accurate discrimination of what sort of message
   is being communicated is *essential to survival.*

2. The individual is caught in a situation in which the other person in the relationship is expressing *two orders of message,* and one of these denies the other.
3. He is unable to comment on the messages being expressed; that is, he cannot make *a metacommunicative statement.*

Obviously, it is far from easy to grasp this complex phenomenon, especially when one considers that over time most of the relatively explicit ingredients in the double bind become superfluous but remain in effect all the same. This is probably the main reason why it has been so difficult to objectify the theory and make it operational. One of the original coauthors, Jay Haley, stated in 1978 that the theory was too complicated to be useful in therapy; other researchers such as Scheflen have disputed the usefulness of some of the elements in the theory, claiming, for example, that Bateson's central notion of different levels of logic in contradictory communications has led to more confusion than clarification.[26] Yet even Steven Hirsch, a critic of the theory who has said that there is about as much evidence for the existence of the double bind as there is for the existence of unicorns, believes that this does not exclude the possibility of one turning up someday: "The fact remains: The descriptions of the original authors, who were clever and experienced clinicians after all, elicited in all of us who have to do with schizophrenics and their parents a feeling of assent and agreement."[27]

Hirsch concludes his remarks with the observation that such complex interaction certainly does occur in the families of some schizophrenics, but it also occurs in other families; *its pathogenic effect must therefore lie in a very high but unspecific degree of stress,* which is particularly difficult for potential schizophrenics to bear. The fact that double-bind messages of the kind described by Bateson and his colleagues do exist, and that they can literally "drive someone crazy," has been confirmed by the numerous clinical examples of Searles, Watzlawick, Stierlin, and others. One illustration is the oft-cited case presented in the original article:

A young man who had fairly well recovered from an acute schizophrenic episode was visited in the hospital by his mother. He was glad to see her and impulsively put his arm around her shoulders, whereupon she stiffened. He withdrew his arm and she asked, "Don't you love me any more?" He then blushed, and she said, "Dear, you must not be so easily embarrassed and afraid of your feelings." The patient was able to stay with her only a few minutes more and following her departure he assaulted an aide and was put in the tubs.[28]

In their analysis of the case the authors show that the mother (1) covered up her own embarrassment and forced the patient to deny his perception of the situation by accepting her condemnation; (2) demanded that he love her and accused him of not doing so; by shifting the focus from his expressing affection to his alleged inability to be affectionate, she put him further in doubt and filled him with guilt; and (3) suggested to him that he was not normal and could not accept his feelings.

The affective-cognitive dilemma in which the young man was caught consisted in being threatened with the loss of his mother's love in both cases, both when he showed that he loved her and when he did not. At the same time he could neither retreat from the situation nor resolve it with a metacommunicative statement, such as the one which the authors suggest would have been helpful but which was impossible for him: "Mother, it is obvious that you become uncomfortable when I put my arm around you and that you have difficulty accepting a gesture of affection from me."

The main questions that now arise concern the extent to which the double-bind phenomena as described are distinguishable from simple contradiction and paradox, and the reasons for their particularly destructive effect. From the standpoint of affect-logic a genuine double bind as originally conceived represents a very special variation of a contradiction or paradox in which the contradictions are subtly concealed. In order to make this clear, we must consider for a moment what the possible affective and cognitive structure of paradoxes might look like. We saw that in a paradox two equally valid systems of reference—let us call them A and B—collide. Each of these systems has its own emotional coloring, which can only be either mainly positive (pleasurable, pleasant, harmonious) or mainly negative (unpleasurable, unpleasant, disharmonious). In other words, four types of affective-logically structured paradox can exist, depending on whether positively or negatively colored cognitive and emotional components clash:

1. $A+/B+$. Two systems of reference with a mainly positive coloring collide. This constellation occurred in the case of the dolphin being trained in Hawaii, described by Bateson. An example from the

natural sciences is the paradoxical nature of light as both waves and particles. Perhaps the best way to grasp the situation is to analyze the structure of several different kinds of jokes, since—as Arthur Koestler demonstrated in *The Act of Creation*—jokes are usually based on an unexpected joining of two levels of meaning that were previously unrelated and thus appear paradoxical. If both systems of reference have a positive coloring, then the joke may be of the following pleasantly harmless kind:

> Little Johnny learns at Sunday school that all men are made of dust, and to dust they shall return. When he gets home, he runs to look under his parents' bed and asks excitedly, "Mommy, Daddy, is that somebody *coming* or *going?*" (Unexpected linking of the very different but positively colored levels of meaning for the word *dust,* one religious and one ordinary.)

If paradoxes with this configuration represent the only alternatives available for action, then no grounds exist for a pathogenic increase in psychological tension, in contrast to a double-bind situation. In fact the result can be a pleasurably tranquil state of mind. There are only two possibilities, but both are pleasant. (For instance, I can spend my vacation only in Spain or Italy, but either would be nice.)

2 and 3. $A+/B-$ *or* $A-/B+$. One of the two systems of reference has a mainly positive coloring, the other a mainly negative one. This situation may occur when completely positive idealizations of another person or oneself collide, in the event of some frustration, with a totally contrary negative image that is normally split off. According to Kernberg this frequently happens with immature borderline personalities. Paradoxical situations of this kind will not lead to manifest psychological problems as long as the positive system of reference being maintained is not contaminated by the negative system. However, the effort to achieve this may give rise to considerable tension and anxiety. This is exactly what Kernberg means by the splitting of internalized self and object representations into two "all good" and "all bad" extremes. All problems appear to be solved as long as I can maintain the fictitious idealizations of myself or my partner, but the danger threatens constantly that I may suddenly drop into a contrary "underworld" where such unrealistic images turn into their exact negative counterpart.

Once again it is interesting to note how these two "halves" of the

world belong together and how one obviously conditions and constitutes the other. Jokes based on this type of constellation cease to appeal only to pleasant feelings and are directed also at their repressed
opposites (tension, irritation, fear, aggression, sadism, and so on):

> A crusty old Scottish farmer is sitting on the shore of a beautiful
> loch, watching a German tourist swimming in the cold and
> stormy water. The German, losing the battle against the waves
> and in danger of drowning, begins to wave his arms and shout,
> "Hilfe! Hilfe!" The farmer makes no move to go to his rescue, but
> instead just shakes his head and mutters, "That will teach you to
> fool about with foreign languages instead of learning to swim!"

The positively colored side is represented here by the system of reference "Scottish farmer," with which we associate droll anecdotes, and
a strongly rooted sense of identity and locale; the negative side consists of the foreigner, the cold water, the storm, and mortal danger
and death. The unexpected connection that makes us laugh occurs in
the word *Hilfe;* the farmer interprets in genuine double-bind fashion
on a different level of logic from what was intended, on the level of
the word itself rather than its meaning.

4. $A-/B-$. Both levels of reference are negatively colored, that is,
unpleasurable and perhaps even full of fear and anxiety. This fourth
possibility is expressed in the Greek myth of Scylla and Charybdis,
between which dangers so many seafarers perished, and also in the
myth of Sisyphus. Every tragedy, whether on the stage or in life, has
this same inescapable, doubly negative affective and cognitive structure. This can also be illustrated by a joke:

> An old Jew in the Soviet Union finally receives permission to
> emigrate after a long wait. He sells all his possessions and realizes
> his dream of going to Israel. He is bitterly disappointed by life
> there, however, and soon asks to be allowed to return to Russia.
> Permission is granted, but after a short time back at home he
> makes another tremendous effort to emigrate. Amazingly his
> request is granted again—but he doesn't fare any better in Israel
> the second time. When after a second return to the Soviet Union
> he asks permission to emigrate for a third time, the authorities
> demand that he make up his mind once and for all where he likes
> it better. The old man only shakes his head and answers, "I guess
> all I really like is traveling!"

This story, which upon close inspection proves to be both cruel and profound, is structured exactly like a typical double bind, except that the man in the joke appears to have one desperate way out: he could travel back and forth without cease. The Jew is caught in two irreconcilable systems of reference. He cannot endure either one of them, and he cannot escape them, except by choosing an all but impossible compromise, which is neither the one nor the other but a bit of both.

This "way out" for schizophrenics—at least according to Bateson's hypothesis—is the leap into psychotic behavior ("going over the edge"). And in fact we must agree that a dilemma of the kind described is conducive to tension, confusion, and anxiety in the highest degree. When such paradoxical situations occur in areas vital to survival and without any possible alternative, then, the double-bind theory postulates, they must represent potentially explosive "trouble spots." The longer the unbearable situation lasts and the more clearly it is perceived that no way out exists (that is, cognitively grasped but above all *felt* emotionally and physically), the greater the degree of tension and instability that arises. Berger's careful observations reveal that characteristic reactions are feelings of insecurity, confusion, perplexity, mystification, irresolvable contradiction, frustration, guilt, disappointment, hopelessness, helplessness, inability to react, cowardice, self-pity, and a craving for love.[29] The person caught in the dilemma resembles in a manner of speaking a rat in a two-chambered cage, both sections of which have been wired to receive constant electric shocks. As is well known, laboratory animals subjected to such cruel treatment eventually lose all their normal ability to solve problems: they may revert to a cataleptic passivity, show bursts of senseless activity, or display other bizarre forms of behavior. The double-bind hypothesis suggests that herein lies the explanation for the pathological behavior patterns of schizophrenics—either catatonic, paranoid and excitable, or hebephrenic and childish.

Pathogenic paradoxes thus appear as inescapable dilemmas between two equally negative, unbearable, and contradictory possibilities for thinking, feeling, and behaving (that is, affective-logical systems of reference and value systems). One further aspect adding to the complexity of the phenomenon should also be emphasized, without which the entanglement represented by the typical double bind cannot be fully understood: The paradoxical contradictions of a genuine double bind are usually not manifest but are concealed so subtly that it takes great efforts of logical (or affective-logical) analysis to uncover them, and sometimes even that does not succeed.[30] Many different strategies for concealment exist, from vagueness and ambiguity in communications on all relevant topics, through evasive tactics, to taboos about touching on certain subjects at all. Using a modified Rohrschach test, Singer and his associates were able to identify thirty-two significant contradictory modes of communication in families of schizophrenics, which they placed under the following six headings:[31]

Remarks that are unintelligible, not to the point, or ambiguous
Distracted and distracting behavior
Unstable perceptions and thought processes
Nihilistic devaluation of tasks to be performed
Inappropriate, illogical, and contradictory commentaries
Abstract, diffuse, and discursive vagueness

Family researchers have described the confusing and unauthentic patterns of relationships resulting from this type of communication in terms such as "pseudo-community," "mystification," and "structural displacement"; they have also uncovered the method behind such contradictions, namely that attempts by any family members to break out are rendered impossible by repeated (mutual) devaluation, disqualification, and denial of the content of clear messages. All these communicative maneuvers have one feature in common: covering up and avoiding any open conflict. We shall go into the reasons for this in greater detail below. For the time being we should note that such tactics block the creative potential that was shown above to be innate in contradictions and paradoxes. We shall see that the underlying meaning of many double-bind messages lies precisely in the blocking of children's separation from narcissistic parents with whom they are symbiotically fused. The double bind is thus revealed as a defense mechanism designed to prevent the transformation of hidden contradictions into open conflicts that could, once exposed, be resolved.

In my view, *mixing different logical orders* in the typical double blind is one tactic for avoiding conflict. Even simple linguistic tricks can suffice to confuse logical classes, and thus can be used quite effectively to mask contradictions:

If I say, "All cats are black, but all cats are white," then the paradox is undisguised, and its impossibility strikes one immediately. However, if I phrase it as "All cats are black. But two are white," then I have already begun to disguise the paradox by mixing two different levels of logic. Instead of comparing the class of "all cats" with another class of the same order (such as "all dogs"), which would be the only correct procedure, I have falsely compared "all cats" with "two cats." I can now go on to make these contradictions even subtler, by continuing to say, "All cats are black," but adding all kinds of ifs, ands, or buts, and providing elaborate but unintelligible explanations. I can add facial expression or gestures to imply the opposite of what I am saying, or give an almost imperceptible but nonetheless significant signal to the same effect; I can shake my head, raise an eyebrow, move my hand, twitch a corner of my mouth, or assume a certain stance. All of these means can help to cover up the manifest content of my verbal message, to the point where a state of total affective and cognitive confusion has been reached.

From this perspective, the mixing of logical classes in the double bind appears to me as just one of many defense mechanisms—albeit a particularly effective one—for preventing the emergence of family conflicts and the possibility that a family member might break out of the pseudo-community. But I do not share Bateson's position that contradictions on different logical levels are an essential component of an affective-logical dilemma—only that they are possible (and admittedly frequent). Nor can I agree with authors such as J. S. Kafka who postulate that every paradox conceals a confusion of logical classes. In my opinion paradoxes and contradictions of the double-bind type may certainly occur on one level, as one of Kafka's own examples shows:

The father of a schizophrenic girl . . . had made major changes in his career in order to pay for her treatment in a private hospital. Despite a recent heart attack, this clergyman has left his pulpit, has become a hard driving nationally prominent lecturer and author. During a visit to the hospital he explains both to his daughter and to the staff that he owes his new-found energy, this renewal in his life, to the financial needs of her expensive hospitalization. One could say, on the basis of these data, that the patient is caught in a double-bind. If she makes successful efforts to recover rapidly, she deprives her father of the reported renewal in his life. If, on the other hand, she fails to improve sufficiently to be discharged from the hospital, the associated financial need imposes a "killing" workload on father. On the face of it she is in a no win situation.[32]

I fail to see how two *different* levels of abstraction are involved here, as Kafka asserts—on the one hand that of life and death, on the other that of the "quality of life." The two seem to me to be on the same level in terms of formal logic. In contrast to many authors who have taken over Bateson's postulates on logic too uncritically, I believe that we can come a step closer to clearing up what is undoubtedly an extremely complex situation if we consider the mixing of logical classes to be only *one* (particularly impenetrable) strategy among many for avoiding conflict. This fits in with all the ideas discussed previously and also with many observations from recent schizophrenia research: apart from acute and disruptive phases in which repressed conflicts often emerge openly, the avoidance of conflict appears to be *the* central characteristic of schizophrenic behavior, as psychoanalysts, communications theorists, and academic psychologists all agree. It represents a particular method of escaping stress, as Lilo Süllwold recently demonstrated for many schizophrenic symptoms;[33] and in addition it serves, sometimes in grotesque ways, the pathological homeostatic tendencies that repeatedly sabotage any possibility for change and progress.

> In a seminar[34] Gottlieb Guntern presented the striking case of a thirty-five-year-old intellectual who had been diagnosed as "schizophrenic" and unemployable and who had been living off his divorced mother for the past 15 years. He spent his days riding his bicycle and reading. Both partners in this pathological symbiosis were able to communicate perfectly normally with a family therapist as long as the topic remained neutral. Whenever the subject turned to their manner of living together, their financial situation, and the son's life as an aimless parasite, however, both the "designated patient" and his mother began to babble incoherently.

The question of logical levels is also related to that of relevant levels of communication in double-bind phenomena, where considerable lack of clarity still prevails: on the one hand many authors discuss narrowly defined, contradictory message sequences limited to a few sentences and gestures, as in Bateson's first example. On the other hand Kafka's example is concerned with global patterns of behavior that in extreme cases can encompass a person's entire life situation. Certainly short fragments of conversation that can be videotaped in family therapy sessions can be more easily objectified, and they may occasionally reflect larger contradictory constellations adequately, with the part standing for the whole. But the original formulation of the double-bind theory (in particular points 2 and 6) suggests that the form of communication central to a correct understanding of the phenomenon is very broad indeed: It is a matter of the fundamental positive or negative messages communicated to one person by the entire attitude of another, which can best be expressed by general polarities such as like/dislike, trust/mistrust, openness/reserve, and object love/ self love. *These,* and not single verbal or nonverbal elements, constitute the effective factors in the destructiveness of communicative dilemmas and double binds. In this sense *all* interpersonal dealings and events are obviously part of the "relevant" information or communication, relevant in that they affect behavior. This can be a case of help offered or withheld at a critical moment, a promise kept or broken, a quarrel about material possessions, an acceptance or refusal of a marriage proposal, the decision of a couple to have a child or an abortion, an instance of marital infidelity, and so on. Differentiation of logical classes in Russell's sense appears quite impossible here. This complex state of affairs no doubt explains the enormous difficulties involved in trying to establish scientific categories for the various kinds of affective-logical binds. It becomes clearer and clearer that these global patterns of communication and behavior represent systems of a higher order containing all the single elements of communication. In other words, such "fundamental messages," as we may legitimately call them, are communicated by means of an endless variety of single facts and ways of behaving, both verbal and nonverbal.

In combination with the issue of logical classes, this point may shed some light on a problem that the preceding discussion has shown to be central, namely the *role played in double-bind phenomena by cognitive elements on the one hand and affective elements on the other.* The view of the psyche as a cognitive-affective double system assumes that under normal circumstances these two components are inseparably linked: they are congruent and validate one another. This is the case when I emphasize a command by striking the table with my fist, or when I accompany affectionate words with a corresponding gesture. In such cases of congruency we can hardly speak of different logical classes, as if the verbal expression possessed a higher degree of abstraction, for example. In some circumstances an expressive gesture may represent a much greater condensation than a word. Certainly such fundamental messages are more often communicated in a non-verbal and largely unconscious manner than by the spoken word; it is well known that animals respond to them quickly and sensitively.

No doubt this is connected with the fact that body language—including facial expressions, gestures, and posture—and action in the broadest sense are the most important indicators of affective motivation and mood; they convey an essential part of the fundamental messages being discussed here, whereas spoken language conveys mainly cognitive messages, which change continually and are much easier to manipulate. It has been clearly demonstrated that confusing divergences can occur between these normally parallel channels of communication in double-bind situations. The result must be a state of disharmony between thinking and feeling: the cognitive, intellectual pole and the affective, physical pole of the psychic double system cease to validate each other. The system as a whole works less and less efficiently; the ambiguities and contradictions existing between affect and cognition require constant sifting of much more information than usual, under more difficult conditions. As a result, internalized affective-cognitive schemata and systems of reference lose much of their clarity and distinct contours, creating a vicious circle in which more of the capacity to process information is lost. Such circular processes can lead only to a considerable increase in intrapsychic tension and confusion. As I have mentioned earlier, there are obvious connections between such phenomena and "ego weakness," as it is called, meaning a general insecurity, vulnerability, and inability to withstand stress. In addition, there are links to specific disturbances in the processing of information that are often regarded today as central to the clinical picture of persons at risk for psychosis. It is clear that this must have an effect on many different situations of great psychological and social stress, particularly in the phase of adolescent and post-adolescent adjustment. Another interesting fact in this connection was mentioned by which Piaget in his early article on children's thinking: small children are bothered very little by contradictions; they have no difficulty in allowing very large contradictions to exist side by side.[35] This tolerance changes, however, as cognitive (and affective) maturity increases, since such maturity consists precisely in learning to recognize contradictions better and finally to harmonize them by means of an optimizing extraction of invariance. Normally the complete reversibility of all intellectual operations is established in adolescence. It may be for this reason that adolescents react with extreme sensitivity to contradictions of all kinds, as we know from everyday experience. It appears quite likely that this circumstance contributes to the unusually high incidence of psychosis in this age group, particularly since the latent contradictions we have been speaking of often show a marked increase at the same time.

It is also significant that both body language and, more broadly speaking, all behavior effective in transmitting fundamental messages are largely *unconscious;* that is, they can be controlled or disguised only with great difficulty. They give away what we really mean more than all our words, and thus represent a different and *deeper* level of communication in an existential rather than in a formally logical sense. But it is important, as we try to gain a clearer understanding of a complex problem, to see that these statements are correct only in a general way. In individual cases it is of course perfectly possible for a fundamental feeling to be expressed verbally, or for superficial messages to be expressed nonverbally, perhaps with a gesture. This fact suggests once again that the issue is not so much one of verbal or nonverbal communication and not one of *formal* logical classes, but rather a matter of deeper and broader contexts of affect and cognition, or affect-logic. We must seek the crucial hierarchies there, in fundamental interpersonal "messages," and there we will also find the contradictions essential for an understanding of double-bind phenomena.

Despite all methodological difficulties, it thus appears more and more plausible that the notions of contradiction, paradox, and double bind as first proposed by Bateson contain some highly interesting clues about a number of pathogenic phenomena. Although these much-discussed ideas have not yet led to a complete understanding of the problem, it does seem that the reflections presented here can shed some light on the relationship between contradictions and some of these pathogenic circumstances. One further important link in the chain of my argument is still missing, however. This is the relationship between interpersonal, familial processes and intrapsychic processes. This is at the same time also a question of narcissistic fusion between parents and children.

Connections between Intrapsychic and Interpersonal Contradictions

After Frieda Fromm-Reichmann first referred in passing to a "schizophrenogenic mother" in 1948,[36] psychoanalysts and family therapists spent a long time concentrating almost exclusively on the relationship between mother and child in their search for a key to the connections between intrapsychic events and events in the family. At the beginning they found some considerable evidence for the hypothesis that many mothers were responsible to a degree for their children's psychoses. However, the last years have seen a growing modification of this idea, on practical as well as theoretical grounds. In essence the previous view was of the schizophrenic child as a victim of a narcissistic, exploitative mother, often in conjunction with a weak father; the mother came to be regarded as the cause of all the misery of these families. Therapists were often unable to avoid an accusatory undertone as a result, which did far more harm than good.[37] It proved far more useful as a therapeutic technique to place the accent on positive forces and strivings, in the mother's case as well, even if these forces were hampered in particular ways that we shall look at below. And in the area of theory, growing psychoanalytic insight into the nature and origins of narcissistic object relations led to a new and more differentiated understanding of many phenomena observed by communications theorists in "families with schizophrenic transactions." Lidz, Wynne, Stierlin, and Boszormenyi-Nagy were among those who attempted to bridge the two disciplines, but despite these attempts, no one to my knowledge has yet integrated the approaches of systems theory, family dynamics, and psychoanalysis into one unified theory of schizophrenia that would relate intrapsychic and interpersonal processes in the way in which they must obviously be connected in reality. Instead, the proponents of each theory would deny the validity of the other theory, as if it were a case of irreconcilable paradoxes. There may be sound enough practical reasons for this attitude: many therapists argue, and not without reason, that the two approaches are too different to be used jointly in treatment. And a certain polarization, an establishing of sharp contrasts, was no doubt necessary if real progress was to be made. Nevertheless, for a more general grasp of the problem, one that is not yet directly aimed at practical goals—and such is the main concern of this book—such one-sidedness is less of a help than a hindrance. I am convinced that every new insight into "the nature of the beast" will prove to be practically useful in the long run, and I will attempt to demonstrate this in the final chapter, which is devoted to issues of therapy.

Returning to our present problem, however, I think the relationship between intrapsychic and interpersonal, familial processes must resemble that between atomic and molecular processes and structures:

each conditions, completes, and explains the other. Here as elsewhere the task is to acquire the degree of flexibility and Piagetian reversibility in our thinking that will enable us to grasp two apparently contradictory aspects as the opposite poles of *one single* structure. In what follows I shall try to suggest, at least, how such a double perspective might look.

All the ideas developed so far point to a view of intrapsychic, affective-cognitive systems of reference (which have also been labeled "representations," "concepts," "schemata," and so on) as crystallizations of experience in the broadest sense—that is, as crystallizations of the total sum of all information that has been processed and integrated. This offers a fundamental perspective (one in full accord with the postulates of many psycho- and sociodynamic theories) from which to understand the relationships existing between constellations and processes on both the familial and individual level: *The cognitive-affective, intrapsychic structures internalized in childhood (above all) represent the result of actual events within the family. Conversely, these events are decisively influenced by the intrapsychic organization of all family members, particularly the parents.* In other words the psyche appears as a kind of synchronic cognitive-affective condensation of the continuing diachronic external and material reality. At the same time the psyche, by virtue of its structure, "develops" and actualizes this internalized synchrony in new diachronic processes. It thus bears a certain resemblance to the genetic code, representing on another level an extremely useful apparatus for preserving and reproducing those previous experiences that have proved to be important for maintaining life. The type of information relevant to this task appears in the case of human beings to be established in innate reflexes and instincts only to a relatively small degree; large amounts of relevant information are stored in channels of acquired associations, which are formed through action and interaction with the environment and passed on from generation to generation. They are probably fixed anew in each individual by the creation of the necessary neuronal or synaptic links. The internalized representations of the self and objects so central to psychoanalytic thinking—our images of mother and father, ourselves, but also siblings, other important figures, animals, plants, inanimate objects, and, above all, the dynamic interplay of forces between all these elements—appear first and foremost as an abstraction and consolidation of what we have actually experienced. They are thus an abstraction of *reality* (and not only of childishly distorted inner "fantasies"), whereby this reality can be defined in terms of affect-logic and information theory as *"everything that has an effect."** This fits well with Kernberg's description of self and object representations:

> The self is an intrapsychic structure consisting of multiple self representations and their related affect dispositions. Self representations are affective-cognitive structures representing the person's perception of himself in real interactions with significant others and in fantasied interactions with internal representations of significant others, that is, with object representations.[38]

From another perspective, the communications researcher and psychiatrist Albert Scheflen has this to say on the same subject:

> In the process of maturation, the learning of social skills will be accompanied by cognitive development. Each of these signals, activities, and patterns will come to be represented by cognitive images of their form and by motor plans for executing a part in them. And skill in participation will bring about self confidence, an adequate self image, and so on. In neurophysiological terms, each acquisition will be coded in a system of neuronal and glial connections.[39]

Typical family structures, whether clear and stable hierarchical relationships or diffuse and contradictory ones, must be reflected, in the sense of the fundamental messages described above, in corresponding intrapsychic constellations. The same holds true for definite or blurred boundaries between individuals, open or hidden conflicts, healthy or pathological alliances, antipathies, sympathies, relationships of love or hate, and the specific actions corresponding to them. They will not be reflected as clearly as in a mirror, to be sure, and various distortions and heterogeneous elements will be incorporated, but all the same the reflections will be such that the most important *relations* between the single elements are preserved.

Helm Stierlin recently made a distinction, in a related context, between "hard" and "soft" reality, with the latter category including perceptions, interpretations, emotions, and fantasies.[40] The category of "hard" reality would then include all factual and physical events (meaning also those that have a direct influence on affects and are

---

* *Translator's note:* The German "Wirklichkeit ist alles, was wirkt," contains an untranslatable pun on *Wirklichkeit,* meaning "reality" (from *wirklich,* "real"), and *wirken,* meaning "to have an effect, be effective."

thus always concrete and *material* in the last analysis). To this category belong, among other things, the quality and consistency of the mother's care, the rhythm of her comings and goings, illnesses (including psychological disturbances in particular, such as depressions) occurring either in parents or in children, constellations among siblings, the general atmosphere in the family (whether relaxed, tolerant, and cheerful or tense, hostile, and envious), the experience of mutual support, injustice actually suffered or inflicted, and so on. "Soft" reality, on the other hand, would consist of the internalized representations, cognitive-affective schemata, and systems of reference in which these external events are condensed by the individual psyche. (Stierlin borrows the term *relational reality* from Bateson. It is interesting, and a little unsettling, to note that these views bring us quite close to the old Platonic dichotomy between world and idea.)

The highly plausible connections between internal and external reality have been strangely neglected by psychoanalysis, virtually the only discipline to have developed a truly differentiated picture of intrapsychic structures and processes. Ever since Freud's traumatic disappointment with reality as reported by his mythomanic hysterical patients, psychoanalysts have tended to concentrate on internal fantasies only. In her recent book *Freud and His Father* Marianne Krüll presents the hypothesis that this striking shift away from real events (both present and past) was also motivated by Freud's massive repression of actual occurrences in his own family.[41] As a result, psychoanalysis for decades cultivated a defensive attitude with regard to all so-called objective facts; this attitude not only was detrimental to the development of psychoanalysis itself but also tended to isolate it from its neighboring scientific and medical disciplines, in a manner quite contrary to the original intentions of its founder. Modern analytic ego psychology, the doctrine of narcissism, and theories of family dynamics all share the credit of having helped to break down some of these barriers and initiated the possibility of a new, constructive dialogue among the disciplines involved.

The psychoanalytic doctrine of narcissism concerns itself primarily with the conditions under which a stable sense of one's own identity gradually develops. This occurs in interactions with the environment and parallel to the formation of object representations. The important aspect of this doctrine for our discussion is the fact that this differentiation takes place in a typical affective-cognitive *mirroring process* with the child's significant others, above all with the mother, as was emphasized by Winnicott, Kohut, and others.[42] In his playful experiments with new ways of behaving, thinking, and feeling in different areas of life, the child takes his orientation from the positive or negative emotional reactions of the people nearby. They may encourage and confirm its discoveries by reacting to them with pleasure (especially by the well-known "light in his mother's eyes" described by Kohut) or on the contrary discourage them by signs of displeasure, ignoring, devaluating, or disqualifying. One can almost claim that children learn from pleasure. It thus becomes clear why and how the internalized affective-logical schemata of the child's significant others—first those of his parents and later those of his older siblings and playmates—are continually "communicated" to him through innumerable concrete instances of behavior that are then internalized and thus passed on from one generation to the next. A central aspect of this "tradition" consists of internalized self and object representations.

It is of great significance that this mirroring process displays a characteristic asymmetry. For a long time the schemata, concepts, and systems of reference of the parents—their world view—dominate in it, representing by far the "more powerful reality," as Stierlin puts it.[43] Each generation teaches the next one to see the world through the eyes of its elders, in a manner of speaking, a process that is no doubt necessary if any cohesion and continuity are to exist in a society. As a rule it is only from the age of puberty onward that the presence of new information (in an affective-logical sense) will lead adolescents to question and revise parts of this world view. This also applies to the relationship between parents and children. The parents' "more powerful reality" thus means that they provide a very inclusive "definition of the relationship" in the sense in which the term is used in communications theory.[44] This is at the same time a prime example of a "fundamental message." Pathological double binds and dilemmas can now be characterized as situations in which *a weaker partner is trapped in a covert affective-cognitive relationship and system of reference from which he or she cannot escape; this system of reference hinders development and is therefore detrimental in the long run.* The insidious part of this situation is the child's inability to question what is happening to him, the impossibility of "metacommunication" to which Bateson and his coauthors refer. If the parents', and especially the mother's, sense of identity reflects a narcissistic disturbance as a result of formative influences in their own families—that is, if their thinking is dominated by immature, poorly demarcated, and unstable ideas about themselves and others—the parents will also experience corresponding fears, self-doubt, feelings of inadequacy, wishes for dependency, inconsistency, and insecurity. Under unfavorable conditions this "more powerful" parental reality will lead to a repetition or even an increase of these same disturbances in certain children. Among these unfavorable conditions we can cite the lack of a father or other family member with enough ego strength to offset the mother, or a constitutional weakness in the child or debility arising from illness or extreme social isolation. In addition other specific characteristics of narcissistic object relations, which are especially important for the questions we are concerned with here, play a pernicious role: people with a basic narcissistic "fault"[45] in their sense of self show a marked tendency to cling to their partners, to "consume" them and suck them dry. The narcissistic object becomes an instrument, perceived no longer as an autonomous being capable of making independent decisions, but rather as an extension of the self (like one's own arm or hand, as Kohut puts it). (It would be even more correct to say "is not yet perceived" instead of "no longer perceived," since narcissistic object relations represent an immature stage before that at which more mature oedipal or genital partner relations become possible.) The narcissistic object is expected to make up for the partner's lack of identity and self-esteem by his constant presence, total subjection, and continual provision of "emotional nourishment," even though this requirement can never be successfully fulfilled, of course. In consequence, all displays of authentic independence must be suppressed and punished, since they threaten the symbiotic relationship. A confusion of identities occurs, which leads to an incapacity for autonomous thoughts, feelings, and actions. The logical result is that internalized self and object representations become increasingly unstable and confused, as do many other affective-cognitive schemata and systems of reference. Many of the phenomena observed in "families with schizophrenic transactions"—such as the typical blurring of the generational boundaries and emotional over-involvement—become quite understandable in this context. First and foremost, however, we can better understand the panic felt at the thought of any open conflict, and the accompanying strategies for keeping issues covered up: all the participants (not only the parents) must see every conflict as a potential threat to the narcissistic symbiosis and thus to their own already precarious sense of identity. A more or less stable psychological balance can be maintained only by careful avoidance of all "differences," at the price of extreme mutual dependency and infantilization. A typical vicious circle ensues, in which the pathological lack of independence serves as an excuse for preserving the unhealthy homeostasis. One grotesque but nonetheless completely authentic clinical case may serve as an example.

> A man who had formerly been employed as an engineer but had been diagnosed as a chronic schizophrenic was recently brought to me for treatment. At the age of fifty-two he was still totally dependent on his mother, who by then was well over eighty. For years he had been playing the role of a gigantic lethargic baby, lying in bed and ordering the exhausted old woman around. His mother, whose relationship to her deceased husband had always been unsatisfactory, had overprotected her only son since his infancy. While he was between the ages of four and sixteen she had personally seen to the cleaning of his anus every day, because of a supposed infection with worms. He had married twice, against his mother's wishes, but left both wives after a short time; his mother referred to both women as "whores." Both mother and son systematically evaded all attempts to confront them with the absurdity of their situation. The mother would merely smile in a helpless, martyred fashion and declare herself incapable of changing anything. The son, though able to respond quite adequately on other topics, would answer questions on his home life in an incomprehensible mumble or else retreat behind a wall of silence.

This case history illustrates clearly the point emphasized by family therapists: The relationship between the "victim" and the "instigator" of a pathological symbiosis is definitely a circular one. Not only does the original instigator (usually a parent) dominate the narcissistic object (usually a child) until it becomes totally dependent, but also the reverse holds true: the child takes on such vital significance for the fragile self-esteem of the adult that the child's infantile narcissistic megalomania is insufficiently corrected or even furthered; the parent becomes dependent on the child, and the child acquires power over the parent. In the light of such relationships of mutual dependency and dominance it is easier to understand why one of the main difficulties in treating such cases is the *united front* presented against any change.

This example also displays with unusual clarity the content and character of the fundamental messages that function as a double bind in narcissistic object relations over and over again. A first negative injunction clearly runs "Don't hurt me by leaving me, don't grow up and become independent!" This corresponds precisely to Scheflen's "single bind" (a simple symbiotic relationship) and is unbearable, since it runs counter to all developmental tendencies, preventing genuine psychological growth in the son *and* the mother and making both deeply unhappy in the end. The second and contrary message runs: "Give me pleasure by growing up, becoming independent, leading a normal and successful life!" It is usually transmitted through social conventions, guilt feelings in all participants, and expectations with a narcissistic coloring ("Be grown up, capable, and outstanding, so that I can be proud of you; that will make me feel good and strong at long last"). On a deeper level this same message is also transmitted in hundreds of subtle ways by the healthy tendencies that are never entirely lacking in the environment. This message is also unbearable, or rather *becomes* so as a consequence of the single bind, for by contradicting the first message it mobilizes both massive guilt feelings and existentially threatening separation anxiety. With time this anxiety can come to have a real basis in fact, because of the increasing ego weakness of those trapped in symbiotic relationships. The failure to make psychological progress is often connected with lack of success at school, at work, and in social situations. To such individuals the leading of an independent life thus appears more and more as a demand fraught with anxiety and tension, impossible to fulfill. Thus the tragic circle that creates a true double bind is closed (although especially unfavorable circumstances are necessary and not every symbiotic relationship must develop in this way): the victims are trapped in a situation that permits no constructive move in any direction; whatever they do, the simultaneous but contradictory demands inherent in it will lead to more discomfort and arouse growing feelings of inadequacy and guilt. This situation is of vital importance to all participants—a fact that explains its insolubility—and tends to become more and more firmly established.

In the first chapter I summarized the message of the double bind, which is based on narcissistic object relations in another way, namely

"I (don't) love you" $\rightleftarrows$ "I (don't) love myself."

This contradictory formula characterizes the intrapsychic condition of the *sender* of the fundamental messages: he believes that he loves the other person, but he loves him as a narcissistic object essentially for his own sake, as someone who will support and "complete" him. This self-love or "self-service" is also inconsistent, however, since the pathological narcissist is not capable of truly loving or serving himself. In actual fact, then, the sender of double-bind messages is able to love *no one* properly as an object. Having grown up with too little confirmation of his own identity, as an adult he possesses neither a consistent identity nor a stable sense of self-esteem. He can believe neither in himself nor in others and remains deeply unhappy. His *partner* (the "victim") equally trapped in the double bind like the rat in the electrically wired two-chambered cage, can do what he likes and try out every possibility, but he will always run up against the same painful fact: his fundamental nature is rejected; it is unwelcome and unloved; he is not allowed to be as he is, and all attempts to adapt, no matter how well-meaning, will result in failure. Bateson and his associates presented a striking example of this in their description of the hospitalized son who could not please his mother, try as he might. Long before that Franz Kafka described a similar constellation in his novel *The Castle*. Mara Selvini Palazzoli has summed up the paradoxical message of the double bind in the unfulfillable command: "You should not be what you are!"[46]

Obviously this description of the double bind represents a great simplification of the complex and ambivalent relationships that actually exist between people. It should also be clear that it would be a mistake to ascribe responsibility for the complicated double-bind situation to one participant, such as the mother. As Bowen and Boszormenyi-Nagy have shown, the processes at work are largely *unconscious* and *circular*;[47] they usually encompass several generations of a family, and *all* the participants are equally caught up in the dilemma, the "instigators" as well as the designated "victims": The totality of events in a family, the result of all the intrapsychic "behavioral programs" involved (which is much more than their mere sum) leads to the formation of a contradictory affective-cognitive system of reference that casts itself over the participants like an inescapable net. The case of the schizophrenic engineer described above provided a radical illustration of this; here is another striking example.

The members of a highly educated family have come to me seeking treatment. The sensitive mother suffers from severe narcissistic problems and low self-esteem as a result of her own very problematic upbringing. She has fled from a frustrating relationship with her husband into a symbiotic one with her only son. The son has been assigned the role of his mother's comforter, the little darling who is not supposed to grow up and leave her. Yet at the same time he is under pressure from his ambitious, authoritarian father to emulate the latter's brilliant career. The son has developed into a clumsy, insecure scapegoat; his parents pushed him to enter a university, but his studies were ended by the outbreak of a psychosis marked by delusions and hallucinations in which the contradictory voices of both his parents constantly pursued him. A younger sister, with whom the father had closely allied himself, had several attacks in which she became excited and aggressive; these were diagnosed as hebephrenic. In this state she pointed to massive but hidden family conflicts in the most unmistakable manner. Two other sisters suffered from serious neurotic disorders, and the mother had to be hospitalized repeatedly for depression.

This tragic constellation revealed in family therapy sessions a whole list of the disturbances described in "families with schizophrenic transactions" with a clarity seldom met with. Quite apart from the terrible suffering of *all* the participants, there were double-bind paradoxes and contradictions of all kinds, pseudo-incestuous alliances across generational boundaries, a blurring of hierarchical structures, emotional overinvolvement on all sides, an inability to communicate unambiguously, and a number of other cognitive and affective disturbances that have been repeatedly described by family therapists of all schools. The case also illustrates the fact emphasized by Weakland that under certain circumstances the contradictory messages may emanate from *different* family members.[48] Behind a façade of polite reserve that the members of the family were barely able to maintain, events resembled an all-devouring whirlpool. Archaic, poorly demarcated "all good" and "all bad" self and object representations alternated with one another in unrealistic idealizations, depressive bursts of self-reproach, and bitter aggression. The unfulfillable paradoxical demand that every participant seemed to be making of all the others, implicitly or even explicitly, is summarized in Selvini Palazzoli's phrase, "You should not be what you are!"

Here, as in many other similar cases, it is obviously the narcissistic element that poisons human relationships; opposed to all development, it represents the exact opposite of loving care for someone according to that person's *own* needs. One could perhaps even say that one form of emotional immaturity, pathological narcissism, is a facet of the universal curse that is passed on from generation to generation.

We have seen that the individual's relation to the family is like that of a small, homeostatically regulated (partly closed and partly open) subsystem to a larger system. The two interact in circular, diachronic processes that become consolidated, over time, into synchronic intrapsychic or familial rules and structures. Intrapsychic and interpersonal constellations will therefore necessarily display certain analogies and isomorphisms. There are of course further analogies between the family and society at large. This suggests new possibilities of understanding: both psychoanalytic and systems theoretic insights can be applied to intrapsychic processes *and* to interpersonal and social events as well. Freud's own numerous applications of psychoanalytic theory to social processes are well known; we need only think of *Totem and Taboo* (1913), *Civilization and Its Discontents* (1930), and *Moses and Monotheism* (1937). Every collective as it develops incurs problems of identity similar to those of growing individuals; like individuals, groups are very sensitive to narcissistic injuries: they are frequently constituted in the face of an external enemy and become capable of mature partnerships only when they have reached a certain position of inner strength. Such psychoanalytic insights into social processes complement the view of systems theory, which sees circular, homeostatic processes between two or more groups at work in the same phenomena. Many social or political movements can be understood as swings of a pendulum. The extremes are of particular interest in this regard; left and right wing extremism clearly equilibrate and *determine* one another according to systems theory. Further reflections and pendular developments may then lead to the formation of intermediate groups such as the moderate left and right. At the same time the terrorist aggression of extremists, such as occurred some years ago in Italy and Germany, corresponds strikingly to Kernberg's description of autoaggressive rage in poorly structured, borderline personalities threatened by internal collapse. In an organism still in a state of relative health, be it an individual or an entire nation, such an "abscess" may sometimes be able to activate powerful defensive and constructive forces. In this case autoaggression becomes—paradoxically—a homeostatic force helping to keep the system alive. It will destroy a rotten and corrupt system like a cancer, however. Such structural and dynamic analogies can be followed down to the level of cells and beyond, for instance in immune reactions. Processes on higher levels, such as in society (between groups or nations), can frequently contribute to a clearer understanding of processes on lower levels, such as intrapsychic ones, if we reflect that they are basically similar, only magnified. This is equally true of structures. The individual "jurisdictions" or functions in the psyche, for example— the ego and superego—correspond to the executive and judicial branches of a national government; the id plays a role analogous to that of an unruly, creative population; the defensive forces that can be mustered by the ego are analogous to an army; and so on. The relations between entities such as the individual, the family, and society can thus be represented, as in Figure 6, by several surfaces of different sizes that interact with one another. (Only one of each subsystem is depicted, with one individual standing for the many that constitute families, and one family standing for the many that constitute a society.)

Each entity has its own pattern of straight, curved, or wavy lines, representing the processes and structures it contains. To a certain degree these patterns are reflected in the other entities, however, and there they become an element of the total structure: the "waves" or structures that we find in a society are, at least in part, the result (the "essence" or invariance) of all the "waves" and structures of all the families or groups that make up this society. Conversely, the basic structures ("norms") operating in the society will shape and influence families and groups. In concrete terms these structures could take the form of value systems, hierarchies, forms of organization, and the

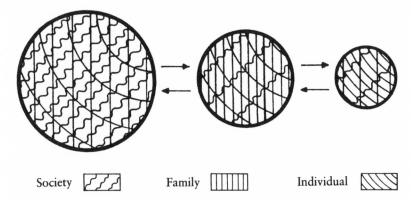

Figure 6.   Relations among entities in a structure.

like, which may then manifest themselves in attitudes on general or personal questions (political and religious orientation, legal issues, contraception, abortion, relations between men and women, decision-making processes, and so on). As we shall see below, such isomorphisms can be demonstrated to exist in thought and language as well. The relations between the individual and the family are similar. It is thus hardly a matter for surprise anymore that recent family research on schizophrenics has uncovered contradictions and inconsistencies not only in the psychological makeup of the "designated patient" but also in his or her total family environment.

In this connection we should next take a closer look at an important psychological phenomenon that corresponds on an intrapsychic level to the contradictory patterns of interpersonal communications: the "ego weakness" that creates a predisposition to psychotic decompensation. Before we do so, however, I would like to summarize the main results of the preceding analysis.

Intrapsychic and interpersonal events are to be understood as complementary phenomena, dependent on each other in a circular process. They correspond to open systems on different levels, which are connected by communicating channels. A child's internalized basic concepts, behavioral schemata, and systems of reference—in particular its self and object representations—are a result of the total of factual events in the family. Conversely, the internalized parental systems of reference represent a "more powerful reality" and have a decisive influence on family dynamics. Clarity and consistency in one area, or alternately confusion and contradictions, lead to corresponding structures and modes of behavior in the other. Both areas can be viewed in terms of both psychoanalysis and systems theory; conflicts within the family, on the one hand, and intrapsychic inconsistencies, on the other, which are related to narcissistic defects and their corresponding self and object representations, will lead to conflictual contradictions in communication and behavior. The narcissistic separation anxiety of family members will require that these contradictions be concealed in a number of ways, one of which is the double bind. This leads in turn, of necessity, to contradictions in the interpersonal "fundamental messages" comprised of all verbal and nonverbal behavior, which we have come to recognize as the truly relevant form of communication: in a context of narcissism the partners make contradictory demands of each other in alternation, first total intimacy and submission (as in the case of parents who demand that their children give up all strivings toward independence), and then development into autonomous adults (whose success will bolster the precarious self-image of the parents). This insoluble paradox creates a degree of tension that, as was implicitly postulated in Bateson's hypothesis, becomes unbearable for certain vulnerable individuals, causing them to "go off the deep end" into psychotic modes of feeling, thinking, and behaving.

The Origins and Structure of (Pre-)Schizophrenic Ego Weakness: An Affective-Logical Hypothesis

On the basis of the preceding discussion we can now turn our attention to the consequences of severely disturbed family communication for individual family members. In cautious terms we can say that the following hypothesis describes the intrapsychic structure of at least *some* potential schizophrenics:

> *Important internalized affective-cognitive systems of reference in (some) schizophrenics or persons at risk for schizophrenia are fundamentally confused, contradictory, and unstable.*

The confusion and instability appear to be the logical result of the unclear and contradictory modes of behavior (or communications in the widest sense) within the family group. (The possibility also exists that some of this instability stems from a predisposition that may be, or in fact probably is, inborn, but this is a subject I would like to reserve for the next chapter.) As Scheflen has plausibly suggested, such instability can be exacerbated by a number of social factors such as isolation, illness, financial problems, and conflicts.[49] To the extent that inferences from neurophysiological research on animals are permissible, we assume that this confusion and instability are reflected in correspondingly unstable neuronal networks and channels of association in the brain. Earlier I compared internalized affective-logical systems of reference to systems of roads or pathways with a structure that has been established by the amount of use it receives. If we now try to visualize these systems in the case of potential schizophrenics, we should picture them as confused in certain sections, as if two or more road systems of equal order were trying to occupy the same space and the roads sometimes ran into one another. Affective and cognitive association processes might veer off along one road or another unpredictably, a state of affairs that would explain why they are not only unconventional but also inefficient and unstable.

The most significant instances in which clarity is lacking are undoubtedly the internalized representations of the self and objects; indeed, according to Kernberg, these are not clearly separated from each other in schizophrenics. It appears quite possible that many other cognitive and affective disorders can be traced back to this first fundamental lack of differentiation between the inner and outer worlds. I am thinking of the frequently flawed ability to categorize things, difficulties in focusing attention on a specific object or topic, sudden associative leaps, instability of moods and feeling—in sum, the lack of continuity that often seems to be the most striking characteristic of schizophrenic thinking and feeling. At the same time it appears only logical that important systems of reference in the members of a family will bear a strong resemblance to each other, if they live in close enough proximity: members of all groups, including families, share a large number of ways of perceiving things and behaving, habits, beliefs, values, language codes, and so on, despite all individual differences. These add up to a certain "mentality" that makes social cohesion possible and constitutes the group identity in a sense. Their communications will correspond to this mentality, by which I mean first their thoughts and feelings, and then the actions and modes of behavior determined by them. Even in families with "schizophrenic transactions," however, not all areas of communication need necessarily be disturbed. On the contrary, observation reveals that they frequently remain limited to certain emotionally loaded topics.

> A twenty-four-year-old technician whom I treated had a severely dependent symbiotic relationship with his mother. He would speak in a peculiar high, childish voice whenever he had to justify a decision to her. In other situations, such as at work, however, he was capable of acting in a decisive manner like a grown man.

In the confused, error-laden instability of important internalized systems of reference we can thus recognize the correlative (and possibly the organic substrate) of the "ego weakness" both of persons at risk for schizophrenia and of members of their families. We can also see them as related to the confused behavior patterns existing in the social milieu of psychotics that are referred to as "enmeshment," "emotional overinvolvement," "schizophrenic transactions," and "narcissistic" or "symbiotic" partner relations, depending on the theoretical orientation of the observer.

Several implications of this hypothesis will be discussed in the next chapter. But several aspects more closely related to the topic of this chapter warrant consideration here.

Let us start by recalling that faulty structuring of internalized affective-logical systems of reference must of necessity make it more difficult to process information and cope with stress, leading to precisely those disturbances that have come to be the focus of schizophrenia research in recent years. Under such conditions, integrating any kind of contradiction becomes an especially hard task: a faulty information-processing system is confronted with a much greater amount of information than has normally has to be processed in the same situation. Genuinely paradoxical and double-bind communications, for example, can virtually double the amount of information that needs to be mastered about a situation. I can thus only agree with Hirsch's claim, mentioned earlier in this chapter, that contradictions that are *not* in themselves specific to schizophrenia may represent an enormous strain under which persons so disposed may rapidly break down. This argument also provides a convincing explanation for one interesting finding made by genetic researchers, namely that the biological children of schizophrenic parents who have been adopted by healthy families will tend to develop psychoses when the patterns of communication in the adoptive family are particularly contradictory and confused.[50] In addition, my hypothesis helps to explain another observation: It is known that persons at risk for schizophrenia are frequently unable to deal with complex information if it reaches them via several sensory organs simultaneously (so-called cross-modal stimuli). This inability is strikingly similar to that of persons who have suffered minimal brain damage in early childhood. A further indication that the proposed hypothesis is correct is our experience that potential schizophrenics are especially poor at dealing with severe psychoaffective stress and thus tend anxiously to avoid every unusual situation: poorly structured systems of reference constantly force them to use increased caution and vigilance, just as poor eyesight might. This leads to a perpetual undercurrent of tension and insecurity, and in turn to the corresponding fatigue and avoidance reactions that have recently been investigated by Lilo Süllwold.[51]

I have already referred several times to the *cognitive disturbances* of schizophrenics, which have been the subject of intense research in the last few years. These include numerous deviations from the normal ability to concentrate attention on something, such as "overinclusion" (Cameron) and "response interference" (Broen and Storms). In

essence these disturbances all result from the fact that opposing cognitive (and affective) components interfere with one another, so that
the focus of attention is either too broad, too narrow, too inconstant,
or too easily distracted.[52] It seems justifiable to assume that these phenomena represent just one more aspect of instability and confusion in
internalized affective and cognitive schemata and systems of reference, and they also appear to be virtually identical with the "thought
disorder" or "loosening of associations" identified by Kraepelin,
Bleuler, and Jung at the beginning of this century as central to schizophrenia. A detailed analysis of these phenomena would take us too
far into a very specialized area, so I will mention just a few particularly important points. Channels of association structured in a contradictory manner must clearly have a considerable negative effect on
the ability to store and recall information. An affective-logical system
of reference determines and orders perceptions just as a system of
roads or canals determines how the traffic or water flow, thus the
hypothesis presented here is compatible with the disturbances in filtering and storing new information postulated in schizophrenia by
Payne and others, as well as with the defects thought by Poljakov to
exist in the selection and activation of experiences from long-term
memory centers.[53] The flickering instability of schizophrenic thinking
and the rapid shifts from one system of reference to another (the main
symptom of schizophrenic ambivalence) can be understood as the result of faulty filtering or exclusion of extraneous elements. Connections also exist between this hypothesis and the formation of categories in young children, a topic to which Lidz has devoted intensive
research.[54] Such categories correspond to the clear separation of self
and object representations.

Lack of clarity in communication and perception are not only the
cause (in the family, for instance) of faulty association systems, but
also their logical *consequence*. Connections with the concepts of Piaget (whom Lidz mentions several times) are quite evident here. The
first (and to my knowledge only) Piagetian article devoted to schizophrenic thought disorders contains a number of observations that fit
very well with the hypothesis of disturbed internalized systems of reference.[55] The authors refer several times explicitly to schizophrenics'
characteristic difficulty in maintaining a stable frame of reference because "parasitical references" constantly interfere. Thus although
they possess certain schemata, they have trouble actualizing them. In

general, the disturbances observed are interpreted as an "inequality between assimilation and accommodation," that is, between already internalized schemata and new information. The authors lay particular emphasis on the influence of *affective* components as well as cognitive components and even use the term *affective schemata*.

Finally, the idea of "fundamental interpersonal messages" provides an excellent illustration of the way in which internalized affective-cognitive systems of reference can become confused and lead to the thought disorders observed: if the totality of events in a family, in early childhood represented above all by the mother, continually gives contradictory messages about the mother and her relationship to her child, about her wishes, expectations, instructions and prohibitions, systems of values, and so on, then the child's corresponding internalized schemata must become confused. We may assume that the child may defend himself by splitting them into two opposed and often competing complexes of ideas, similar to Kernberg's "all good" and "all bad" self and object representations. The entire system of reference related to the mother (or the internalized system of *relations* between mother and child acquired through experience) then becomes ambiguous and unstable. Although the child must now process double the amount of information where the mother is concerned, he still lacks a secure basis on which to interpret new experiences. From this vantage point it is not hard to see that the resulting insecurity and instability in affective, cognitive, and social areas—which has been labeled "ego weakness" and studied in detail by Bellak and others[56]— offer especially fertile soil for the development of psychosis.

An impressive amount of evidence thus fits together to lend support to the system-of-reference hypothesis. This theory enables us to assemble under one heading a large number of problems that have previously been viewed in isolation or even divided among rival disciplines. We can now view both intrapsychic and familial conflicts, contradictory patterns of communication, numerous cognitive and affective disorders, and disturbances in internalized affective-logical systems of reference as all related, though in a complex manner. They influence and reinforce one another via various circular processes, forming in reality *one single phenomenon* with many different facets. This would represent an interesting example of a structure as it was described in general terms in Chapter 3; in this case we have an extensive psychic structure displaying both the required invariance (the contradictory character of all the elements involved) and variance (the different specific manifestations of this contradictoriness). The relationship of the main components is shown in Figure 7.

Depending on the phenomenon being studied and the theoretical orientation of the observer, any one component of this system may become the focus of investigation. As long as the approach remains limited to this one aspect, it will continue to be seen as the "actual" or "fundamental" disturbance. Unfortunately, the various disciplines that cover this general field tend to fall into such methodological reductionism over and over again, including systems theory with its supposedly nonreductionist approach.

The diagram suggests that within such complex affective-cognitive structures and systems of reference what begins as a pathological imbalance (up to and including psychosis) can, in unfavorable circumstances, establish a new balance and become stabilized. Before we turn to this subject, however, I would like to summarize the findings of this chapter.

Conclusion

In exploring contradictions, paradoxes, and the double bind in connection with the ideas presented in earlier chapters, we uncovered the following important aspects:

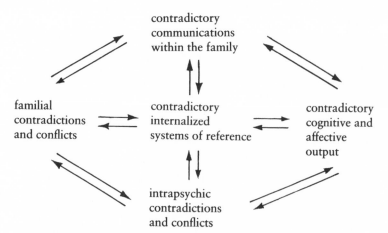

Figure 7.   Interactions among faulty systems of reference.

- All the types of contradictions discussed can be seen as a collision of different affective-logical systems of reference, which may vary in comprehensiveness and importance. In the case of a simple contradiction, a limited system of reference collides with a larger one; in the case of a paradox, there is a collision of affective-cognitive systems of reference of the same order. The double bind represents the most unpleasurable possible variant of a paradox, in which two irreconcilable components, both with a negative affective coloring, collide in a hidden manner, preventing a resolution by means of "metacommunication."

- All of these phenomena create affective-cognitive tension and confusion; above all they can interfere with the normal harmony of feeling and thinking in the bipolar system of the psyche. On the other hand they contain enormous creative potential: under favorable conditions similarities (invariances) can be discovered in two systems of reference that at first seemed irreconcilable and can lead to the formation of structures of a higher order. This mechanism forms the basis of Piaget's "optimizing equilibration"; it also represents a very general principle of development based on the occurrence of fundamentally new "interferences" in the area where two contiguous systems meet.

- The malign double bind is characterized not so much by single contradictory communication sequences on different levels of logic, such as a contradiction in the verbal and nonverbal content of one message, but rather by sweeping contradictory "fundamental messages" in vital areas transmitted by the totality of interpersonal events. In the family these consist above all of the contrary affective needs of children and parents whose sense of their own identity is disturbed. The relations between such parents and children can best be understood in terms of the psychoanalytic concept of narcissistic object relations. A fundamental contradiction in this constellation consists of the demands placed on children who become "narcissistic objects" not to develop any autonomy and still to grow up into successful adults. In a typical double bind this paradox remains concealed; the avoidance of conflict characteristic in such families blocks the creative potential that could bring about a resolution of the pathological symbiosis.

- The internalized affective-cognitive systems of reference, in particular self and object representations, form the basis of intrapsychic dynamics, which can be interpreted within a psychoanalytic framework. At the same time they represent a condensation of the totality of actual events in the family and can thus also be interpreted within a framework of systems theory. Between these intrapsychic and familial structures there exist many isomorphisms, which in principle are accessible by the approaches of both psychoanalysis and systems theory. Family events are determined in large measure by the parents' affective-cognitive systems of reference (which they have acquired in the course of their own development) in interaction with the children's modes of feeling, thinking, and behaving.
- Intrapsychic and familial conflicts, confused and contradictory modes of behavior and communication between family members, and cognitive and affective disturbances in individuals can all be regarded as different facets of one phenomenon. From the perspective of this comprehensive hypothesis, poorly structured and unstable internalized cognitive-affective systems of reference are seen as the basis for a specific "ego weakness" and a predisposition to psychotic reactions.

Readers familiar with the literature in the field will be aware that most of the individual elements in this line of thinking are not new. What is new is the regarding of these ideas as part of a coherent whole, so as to shed some light on the pathogenesis of schizophrenia. We may now ask again: What have we learned about the general structure of the human psyche? Some further progress toward an answer is observable. The first two chapters established an approach for arriving at a more comprehensive understanding of psychic structures; the third and fourth investigated the general nature of these structures. Now these quite abstract ideas have been applied to the specific conditions under which schizophrenia possibly develops. Once again pathological elements have served as an opposite pole or mirror, in which we can better recognize what is normal—and for just that reason often not apparent. We have come to see that the psyche consists of a great number of "programs" or systems of reference, with inseparably linked affective and cognitive elements; they are formed through the totality of experience and structured in a hierarchical order. The most important of these structures for interpersonal relations are the self and object representations whose origins have been studied by Jacobson, Mahler, Kohut, and in recent years above all by Kernberg. He has demonstrated convincingly that these representations are "organized" or *ordered,* matching affects: *Affect ("mood") is the fundamental invariance in affective-cognitive psychic structures.*

These structures, including those of a high order such as the self and object representations, represent dynamic *states of equilibrium* comparable to the motion of waves in a pool of water. These states become equilibrated in interaction with the environment, and they help us to respond to and master this environment at the same time. If different, possibly contradictory messages are sent, several different concepts may be formed for one and the same thing or person, such as the mother or a significant other. These concepts will then have contrary affective colorings; they may be split and kept strictly separated, and in that case will possess only limited stability. We shall see in the next chapter that rapid fluctuation between systems of reference is typical of preschizophrenic states and contributes to the outbreak of psychosis. In other disorders such as mania and depression, the dominant affective-logical systems (the moods dominating the affective hierarchy with their corresponding cognitive contents) are clearly characterized by too much rigidity. The psyche is thus truly "healthy" and in equilibrium—that is, capable of optimal functioning, adaptation, and development—when it steers a middle course, and when shifts from one system of reference to another are moderate in flexibility, amplitude, and speed. This middle course appears to have its origins in a kind of relativization, in which affective experience is held in check by an opposite cognitive pole, and vice versa. It may also be connected with the "filter effects" mentioned previously, and also with certain biochemical influences ("buffers"). This type of regulation must play an essential role if the affective and cognitive poles of the affective-logical double system of the psyche are to resonate together in harmony.

These admittedly incomplete conclusions should enable us to tackle the puzzling phenomenon of schizophrenic psychosis (or "disorder," as I prefer to call it) with considerable prospects of success.

6   On Schizophrenia

Since Emil Kraepelin first isolated the disorder that he named dementia praecox from a confusing array of psychotic disturbances about eighty years ago, and Eugen Bleuler introduced the broader term *schizophrenia* (a splitting of the psychic functions) some years later, an immense amount of data have been amassed on the subject. Nonetheless, the state of our knowledge remains far from satisfactory. Generations of researchers in every conceivable discipline—brain anatomists and physiologists, geneticists, students of constitutional types, biochemists, psychopathologists, psychoanalysts, and sociologists, to name only some of the most important—have labored to fathom the nature of this new "disease entity." Waves of empirical methods of treatment accompanied their efforts, from sleep cures, through insulin and shock therapy, to the neuroleptics. But despite all this, specialists today are less able than ever to agree on the fundamental issues. Not only do they disagree on what schizophrenia is; they are also highly uncertain about what causes it. In addition, an unbiased observer cannot help noticing that we have made no really decisive progress in forms of therapy either.

Striking fluctuations still occur even in the *definition* of schizophrenia. In the DMS-III (*Diagnostic and Statistical Manual of Mental Disorders,* third edition, 1980) the American Psychiatric Association introduced an extremely narrow and rigid definition after decades during which a very broad concept had prevailed. Stephens criticized this inclusiveness as early as 1969, remarking that "practically every functional psychosis which was not obviously manic or depressive was diagnosed as schizophrenia."[1] The new, narrower definition of schizophrenia is based chiefly on the presence or absence of massive delusional or hallucinatory experiences in the sense of Kurt Schneider's "first-rank symptoms," that is, on the same phenomena that suggest the idea of "insanity" to laymen. Such a definition is problematical, however, since even Eugen Bleuler regarded most of these spectacular manifestations as merely superficial, "secondary symptoms" arising from much deeper "primary disturbances." Several present-day authors also surmise that "true schizophrenia" is not defined by such psychotic productions, which have been recognized to be reversible in many cases, but rather by more covert and permanent "basic disturbances." These latter consist, in their view, of certain characteristic types of thought and behavior, as well as of a general "reduction of energy potential."[2] The problem here lies in the unspecific character of such symptoms and in the great difficulty of determining to what extent they deviate from the norm: reducing the definition of schizophrenia to these terms would provide not more clarity, but less.

A further difficulty stems from the fact that many German, French, and Scandinavian adherents of the traditional school of psychiatry will speak of "genuine" schizophrenia only in cases of a chronic course of decline; for psychotic conditions that appear similar at first but show improvement in the short or long run they prefer to use terms such as "reactive psychosis," "schizophreniform psychosis," "bouffée déliriante," and "affective psychosis," considering them to be forms of pseudo-schizophrenia. However, other researchers (including myself) in these countries, the United States, Switzerland, and elsewhere believe that such a limitation of the diagnosis to the least favorable cases should be avoided: not only is it not particularly sound scientific theory, but it is also disastrous in practice. Several long-term studies (including one conducted by my associates and myself with the longest follow-ups available to date)[3] have pointed to the same conclusion, namely that this complex disease has an enormous potential for development over a long time and can take extremely disparate forms. Manfred Bleuler and my coauthors and I still distinguish among eight different developmental paradigms even though we tried to create the broadest possible categories, and Huber and his associates recognize fifteen. We have observed extraordinary instances of improvement in a number of patients who had reached an advanced age and been severely affected for many years. In addition, the rates of improvement and recovery in all the studies cited, in which almost two-thirds of the patients showed rather favorable developments over the long term (approximately 25 percent recovery and 30–40 percent improvement), were found to be significantly higher than had previously been supposed. None of these data could be reconciled at all with the original concept of the disease as a pathological organic process in the brain marked by inevitable progressive deterioration. On the contrary, the cases followed over several decades suggested that we should view the disorder as a life process open to the influence of a large number of variables (analyzed in more detail below). An inherently plausible alternative hypothesis, considered repeatedly since Bleuler's time, assumes the existence of a heterogeneous "group of schizophrenias." This hypothesis, however, does not affect matters decisively, for it is still not possible to establish stable subgroups with clearly predictable courses of development. Our own follow-up studies have shown that no categories are clear-cut and that every imaginable intermediate or transitional form occurs.[4] We could find only very few statistically reliable criteria for prognosis, and even these often proved inadequate for individual cases.

Acceptance of a diagnostic framework based on unfavorable development would require clinicians to wait until patients reached old age, or even died, before they could make a correct diagnosis. In practice, of course, rapid diagnosis is essential. Defining schizophrenia as a disease with an (almost) inevitably bad outcome causes many patients to be labeled, completely incorrectly, as incurable, year after year. It creates a basis for negative expectations that may contribute to negative development in a kind of self-fulfilling prophecy. In the long run such a negative concept can set in motion a vicious circle with the worst consequences. Social discrimination, enforced hospitalization for long periods, aggressive forms of therapy, prejudices of all kinds (including the erroneous belief that schizophrenics are especially dangerous),[5] lack of understanding or even ridicule from those around them, increasing isolation, disorientation, loss of self-esteem, and resignation of patients and their families are all possible long-term results of a negative definition of schizophrenia. The interrelatedness of these factors has become so clear in recent years that even traditional academic circles have begun to discuss the questions raised by the school of "antipsychiatry." Laing, Basaglia, Foucault, Szasz, and others initiated this discussion some time ago with their claims that all chronic conditions—which, as we have seen, constitute the essence of "true schizophrenia" for many adherents of traditional psychiatry—represent a "social artifact." In other words, an acute psychosis is transformed into a chronic state mainly by social and psychological influences in the patient's environment. I shall come back to this highly controversial issue, which I dealt with in a recent article.[6]

Not only is our understanding of the nature and progressive course of schizophrenia not very profound; we know no more, and probably less, about its *causes*. Kraepelin and Bleuler assigned it to the category of "endogenous" psychoses, meaning those that occur "from within" for unknown reasons; today, despite all the spectacular discoveries of brain researchers, the tireless efforts of psychoanalysts, and the feverish search of biochemists in the last few decades for a breakthrough (which will certainly earn a Nobel Prize when it comes), we know little more about schizophrenia than that hereditary factors must be involved. Even this fact—which an earlier generation of researchers took for granted—could be established beyond doubt only within the last ten or twenty years, because of the immense difficulty of distinguishing between environmental and hereditary factors. It took the efforts of large research teams and extremely complex methods of comparative investigation in studies of monozygotic and dizygotic twins, as well as of children of schizophrenic parents who were adopted by healthy parents soon after birth.[7] Nevertheless the exact nature of these hereditary components is still obscure. Schizophrenia does not progress according to any known pattern of genetically transmitted diseases; the genetic influences do not take the form of any specific anatomical or biochemical "defect," and the role played by heredity in the whole range of possible variations that the disorder can take appears today to be much smaller than was previously thought, as I shall try to show in more detail below. Furthermore— and we will see that this point is of great significance for the entire discussion—geneticists now agree that it is not the disease itself that is transmitted by heredity, but rather a quite intangible form of vulnerability, which may be a disharmonious personality structure or another pathological predisposition. According to the stress diathesis model (diathesis = an inherited predisposition), which is quite plausible, the disease occurs only when the predisposition *and* certain environmental factors are present. Psychophysiologists have turned up some clues about the nature of this diathesis; taken together, these suggest that schizophrenics possess a heightened nervous excitability, vulnerability, and hypersensitivity.[8] These qualities, if they were to be confirmed by further research, would reduce schizophrenics' capacity to withstand stress of any kind almost in the same way as does the confusion in internalized systems of reference postulated in the last chapter. Such a theory restores environmental conditions to the center of interest; it indicates that we should look to research on families and communication for further progress. In particular, the modern schools of crisis intervention and life-events research appear promising. In the meantime we can say only that the various elements of our knowledge about the causes of schizophrenia seem like pieces of a difficult puzzle that we cannot yet put together; indeed, the most important pieces may still be missing.

As far as the *treatment* of schizophrenia is concerned, optimists are inclined to assume that we have made tremendous progress in the last twenty or thirty years. It is certainly true that many aspects of treatment have improved. The possibilities for drug therapy have expanded in ways that no one could have foreseen; many—though by no means all—psychiatric hospitals are smaller, more modern, and more open than they used to be; and an entire range of alternative and transitional institutions has come into existence, providing for the social and medical needs of patients: day clinics, night clinics, professionally staffed halfway houses, and job-training centers. Nevertheless, the effect of all these measures has not been overwhelming. Kraepelin and Bleuler reported a recovery rate of 15 to 20 percent in their own day; today we reckon with a rate of approximately 25 percent. Our own long-term study (which admittedly in this respect contains a number of uncertain variables) reflected no statistically significant improvement from the beginning of this century to the 1950s.[9] The neuroleptics introduced since that time can bring about rapid short-term improvement; however, these benefits may be offset by subsequent side effects of the most serious kind, such as irreversible motor disturbances, which occur with alarming frequency. And although certain indications suggest a considerable increase in "social cures" (successful social reintegration of patients despite some continuing symptoms), the eminent British social psychiatrist John Wing has pointed out that the "moral treatment" in vogue a hundred years ago resulted in almost as many schizophrenics returning to the community after institutionalization as is the case today.[10]

Since there can be no doubt about the importance of the subject—

in Switzerland and its neighboring countries psychiatric patients occupy almost one of every four hospital beds, and a large proportion of them are schizophrenics—and since medicine has made such spectacular advances in other fields, how can we explain the insufficient state of our knowledge? I think there are many reasons, foremost among them a lack of cooperation among specialists and a tendency to overgeneralize one-sided organic or psychosocial theories and to indulge in polemics in their defense. The lack of interest in psychiatric problems long displayed by both the general public and traditional somatic medicine has no doubt also played a role. But the real causes lie deeper, in the nature of the subject itself: there is no more complex phenomenon than the human mind or spirit with which we are concerned here, and no subject that presents greater problems for research. However, of all subjects it is also the most fascinating. Since immense gaps still exist in our understanding of fundamental processes within the brain, we cannot help but be at an even greater loss in the face of the higher mental and intellectual functions. Nonetheless, our insight into the whole complex of these problems is constantly increasing, and we can probably expect major advances to occur in the near future. Brain research has made great strides in recent years; it has cast light on the different functions of the two hemispheres and on the plasticity of the brain when confronted with new experiences, and it has also developed new techniques such as transaxial tomography.[11] Nor have researchers in psychology, sociology, and psychoanalysis by any means exhausted the possibilities of their fields. In the case of schizophrenia in particular, it seems very likely that important new syntheses lie just around the corner. So much detailed information has been compiled over the years—more than any one person can now absorb—that we appear to have reached a critical point at which a leap to a higher plane of understanding is positively *demanded*. In fact we are perhaps closer to a definitive breakthrough than the recent tempo of events has led us to expect. Wherever creative thinkers have been occupied with the problem of schizophrenia—I am thinking of Bateson, Wing, Wynne, Scheflen, Stierlin, and Selvini Palazzoli, for example—the atmosphere has been electric. Wing called the book he edited in 1978 *Schizophrenia: Toward a New Synthesis;* Wynne and his associates named theirs simply *The Nature of Schizophrenia.*[12] Both works contain a compilation of all the most recent data, assembled by renowned specialists, and both clearly aim at a comprehensive synopsis. New publications with a similar approach have appeared on all sides: In the two months be-

tween completion of the preceding chapter of this book and com-
mencement of work on this chapter (February–March 1981), Albert
Sheflen's impressive survey of schizophrenia on eight different levels
appeared posthumously, Otto Kernberg's book on the relationship
between internal world and external reality was published, and the
Swiss analyst Henri Schneider published his interesting investigation
of the relationship between the thought of Piaget and psychoanalysis,
in which he touches on many of the same issues that I am concerned
with here (particularly in Chapter 2).[13] There can be no question but
that systems theory has served as an important integrating force in
this movement toward synthesis; both Scheflen and Schneider make
explicit references to it. In my view, however, systems theory represents only one modern variant of a mode of thought with a long tradition. This holistic tradition runs counter to and complements analytic and deductive concern with isolated phenomena. Some time ago
the French structuralist school appeared as one manifestation of this
mode of thinking, and in recent years, after considerable delay, it has
also entered psychiatry. That such a development should be concentrated in the field of schizophrenia research is certainly no accident.
Everything suggests that this complex but as yet unsolved problem
lies at the critical meeting point not only of affect and intellect, body
and mind, but also of the sciences and the humanities. It thus presents
itself as a key area in the growth of human knowledge, predestined
to call forth the best efforts of researchers in many disciplines.

It is in this general framework that the concept of affect-logic belongs, representing as it does my own attempt to contribute to our
understanding of how the cognitive and affective components of the
mind interact. Such an approach should have particular value in our
search to learn more about the nature of schizophrenia, since this
disorder is characterized by inextricably linked disturbances of both
feeling and thinking.

I see the development of schizophrenia as a process with *three
phases.* Each phase presents a distinct group of symptoms, and each
probably has distinct causes, at least in part. These three phases are:

The premorbid phase (from birth until the outbreak
    of the disease)
The phase of acute psychosis
The chronic phase

I proceed from the basic premise that a (more or less) acute psychosis is a necessary condition for us to be able to speak of schizophrenic illness at all;[14] by contrast, both the premorbid phase and the chronic phase appear to be less specific categories (each in its own way, of course). It should be emphasized that these phases cannot always be sharply differentiated; many transitional and combined forms occur, particularly in the acute and chronic stages as they are defined below. I hope to show, however, that this circumstance does not invalidate the case I am arguing here. This concept of three-stage development allows us to resolve a number of problems mentioned at the beginning of this chapter, especially if we combine it with the hypothesis of the internalization of very unstable affective-cognitive systems of reference.

Briefly summarized, my argument runs as follows. In the long *premorbid phase* preceding the outbreak of actual psychosis, the groundwork is laid for the later illness; a large number of different influences—genetic, somatic, familial, social, and psychodynamic—act in concert (though differently in each individual case) on a person's internalized systems of reference, which are in part innate and in part formed by experience. In the case of schizophrenics, certain essential areas of these systems are set up in a defective, confused, and unstable manner. This results in a characteristic ego weakness and so leads in turn to increased vulnerability and reduced ability to deal with stress in the environment. *Actual psychosis* in a more or less acute form then breaks out in situations of great stress; it may appear only once and be entirely reversible, or it may gradually become an ingrained response to stress and be repeated until it takes the form of specific "residual symptoms." Which course the disease takes depends on the interaction of the patient's vulnerable premorbid personality structure with what is probably a large number of accompanying factors, including important environmental influences. Under unfavorable conditions the mechanisms of a vicious circle may take over and, as they repeat themselves, cement the pathological patterns in the patient's social mileu, in his affective-cognitive functions, and probably even in the physiological activity of his brain. These mechanisms consolidate the disturbance once it has occurred and lead gradually to the typical symptoms of the *chronic phase*. Should we ever become able to categorize these influences and the typical ways in which they act in conjunction, it might become possible to distinguish relatively predictable subgroups for a "group of schizophrenias" after all.

In the view of schizophrenia presented here acute psychosis occupies a central position. It represents the clearly and obviously diseased state, whereas everything else is either preparation or consequence (although these consequences are by no means either specific or inevitable). Quite a large number of recent publications have begun to outline a flexible concept of schizophrenia along these lines; it corresponds much more closely to the living reality than does the rigid idea of one or more "disease entities" handed down to us from the somatic medicine of the last century—even if this older concept, with its single cause, clinical picture, and course, would be more practical for treatment and especially for research purposes. However, modern somatic medicine long ago replaced such unilateral concepts with more differentiated, multidimensional approaches, as for example in the case of heart attacks, hypertension, and diabetes mellitus. In the following discussion I will use this perspective to try to single out the most important characteristics of the three phases of schizophrenia and to suggest how the thoughts on affect-logic presented in earlier chapters can be usefully applied to them.

The Premorbid Phase

The influence of certain hereditary factors is virtually the only characteristic of this stage to have been established with any major degree of reliability. The enormously complex problems of genetic research on schizophrenia are reviewed in a special 1976 issue of the *Schizophrenia Bulletin*. In a survey there of the large-scale studies of adopted children in the 1960s and early 1970s, Gottesman and Shields reach the conclusion—shared today by almost all schizophrenia researchers—that hereditary factors lead to psychosis only in combination with certain environmental conditions, along the lines of the stress diathesis theory mentioned above (in this case the inherited predisposition is a relative inability to withstand stress). They state that both the gene and the environment (even if we cannot yet define precisely what the latter must contain) are necessary, but not sufficient, to cause schizophrenia.[15]

It is a fact that the more closely someone is related by blood to a schizophrenic, the greater the probability is that he or she will also incur the disease; the highest probability exists in the case of identical twins, since their genetic material is the same; but even such twins do not always follow the same pattern. Before World War II, F. I. Kallman, the leading genetic researcher, found a correspondence rate of 87 percent, which would indicate an overwhelming preponderance of genetic influence; however, his methods have since been placed in doubt. According to Gottesman and Shields, the latest figures lie between 14 and 50 percent, or between 35 and 58 percent, depending on the method of calculation used. The authors state that the remaining variance can be ascribed to environmental influences. If we consider that certain factors having nothing to do with heredity (such as prenatal and perinatal defects, milieu, and social and cultural conditions) also contribute to this correspondence rate, then we must give at least as much weight to environmental factors as to genetic ones. The continuing controversy on this issue indicates just how complicated matters are,[16] and so do the results of some interesting recent research. The well-known large-scale studies by Kety and his associates of children of schizophrenic parents who were adopted at an early age by healthy parents showed that such children suffered from schizophrenia at a significantly higher rate than did a control group.[17] This finding seemed to confirm the influence of hereditary factors. However, the family milieu in which the children who developed schizophrenia lived had not been investigated. Wynne and Singer were then able to show that the children who were genetically at risk had a greater tendency to develop the disease in adoptive families whose confused and contradictory style of communication resembled that of "families with schizophrenic transactions." Using this feature alone, the authors were able to predict with 100 percent accuracy which sets of parents would have a schizophrenic child.[18] More recently, Tienari in Finland found that in a population at risk—constituted by adopted-away children of schizophrenic mothers—those who lived in a disturbed family environment much more frequently became schizophrenic themselves, whereas harmonious families had a protective effect.[19] The nature of the genetic factor remains completely unknown, as well as the course it takes and what organic substrate might possibly be involved. Still it is also a fact that schizophrenia often occurs in families in which no history of this disease or other mental illness can be found, despite the most careful investigation. (This last fact has received surprisingly little attention in my view, since in one of our own studies it applied to a full 20 percent of the cases, and in Bleuler's up to 40 percent.)[20] All this shows that many questions on the subject remain unanswered.

If anything we are even more in the dark about nongenetic *further cerebral or somatic changes* that may influence the outbreak of a schizophrenic psychosis. Studies of this particular aspect are still extremely rare, but a few findings suggest an increased incidence among schizophrenics of the psycho-organic brain damage in early childhood known as "minimal brain syndrome."[21] These results are particularly interesting for two reasons. First, if a psycho-organic syndrome incurred in early childhood does in fact increase the risk of schizophrenia, then the correspondence rates of genetic researchers will have to be recalculated to take this new variable into account, since more birth defects occur in multiple births than normally. Second, there are in fact striking similarities between the cognitive disturbances described in schizophrenics and those in minimally brain-damaged children. They both have difficulty keeping their attention focused, can be easily distracted, and seem to suffer from very similar defects in their ability to filter out relevant information. In addition both find it quite hard to absorb complex information (especially crossmodal stimuli reaching several sensory organs simultaneously), and they react to all these difficulties in a similar manner, with increased psychological tension, feelings of insecurity and inferiority, social withdrawal, and other defense mechanisms.

Although there are still too few studies of groups at risk for schizophrenia, such as children of schizophrenic parents, to permit broad generalizations, their findings so far offer particularly interesting possibilities. One such project, by Mednick, Schulsinger, and their research group, has studied the development of high-risk children of schizophrenic mothers in Denmark for more than twenty years.[22] In addition to the expected higher incidence of psychoses and other forms of mental illness, these children also frequently display unusual nervous sensitivity and excitability from an early age, a phenomenon I mentioned above. Other investigations have produced similar results.[23] We have thus found an important clue to the possible nature of the vulnerability and inability to withstand stress that plays such a crucial role in the stress-diathesis theory.

The aspects of family and parent-child relations relating to schizophrenia that contributed to my systems-of-reference hypothesis in the previous chapter are: the central importance of symbiotic ties based on narcissism, faulty identity formation, insufficient demarcation of generation lines, and particularly the contradictory patterns of communication in the family as studied by Wynne and Singer. Many family therapists today regard these as the most significant schizophrenogenic factors. There are also a number of older studies on the connections between schizophrenia and broken homes, but the methods used were problematical and on the whole they failed to produce convincing results. According to Manfred Bleuler, broken home situations occur with hardly any greater statistical frequency in the childhood of schizophrenics than among alcoholics, people with other forms of mental illness, or even the general population.[24] It appears that questions on such matters as the loss of a parent, divorce, or break-up of the family for other reasons are not specific enough to be of real value in schizophrenia research. Most probably a great deal depends on when such events occur, how they are dealt with, and so on. In any case studies of family communication patterns seem to be far more fruitful.

Scheflen also notes the negative influence of social isolation, which may occur among immigrants or otherwise poorly integrated families. It is known that immigrants face an increased risk of schizophrenia during the first few months in new surroundings, especially if ties to their own ethnic group have been broken. However, there is virtually no likelihood of a direct causal connection between lower-class status and the incidence of schizophrenia. The so-called drift hypothesis shows instead that schizophrenics tend to drop in social status, or fail to rise in status as a consequence of the illness. There is also no clear evidence that schizophrenia occurs more often in any particular country, type of society, or race, although highly interesting studies by the World Health Organization indicate that the prognosis for recovery is better in the Third World than in industrialized nations.[25] This circumstance has been attributed to patterns of life in the extended families that often prevail in these countries, since they are cohesive and tend to provide a strong support network. The idea of social solidarity may also explain why the incidence of schizophrenia tends to drop in times of crisis or war. These phenomena indicate that social feedback mechanisms are important in maintaining and validating internalized affective-cognitive systems of reference, a point to which I shall return later.

Finally, several authors such as Janzarik and Huber have identified a number of conditions on the borderline between sickness and health which quite often appear to precede the outbreak of acute psychosis.[26] Some are symptoms corresponding in large measure to the "reduction of energy potential" observable in the later chronic stage; others are vegetative, often hypochondriacal physical ailments or mood changes such as depression. Wing speaks in this connection of "neurotic symptoms," including depression, anxiety, tension, irritability, absent-mindedness, and hypochondriacal complaints that can appear before, during, and after acute psychotic episodes.[27] Scheflen describes a condition he calls "nonpsychotic schizophrenia," which is characterized by (1) problems with sequential psychomotor activities and with thinking and speaking sequentially; (2) abnormal, rapid shifts of mood, tone, and attention; and (3) overdependency on one partner, accompanied by loss of contact with other people.[28] He does not make it entirely clear, however, whether these symptoms are observed before the first onset of psychosis. These nonspecific "prodromes" and intermediate and post-acute stages are of great theoretical interest. Some authors, such as Huber and, more recently, Scheflen, are inclined to consider them as connected with a form of organic brain damage, the "underlying pathology" of schizophrenia. In my view, these nonspecific symptoms are an interesting aspect of premorbid vulnerability. They reflect an increasingly destabilized "terrain," which under some circumstances will lead to actual psychosis, and they can be understood at least in part as a defensive retreat from stressful situations and/or as one aspect of the disturbed communications occurring within a family.

In summary, the evidence indicates that persons who later become schizophrenic frequently manifest great vulnerability and hypersensitivity. These traits have their origin in both inherited and acquired factors, which are inseparably linked and will also vary from case to case. Many studies have shown that one striking characteristic of persons at risk for schizophrenia is their difficulty in processing complex information—in other words, their clearly reduced capacity to withstand stress. In my theory of poorly structured and unstable affective-cognitive systems of reference, developed in the preceding chapter, I brought together various aspects of this ego weakness (a characteristic of persons at risk also emphasized by psychoanalysis). There is nothing in the literature, and certainly not in the results of genetic or psychophysiological research, that seems to me to contradict this hypothesis; on the contrary, it has room—perhaps for the first time for this type of theory—for all kinds of influences, both hereditary and acquired—that is, for genetic, somatic, biochemical, psychophysiological, psychogenic, and sociogenic factors. This hypothesis appears to fulfill Wing's requirements for a theory of schizophrenia better than many more one-sided explanations: "What will eventually be needed is a set of linked theories, relating epidemiology, genetics, biochemistry, pathology, psychopathology, and therapeutics, to the development of . . . specific clinical syndromes."[29]

Two remaining points are also quite consistent with the systems-of-reference hypothesis. First, almost all of these premorbid symptoms are *nonspecific;* they occur in similar form in many sensitive people who are by no means schizophrenic and who do not incur other forms of mental illness. Nonetheless instability and vulnerability of this type are clearly more pronounced in the near vicinity of schizophrenia, in borderline cases and in persons with a tendency to develop psychotic disturbances. To put it another way, inner confusion and instability can occur in varying degrees; they can lead under certain circumstances to a psychotic disorder, but they do not have to. Whether this happens or not probably depends on the interaction of a great many complex factors, some of which may be somatic and some related to an individual's social situation or personality.

Second, the existence of the premorbid "terrain" is of tremendous importance. Our own and many other long-term investigations have shown again and again that in following the course of the disease over a long period—in our study until old age—the more balanced and normal the patient was before the outbreak of psychosis, the better was the long-range prognosis.[30] Interestingly, some older notions on this subject proved to be largely irrelevant, such as the close connection long suspected to exist between an asthenic or leptosomic constitution, so-called schizoid character traits (reserve, an even temper, sensitivity hidden behind apparent coldness, ambivalence, introversion), and an unfavorable prognosis. In fact *any kind* of premorbid symptom worsens the long-range-prognosis, and a lack of them improves it. These findings are of general importance because almost no other predictors exist that could be traced with any regularity in the different studies. The few that do exist—such as a sudden onset of the disease, the severity of initial symptoms, and an episodic rather than a steady and continuous course, all of which are statistically related to a favorable outcome—are probably all closely connected with personality-specific patterns of reacting.

Acute Psychosis: An Affective-Logical View

In my view the central and decisive phase of schizophrenia is the acute psychosis. At first glance it does not seem especially difficult to say what an acute psychosis is; clinicians, just like laymen, associate this term with a picture of complete confusion, agitation, delusions, hallucinations, jumbled speech, and strangely inappropriate behavior. On closer inspection, however, this description presents difficulty after difficulty. It is not at all easy to give a precise definition of psychosis, and the term *acute* is almost as unclear. There are at least three or four different classification systems for acute psychotic symptoms, which overlap to some extent but also contradict each other in places, reflecting different views of the same phenomenon. The difficulty of distinguishing an acute schizophrenic condition from other psychoses or forms of mental illness remains an unsolved and controversial problem, and there are further questions about its origins and whether or not it is "endogenous." There is also no general agreement yet about the relative weight of genetic, somatic, psychological, and social factors.

The details of all these problems would fill a book of their own. I will therefore select a few points and concentrate on outlining the theory of acute psychosis that suggests itself as the logical consequence of my discussion so far.

The concept of *psychosis* is rarely defined precisely in the literature on the subject. Originally the word meant simply any disease of the psyche, analogous to "neurosis" (a disease of the nerves). Today it is normally used to refer to a gross impairment of reality-testing functions, that is, incorrect inferences concerning external reality. Other types of psychosis exist besides schizophrenia, such as psychotic disorders caused by organic brain damage or toxic substances. When I use the word here it will be in this conventional sense (although it begs an important question about what "reality" is).

The word *acute* usually has two implications, which sometimes but not always occur in combination. The first is qualitative and denotes a particular intensity or severity; in this sense one often speaks of "acute symptoms." The second is related to the aspect of time and refers to symptoms that are sudden in onset and relatively short-lived. Various suggestions have been offered for an operational definition of this second meaning; an "acute onset" of psychosis has been used to mean occurring within one, three, or six months, for example, without any reference to the severity of the symptoms.[31]

The main difficulty lies in the fact that "acute" symptoms in the qualitative sense may last for years or may flare up repeatedly, in a "chronic" manner. For this reason the British school of psychiatry led by Wing has urged the adoption of new terms, which provide useful clarification in many respects. They suggest that *acute* should be replaced by the term *productive* or *positive* when it refers to the severity of symptoms, and that *chronic* should be replaced by *unproductive* or *negative*.

Since the days of Kraepelin and Eugen Bleuler, acute schizophrenic psychoses have usually been divided into four classic types, although many overlappings and shadings occur. Depending on whether delusional, psychomotor, childish, or merely "primary" disturbances in behavior predominate, the psychoses are labeled paranoid, catatonic, hebephrenic, and "simple" ("schizophrenia simplex"). As long-term studies have shown, these differences tend to disappear if the disorder becomes chronic, giving way to uniform, typically "negative" and "unproductive" residual conditions. Eugen Bleuler saw "primary disturbances" as consisting of ambivalence, a typical "loosening of associations," a blunting of affect, and autism (the famous "four A's," which are frequently cited in the American literature on schizophrenia). In addition he mentioned experiences of depersonalization and unreality, loss of contact with the outside world, and affective withdrawal. Phenomena such as delusions, hallucinations, psychomotor agitation or immobility, and childish clowning, which gave each type its characteristic stamp, were regarded by Bleuler as relatively superficial and changeable "secondary symptoms."

Since it often proved difficult to distinguish schizophrenic disorders from other forms of illness both for treatment and reserach purposes, Kurt Schneider later attempted to isolate a number of frequent and recognizable "first-rank symptoms." By proceeding on a purely pragmatic basis and avoiding theoretical constructs he hoped to facilitate the diagnosis of schizophrenia. These first-rank symptoms are:

Thought broadcasting (the feeling that one's thoughts
   have become audible to others)
Auditory hallucinations (hearing voices as conversations)
Hearing voices commenting on one's own actions
Experiences of being physically controlled from outside
Spreading of meaning
Delusions
The feeling that one's emotions, strivings, and will are controlled
   from outside

"Where one of these modes of experience is clearly manifested and no evidence of underlying somatic illness can be found, with all modesty we speak clinically of schizophrenia.[32] In recent years this concept has been taken up largely for methodological reasons, by Anglo-American psychiatry, and used in the computerized "Catego system" diagnosis based on the "Present State Interview" (PSI).[33] Schneider's first-rank symptoms do not appear, however, in all acute psychoses diagnosed as schizophrenic: in recent British and American PSI studies they were found in only about two-thirds of the cases.[34] Despite the supposed lack of any basic theoretical concept, they do point to something most typical of such conditions: just as the definition of psychosis above implies, they all share a sense that the patient's own experience has been invaded by an external, alien force. In other words, a profound disturbance of identity has occurred, with a blurring of the limits of the self and a loss of distinction between internal and external reality. When the symptoms classified by Schneider as secondary—other perceptual delusions, hallucinations, ambivalence, depressed or elated moods, blunted affects—occur, they do so only partially or in less definite form.

In addition to this approach, another classification system has become increasingly useful, namely the distinction between acute, positive, or productive symptoms (sometimes also referred to as "floridly psychotic" symptoms), on the one hand, and chronic, negative, or unproductive symptoms on the other. The first type overlaps somewhat with the indications established by Bleuler and Schneider and consists of anxiety, tension, agitation, affective-cognitive confusion, experiences of depersonalization and unreality, delusions, and hallucinations.[35] The latter type consists mainly of blunted affects, apathy, a slowing down of thinking and psychomotor activity, a narrowing of interest, social withdrawal, and impoverishment of speech, all of which usually predominate in chronic schizophrenics after long hospitalization. Here again overlaps occur, because some "productive" symptoms can also be observed in chronic stages, and "unproductive" symptoms in acute stages. "However, the florid types are usually acute and the negative types usually chronic, and so they will be called the acute and chronic syndromes, for brevity and convenience."[36] The studies by Wing and his associates have pointed to some significant correlations; they associate acute or productive states with psychosocial overstimulation, and chronic or unproductive states with the kind of understimulation that can be met with in the rigidly run, neglected closed wards of old-fashioned mental hospitals. For this reason the authors also relate typical negative symptoms to the concept of institutionalism that takes the form of the "clinical poverty syndrome."

Scheflen offers another interesting approach to the same acute states: he suggests classifying them according to their degree of severity.[37] The classic subgroups of schizophrenia have usually been regarded as of an equally severe order, but Scheflen proposes different categories, beginning with the relatively unspecific initial condition characterized by tension, anxiety, insecurity, identity disturbances, and general disharmony, which would correspond in large measure to the traditional "schizophrenia simplex" syndrome. As the psychosis increases in severity, these escalate in a second stage to become delusional and hallucinatory (paranoid); in a third stage, hebephrenic; and in a fourth, a trancelike catatoniform state usually marked by stereotyped actions and physical rigidity or immobility. Strikingly similar ideas are contained in a work by the German psychiatrist Klaus Conrad, with which Scheflen does not seem to have been familiar. Written almost thirty years ago, Conrad's book on the early stages of schizophrenia uses a phenomenological approach. He distinguishes three phases: an initial *trema* (a Latin term used in the context of theater), characterized by anxiety, tension, and a sense of expectancy; usually followed by *apophenia,* a delusional and hallucinatory "revelation" of the real meaning of things; and the "apocalyptic" stage, the progressive disintegration of all psychic functions until dreamlike and catatonic states occur. In Conrad's view, "according to the laws of the disease's progression" the catatonic stage can occur only after the individual has passed through the paranoid phase: "A short phase of paranoia occurs before the catatonic phase is entered; this paranoid phase also may occur briefly at the end of a catatonic psychosis, as the illness recedes. Thus, from a phenomenological point of view, *the catatonic experience represents an intensification of the paranoid experience.*[38] According to Conrad the disease may run its course through all three stages, or it may be arrested at any point. "Consolidation" (recovery) may occur, or there may be a partial recovery with different residual features of varying severity. Both Conrad and Scheflen believe that underlying these progressive stages are different modes of cerebral functioning that would correspond to a gradual loss of functional differentiation. These stages match rather well the progressive disturbances described in recent research on the phenomenology of crises; they occur when a "coping system" of a given capacity is progressively overtaxed—something which Conrad could not have known and which Scheflen appears to have overlooked.

Wing also suggests that a progressive escalation of acute pathological symptoms may exist; he mentions in passing that phenomena such as thought broadcasting, the feeling of outside influence on thoughts, spreading of thoughts, and auditory hallucinations first perceived as coming from within and then from outside form a continuum.[39] He does not elucidate this idea, but we do in fact often see the *successive* appearance of such symptoms in the early stages of psychosis. We need only place the initial stage of self-absorption accompanied by strong emotions—which is frequently observed and in which the person may carry on conversations with himself—at the beginning of this list in order to arrive at a virtually continuous spectrum of phenomena ranging from the perfectly normal to the pathological. This spectrum reflects a progressive retreat from the shared world of external reality into a private inner world, and at the one end we find the same phenomena that can occur in states of intense agitation or concentration (as in yoga exercises or autogenic training). It is still a matter of debate whether the modes of psychic functioning and experience occurring in psychoses are different from healthy modes only in degree and quantity, or whether they actually differ in *quality*. However, the existence of such transitional states can be observed in many other areas, such as difficulties in speaking or focusing attention, in psychomotor phenomena, and in exaggerated ideas that have not yet reached the level of delusions. All of this suggests that the gulf between ordinary experience and schizophrenia is not as great as we often tend to assume, and as one school of psychiatry characterized by distancing and defensiveness also teaches.

These observations on gradual increments in a progression toward mental illness can be connected with a number of other facts that are usually viewed in isolation, both in clinical experience and in the professional literature. Besides the British studies on psychosocial under- and overstimulation already mentioned, I am thinking of the findings of crisis-intervention research, life-events research, and older studies on sudden conversions or shifts from one mental state to another. Despite the fact that current concepts about acute schizophrenia are anything but uniform, if we take all of these observations into consideration we arrive at a coherent total picture that fits very well with the other ideas developed in this book: *Acute psychotic decompensation can be understood as a critical disturbance in the area of information processing, that is, as the overtaxing of certain affective-cognitive systems of reference or information-processing systems, which in highly sensitive and vulnerable individuals were already unstable and partially defective.* A predisposition in combination with circumstances at a particular time may affect individual cases differently.

The most important arguments in favor of this assumption are the following. In a series of excellent studies Wing and his associates were able to prove beyond any doubt that flare-ups of acute, productive psychotic symptoms are connected with psychosocial overstimulation in a statistically significant manner, whereas negative, unproductive symptoms are connected with understimulation.[40] Psychosocial overstimulation should be understood here in relation to the reduced capacity of the person at risk to process information; it may consist not only of familial, professional, and social demands, visits, trips, and other events that imply change or the need to adapt, but also of all information in the broadest sense with which the individual must contend. At the same time Wing confirmed the results obtained by other research groups that outbreaks of acute psychosis are significantly higher among those who have experienced a major life event in the recent past (specifically in the preceding three weeks) than among healthy control groups. Such life events include a change of job or city, marriage, the birth of a child, illness, accidents, or a serious loss.[41]

The crisis-intervention research pursued in the United States by Lindemann, Caplan, and others over the last thirty years has shown that every crisis must be understood as the acute overtaxing of a coping system—which could also be described as an information-processing system. The point at which this occurs will vary widely from individual to individual, but when it does occur it is regularly accompanied by a loss of normal behavior patterns. These are replaced by a variety of phenomena that may resemble the initial stages of psychosis and sometimes even more advanced stages. At the beginning we find in both instances a general increase in tension, anxiety and uncertainty, ambivalence, confusion, and possibly also irritability, depression, and agitation. If the pressure continues, even previously healthy individuals will experience feelings of depersonalization and derealization; aggressive or autoaggressive outbursts may occur, as well as delusional projections and introjections (of one's own aggressive feelings onto others, as feelings of persecution), cognitive and speech disturbances, and finally even hallucinations.[42] We can thus regard acute psychotic manifestations in large measure as reactions of sensitive, vulnerable individuals to stress that has become too great for them. These symptoms are indeed pathological, but the potential for developing them exists in every healthy person, just as everybody has the potential for developing epileptic seizures.

Further crisis-intervention research has shown that at the height of a crisis a particularly unstable phase occurs, in which an individual is highly suggestible. Minor events (such as external influences and situational elements) may have a disproportionate effect. Small alterations during this phase may easily lead to significantly different behavior patterns, which then become stabilized and can be reversed only with great difficulty. Modern family therapists emphasize that a physician's diagnosis or the hospitalization of one family member may be enough to set a family crisis in motion, and the family member who has been designated as the scapegoat will often embark on a long career as a mental patient. Intervention with the proper family therapy techniques can prevent this from happening right from the start. Similar observations were made years ago by the British psychiatrist Sargant, whose book on religious conversions, initiation rites, war neuroses, and brainwashing techniques has been unjustly neglected.[43] Sargant identified the same fundamental mechanisms at work in all these forms of psychic disorder that occur under conditions of extreme stress: an individual's system of opinions, values, modes of perception and behavior (that is, a comprehensive affective-logical system of reference) is first systematically placed in doubt by means of contradictory, devaluating messages; the pressure on the individual is then increased on all levels simultaneously, both emotionally (through threats and promises) and physically (through hunger and sleep deprivation), until finally a crisis is reached and the existing system of reference has been totally destabilized. At this critical point the subject is acutely sensitive, suggestible, and confused and may even display psychotic behavior, with the result that new beliefs or values may be implanted in him with relative ease. These remain stable later, especially if brief repetitions of the traumatic conversion conditions are provided as a reminder from time to time. Sargant suspected that quite similar processes were at work in Pavlov's experiment on conditioned reflexes in dogs; in this connection it is interesting that the animals' individual temperaments made a significant difference in their ability to withstand stress. He also recognized similar factors in successful psychotherapy treatments when the therapy takes on a particularly intense emotional character.

Even if the interpretation of all these observations may not be correct in all parts, it still seems clear that they are relevant to the subject under discussion here, namely the sudden shift from normal patterns of behavior to the strange patterns that we are accustomed to label "psychotic." The parallels to certain family processes described by Searles in quite drastic terms are striking (see below). But in addition crisis-intervention and life-events theory points to something different but equally significant: *No longer are manifestations that are far removed from ordinary experience regarded as "primary." The older, more traditional view of schizophrenia recognized as "primary" (in the sense of "fundamental" or "first-rank") a number of symptoms that are most foreign to a healthy person's experience. From this new perspective, however, these no longer appear so primary in the sense of "initial," or "original." What does appear primary is rather the ordinary human experience of tension, confusion, anxiety, and ambivalence, which under certain circumstances may become intensified to the point where the peculiar symptoms of psychosis emerge.* Obviously such a revision of our understanding of schizophrenic symptoms, if correct, has tremendous implications: the schizophrenic ceases to be the radically alien, deficient, and incomprehensible creature he has often been seen as, both within and outside the domain of psychiatry, and instead we might at last be able to recognize him for what he is, and presumably always has been—a fragile, confused human being who is sensitive and thin-skinned behind his strange defenses. He has sought refuge from unbearable tension in his psychosis, but this has only created more difficulties, in the end becoming both his prison and his undoing. As I try to show in the following pages what consequences such an altered view of schizophrenia has for therapy and for dealings with such patients in general, my version may not be correct in all details, but it can hardly cause more damage than was inflicted in the name of our former, misguided theories.

Both the results of crisis-intervention and life-events research and Sargant's findings indicate that sudden, major shifts in the functioning of psychic systems can occur under the most varied conditions, and that these may occur far outside the limits of an actual psychosis. We are certainly justified in seeing them as a kind of "dis-order" or as shifts of balance within formerly equilibrated affective-cognitive systems of reference established on the basis of all previous experience. The likelihood that fundamentally similar mechanisms play a role in all these phenomena would imply that we ought to be able to recognize certain structural analogies in all mental "disorders" or forms of mental illness.

We can pursue this idea by first examining some specific cases of disorder and then following up what they suggest.

The Structure of Mental "Dis-Orders"

If we ask ourselves what is usually meant by the term *craziness* or *mental disorder,* we realize at once that it includes a wide range of ill-defined phenomena. Whether behavior is deemed to be "crazy" or not will depend on the point of view of the observer; it may extend from ordinary but eccentric actions of healthy individuals to the definitely pathological and schizophrenic. Does this interesting term *disorder* actually imply that these extremes have something in common, and if so, what distinguishes "normal craziness" from the pathological kind?

Let us consider a few examples from everyday life. In the preceding chapters we have already encountered examples here and there of what is commonly called "crazy" behavior. People who purposely expose themselves to danger, such as mountain climbers, deep-sea divers, and spelunkers, are often thought to be "out of their minds." One can be out of one's mind with joy, rage, pain, or fear; collectors may be "mad" to acquire a certain object for their collection, and lovers may be "crazy" about another person. From a certain perspective an eccentric Englishman, a teenager, or an obstinate old man might be considered to be behaving strangely enough for the observer to doubt his sanity. In short, the man in the street tends to consider "crazy" all forms of behavior that appear unusual to him, even though—and this is the important point—they are in fact usually as appropriate and equilibrated in their own context as his own. The use of the word *crazy* thus always implies a reference to what is considered as ordinary, that is, to whatever is the norm in a particular system of reference. Such a norm is both highly relative but also extremely useful, since it represents an optimal adjustment to average experience in a specific context.

Certain everyday instances of "craziness" are of special interest to us here. Sudden fits of rage and the experience of being in love resemble pathological conditions in many respects: they may lead to unusual forms of behavior, and like psychosis they can take hold of someone's whole being, all his feelings, thoughts, and perceptions. These states thus bring about a fundamental change not only in a person's values but also in his grasp of reality. In Plato's "divine madness" of love, lovers are in seventh heaven, or in the clouds; a special aura surrounds the world, themselves, and, above all, the beloved, investing them with a significance and intensity that they otherwise lack. The mood of lovers is exalted but likely to swing from one extreme to the other. In a manner of speaking their thoughts and feelings are polarized, directed only toward the loved one. All that counts is this special relationship, and the rest of the world may cease to exist—it has become as irrelevant to the lover as the normal world is to the psychotic.

A person in the grip of passionate rage is just as lost in a private world for a brief moment; the same may be true for longer periods in the case of the workaholic, the inspired scientist or inventor, or the fanatic.

Let us now look at a few very different conditions, chosen at random but all diagnosed as cases of schizophrenia:

A twenty-eight-year-old former schoolteacher, a small and graceful woman more like a girl of eighteen, roams the halls of our day clinic white-faced, anxious, and agitated; her hands are clenched tightly and her lips pressed together. She is hearing, as she so often has in the past, the voice of her imagined lover speaking to her without cease. She believes firmly in the omnipresence and direct intervention of this man in her life; he is a young doctor who treated her for a physical illness some months ago, and in whose presence she believes in the face of all evidence to the contrary. Now he no longer treats her as kindly as before, however, and he makes disparaging comments about everything she does. He makes fun of her attempts to finish a piece of needlework and has ordered her to kill herself several times. All attempts to distract her with occupational therapy, company, or friendly conversation have little effect, and she reacts to tranquilizers with massive ocular and motor disturbances.

Another case:

A second patient from the day clinic is a tall, blond, twenty-two-year-old man with a malformed appearance. With his fat stomach and contemptuous grin he usually seems to be playing the clown. He never says anything that makes sense, frequently jabs his fellow patients in the ribs for no reason, will obey none of the clinic rules, chain-smokes, does whatever he happens to feel like doing, completes no tasks, always arrives too late if he turns up at all, and takes an interest in nothing. He has failed at everything he has ever attempted and been hospitalized for several weeks on different occasions when his condition worsened. Sometimes he makes vague references to his delusions that he is being persecuted, claiming that people are looking at him strangely or think he is a spy. At other times he claims that he has been or is going to be a racing-car driver. Supposedly he has been looking for a new job for weeks, but without success. It has not been possible to reach him in psychotherapy or group therapy; he remains aloof from the group, and medication just makes him more indifferent. One day, however, when he creates an unpleasant disturbance in a group, the doctor in charge suddenly loses his temper and tells him off in a quite authoritarian manner in front of all the other patients, saying that his laziness just shows that he doesn't take himself seriously and doesn't deserve to be taken seriously by anyone else. The astonished young man appears to listen attentively; two days later the "hebephrenic" has found a steady job as a housepainter, does well for months, is seen no more at the clinic. A year later, however, he reappears in much the same state as before.

Here is a third case:

A woman of about thirty, who has had several episodes of catatonic schizophrenia but manages to work in a laundry in between them without incident, is brought into the emergency room of the mental health clinic. She is extremely agitated, screaming, incoherent, and disoriented. She swears at the nurses, resists being given an injection, and responds to hallucinatory voices that are apparently coming from the ceiling. She is placed in a cell by herself, where she takes all her clothes off. When the doctor comes by on his rounds the next day, she has used her feces to paint a flower on the wall and explains its mystical significance to him.

And a final example:

A divorced woman in her early forties, a sensitive and imaginative artist, has been suffering from strangely erratic and frightening delusions for weeks. Sometimes she can faintly perceive the voice of her dead father and imagines him to be nearby. She feels watched, influenced, altered; a panic will seize her for a few moments as she fears some vague disaster, and she then paces up and down in agitation, mumbling confusedly. Medication calms her considerably, and she responds well when spoken to gently. Her doctor, whom she knows well, is able, in talking to her, to bring her back to reality from acute psychotic anxiety states on several occasions and soothes her completely.

What is happening to these people? What do these cases, apparently so different, have in common? In their own ways, all these people have plunged into an altered, "insane" world; all their feelings, thoughts, and actions are different, as in a dream or a drug-induced "trip." This applies even to the supposedly hebephrenic young man, who does something most unusual: confronted surprisingly with a stern lecture, he suddenly "snaps back" into a normal mode of behavior, indicating that he may have been only feigning insanity. However, he had entered this state of "feigned insanity" for months on end on several occasions, and a diagnosis of hebephrenic schizophrenia had been made without reservation several times. Every clinician is familiar with similar cases of persons who, after numerous attempts at rehabilitation and several discharges, return to spend years in the hospital to the despair of everyone involved. Labeled as "regressed" cases with increasingly "blunted affects," they develop stereotypical mannerisms and finally end up vegetating in closed wards. On the other hand there do exist isolated cases of remission after a sudden shock, such as a fire, an accident, or a severe illness. According to the story told about Jakob Klaesi, a famous professor of psychiatry in Bern who died not long ago at the age of ninety-seven, he cured a severely catatonic patient by taking her out on the Lake of Thun and throwing her out of the boat. He is also alleged to have cured a violently demented woman in Zurich by calling for her at her cell and taking her out to dinner at the most elegant hotel in town. Eventually, shock tactics of another kind have become routine in the form of electroconvulsive therapy, but both are a long way from being regularly successful.

From the perspective of affect-logic, such observations confirm that in psychosis a global system of feeling, thinking, and behaving is thrown off balance, or rather is thrown into a *new* but skewed balance, just as occurs in a person in love or a harmless eccentric, but to a much greater degree. We can compare these affective-cognitive systems to the mobiles of the artist Alexander Calder. His three-dimensional constructions consist of thin metal arms and colored shapes of different sizes and weights; suspended from a fixed point above (which we may think of as another system of a higher order), they balance in midair, offering a nice instance of a dynamically equilibrated set of relations among the elements of a system. If we now imagine that one of these elements is pulled out of its normal position or given an extra weight, we see that all the parts are still present, and still exist in relation to one another, but that the whole has been twisted and distorted. Another example from the field of art might be the limp watches of Salvador Dali, which lie drooping over the edges of his tables like wilted flowers. "The whole world shifted," a young patient reported recently at our crisis-intervention center, toward the end of a schizophrenic episode. "A bird flew by, and that meant: You're crazy."* At other times the same girl heard voices in the rain; "The rain talked to me." She simply "saw everything differently"; for example, she could no longer see herself as "good," and she felt like a village idiot instead. She also carried on "double conversations" with people; as she heard their voices she could also hear within her head their own unspoken commentaries about her: "You are a stupid cow," a voice once said to her. "I talked to my thoughts," she reported. Although she was recovering, for weeks this patient remained unable at times to distinguish reality from psychotic experience. She would be sitting in a café and have the feeling the once again people were talking about her: "She is schizophrenic, you know," she reported hearing, and she did not know if someone had really said this or not. The psychosis had begun in a similarly gradual manner, although the onset of the acute phase had been very sudden. At the beginning she had heard voices only rarely, about once or twice a month, and she was not entirely sure whether she had imagined it or not. At the end, however, they were present day and night. There is some evidence to suggest that megalomania and other delusions occur in a similar way; even though they may enter consciousness abruptly in a sudden vision or revelation, they have often been present for a long time as occasional, fragmentary thoughts or ideas. It is as if the

---

* *Translator's note:* "Du hast einen Vogel," literally "You have a bird," is a colloquial expression meaning "You're out of your mind," "You're cuckoo."

progressive failure of the normal systems of reference were accompanied, beneath the surface, by the gradual building up of another, "insane" system of feeling and thinking that apparently originates from the archaic "all good" and "all bad" self and object representations and other repressed material. It becomes available as a substitute system, should it be needed, and finally this alternative suddenly takes possession of the psychotic individual. One of Klaus Conrad's cases offers a good illustration of how this can occur. (Conrad served as a physician in the German army during World War II; thus the military setting.)

> *Case 10.* Corporal Karl B., aged thirty-two, reported a trema from a long time previously and a gradual, creeping beginning of his delusion, a stage that we shall omit here. In the further exploration of his case he reported: One morning his unit was scheduled to move on. That was when it really started. As soon as one of the officers came and asked him for the key to the barracks, he knew at once that this was a prearranged test. During the bus ride he could tell from the other soldiers' behavior that they knew something he didn't know. The trip lasted three or four hours, and strange conversations took place about the Führer's headquarters, which were supposed to be somewhere nearby in the forest. One soldier asked him very pointedly if he had any bread. When they reached the spot where they were to relieve another unit, about noontime, some of the soldiers were ordered to set up camp. This was of course a trick, in order to give someone a chance to tell them how they should behave toward him, while he had to wait with the others in the bus. As groups of soldiers kept coming and going, it was clear that they were all getting their instructions. When he was assigned to his quarters, a small room where he was supposed to relieve another soldier, he realized at once from this man's strange behavior that he, too, had received instructions. He couldn't explain how he recognized this; he just knew. He put the room in order and went out to buy some cigarettes. He had to go past a garden where all the noncommissioned officers were sitting; the sergeant was there, and a lady. They were obviously very surprised to see him appear suddenly. Probably they were plotting to get him together with her later that evening.[44]

The experiences of our young woman patient, with her "bird" and "the rain that talked to her," was almost poetic; here, in the case of Corporal Karl B., it is even clearer that the characteristic element of his psychotic experience is a sense that everything is significant and "planned," almost as if by magic or spells. At the same time another aspect emerges that can be observed in all cases to a greater or lesser degree: As the perception of the entire world shifts, the patient plays an absolutely central role; everything that happens around him has a special reference to him; it is for his benefit that it has been arranged and is "performed." Conrad writes in this connection about such cases:

> Wherever he turns his glance, he sees something that seems to stand in some relation to himself. His world has been transformed into one large "testing ground," where everything has been "arranged," "set up," and prepared to test him, like the stage set of a peculiar sort of theater. They want to see if he will "tumble to it," if it will "register on him," even though they have "taken pains" to make things "as subtle as possible." They have also used "tricks" and "deceptions"; they are trying to "trap" him. They pretend to be "surprised"; they "conceal" things from him; they do not want him to notice that everyone else has "instructions," has "agreed" on things, has an assignment to carry out. Even the people passing by in the street are part of the act. At the height of the episode he himself gives off a kind of aura, so that everything that meets his eye acquires a strangely distorted expression and is laden with tension (an indication of a sense of omnipotence).[45]

This pervasive egocentricity, this "autistic" shifting of an entire system of reference so that everything in it concerns only oneself, is obviously a central phenomenon. It is present to a degree in the person who is in love or in a fit of rage and clearly is part of the affective-logical structure of schizophrenic pathology. That we can speak of a structure at all, in the sense defined in the preceding chapters, is a striking and noteworthy aspect of the situation. Even though these psychotic states are extremely erratic and changing—this represents their characteristic "invariance"—they nonetheless possess their own coherence and shape. Once again, this means that they form a *system, a certain type of equilibrium that excludes the simultaneous presence of other equilibrations.*

I see in this a parallel to consciousness, and to attention in particular, both of which, it seems to me, can be only "in one place at a time." At those times when we appear to be paying attention to many different things simultaneously, for instance when driving a car or performing another complex task, we have in fact merely expanded the focus of our attention and are making use of a higher-order system of reference constructed from numerous single experiences.

This is particularly well illustrated in an example from Hartwich's book on the attention deficits of schizophrenics.[46] I think that he commits an error in citing, as an illustration of the possibility of maintaining different foci of attention at one time, the case of a gifted chess player who plays several matches simultaneously. In reality, such a player does not play the games all at once but, moving from board to board, plays them *one after the other* in rapid succession. Also, the experience gained from thousands of matches, reading, and studying will have enabled him to develop a system of strategies on a higher level of abstraction, in other words, a higher-order system of reference. He can thus immediately recognize the typical elements in the variety confronting him and be able to dominate dozens, or even hundreds of matches "simultaneously," to the astonishment of laymen.

We could therefore say that, from a healthy person's point of view, in a psychotic disorder everyday reality is overlaid with a strangely distorted perceptual grid or "map," which corresponds to a general shift in affective-cognitive equilibration and consciousness. This places everything in a different light and makes normal perception impossible, just as it is impossible to be in two places at once or to drive a car simultaneously in both third and fourth gear.

But now we must ask what distinguishes the distorted and disordered perception of the psychotic from that of someone who is enraged, in love, experiencing deep grief, or that of the religious fanatic or the mountain climber, all of whom appear to the average person to be out of their minds to some degree.

Obviously all these states of mind are far more flexible and reversible in the basically healthy person than in the schizophrenic. The healthy person can leave this disordered condition behind him at least for certain periods, whereas the psychotic is trapped inside it like a prisoner. Even people suffering terrible grief or the most enamored lovers can usually manage to go to work and carry on with their daily routine; despite their mental state they are able to follow their ordinary paths in a fairly normal manner. When this is no longer the case, when even these routines cease to function, then such people are considered to have completely "lost their heads," or even to be "crazy" in the sense of true psychosis.

The distinction between ordinary "madness" and pathological insanity thus appears to be first and foremost one of degree; all sorts of transitional states exist between them, as the case of the young woman who heard the rain talking demonstrates. Whether someone is truly ill or still healthy depends on how long the disordered condition lasts, how stable it is, and to what extent it excludes other conditions. The quality of the psychotic experience as such is less important.

Further important distinctions do exist, however, although they become apparent only when we shift our focus from the individual to the whole social context in which he lives. Schizophrenic experience takes place in an entirely different context of communication from that of the more transitory "madness" of healthy people; schizophrenic experiences do not elicit any social echo, or if they do, it is a different and strange one. They do not rest harmoniously, like the experience of the healthy, on a shared social foundation that provides constant support and reinforcement. For a long time it was assumed that schizophrenics were completely cut off from their surroundings, living in an "autistic" world without human contact and transference. Now, under the influence of both psychoanalysis and communications and family therapy, we have come to recognize that this contact is not broken off, but just profoundly altered: even a completely mute and immobile catatonic communicates with his environment, sometimes even quite intensively. "One cannot not communicate"; even noncommunication is a form of communication, as communications theory proves;[47] and in a corresponding manner the environment communicates and interacts continually even with a catatonic.

This insight opens up various interesting paths. One of them leads to the well-known experiments with sensory deprivation, which will induce psychosis; another leads to the new ideas developed by systems theorists concerning the role played by the familial and social environment in the development of psychotic phenomena. Both approaches can contribute significantly to our understanding of the normal psyche and of the mechanisms that may operate when it becomes disordered.

Possible Mechanisms of Mental "Alienation"

What factors or influences can cause a normal system of thinking, feeling, and behaving to give way suddenly to a psychotic system? Once more, we have as yet no fully satisfactory explanation. As we explore this crucial question we are forced to rely on speculation, although our current theories are based on several important pieces of evidence.

If we are correct in assuming that a psychic "dis-order" consists in a global shift in a state of psychic equilibrium—a leap from one affective-cognitive system of reference to another, which may have been long in preparation but occurs more or less abruptly—then there must be forces and mechanisms that cause it. Given the strong homeostatic tendency of every equilibrated system, such a shift is unlikely to take place without the intervention of significant forces, which we could call "disorganizers" or "system alterers," for want of a better word.

We are already familiar with several kinds of "system alterers." A *stress overload in a crisis situation,* plays an important part in the destablilization of a system of reference or an information-processing system of a given "channel capacity." In the case of persons at risk for schizophrenia, this seems to be reduced considerably below the norm.

All *intense affects,* such as rage, fear, or joy, function as disorganizers; they can lead for brief moments to the sort of global transformation of feeling, thinking, and behaving that concerns us here. In conditions of more or less constant stress, such as exist in families with "schizophrenic transactions" or "high expressed emotions," they may do so for longer periods.

Similar distortions can clearly be produced by certain mainly *cognitive modifications,* such as *ideés fixes* or fanatically held beliefs. Wing has observed that all the central symptoms of acute psychosis are based on abnormal perceptions (such as changes in the size, shape, or color of objects; a distorted sense of time; or a peculiar clarity of certain impressions). Wing emphasizes that another group of delusional and hallucinatory symptoms is based on *changes of mood.*[48] On the basis of all this evidence it appears likely that every influence can be regarded as a disorganizer that leads to an imbalance between single affective or cognitive elements in the general equilibrated systems of reference that govern our behavior. Apart from psychoreactive and social influences, such effects can also be produced by biochemical or toxic means.

In the category of *biochemical disorganizers,* the dopamine or endorphin hypothesis suggests that endogenous substances play a role in schizophrenia. There are also exogenous hallucinogens, such as LSD, mescaline, scopolamine, psilocybin, and, to a certain degree, amphetamines, cannabis, and alcohol. The former category is definitely associated with the kind of distortions of affects and/or cognitive functions we are concerned with here. However, biochemical research, which has tended to concentrate on microscopic synaptic reactions, has strangely neglected the fact that practically all consciousness-altering drugs appear to influence rather global psychic processes. These have to do with, among other things, the perception of time and space, that is, with basic coordinates for all affective and cognitive functions. It is noteworthy that only slight shifts in such fundamental perceptual grids can cause great changes in the whole manner of our "being in the world" (to use Heidegger and Binswanger's phrase). It is no accident that phenomenologists, and Binswanger in particular, have always viewed distortions in the perception of time as an absolutely basic aspect of mania, depression, and schizophrenia.[49]

It is therefore likely that changing a person's "internal clock" could have a major effect on his entire feeling, thinking, and perceptions: slowing it down would lead to more relaxation, tranquility, and under certain conditions, to depression; whereas speeding it up would lead to more hectic activity and possibly to multiform states. In any case, every significant deviation from the accustomed "psychic tempo" in the direction of one extreme or the other immediately results in an altered relation to others and to reality in general. The same applies to deviations from the normal mobility of affect, or the focus of attention, such as may occur when one emotion persists for too long or when attention remains fixed to an excessive degree on unimportant details. At the other extreme, this applies when emotions change in rapid succession or when attention flits from one thing to another. The latter, combined with a slowing down or speeding up of the perceived passage of time, can be observed both in schizophrenics and in persons under the influence of hallucinogenic drugs.[50]

The ideas above suggest other mechanisms that might be involved in altering the equilibration of affective-cognitive systems of reference through the action of chemicals. One could be the selective activation or inhibition of a cerebral subsystem (such as the dopaminergic pathways); another could be a relatively nonspecific alteration of nervous excitability. (Chemical "system alterers" known as pheromones are probably involved in the "madness" of the passionate lover. Pheromones, aromatic substances signaling sexual receptivity, were first discovered in Central American moths. They are effective in unbelievably small quantities; a single molecule of this substance emitted by a female moth appears to be sufficient to attract a male from up to twelve miles away. In other words, it can alter his behavior—his system of reference—so thoroughly as to make him fly toward the signal, against the wind and any other obstacles, until he reaches the female and can mate with her. Recent research has discovered that such sexual aromas can have an intense effect on many animals and also on human beings.)

The question of how much we can learn about schizophrenia—the biochemical processes involved, its phenomenology, and the subjective experience of it—from drug-induced psychoses remains a controversial one. On the one hand, the fact that some states caused by amphetamines or LSD cannot be distinguished from schizophrenia suggests that the two are closely related. On the other hand, the frequent and apparently correct objection is raised that most drug-related psychoses present a psychopathological picture in many respects different from that of a genuine schizophrenic psychosis. For example, visual hallucinations usually predominate in an exogenous, drug-induced psychosis, whereas auditory hallucinations are more frequent in "endogenous" schizophrenia. Furthermore, the entire personality is clearly more deeply affected in schizophrenia, and the person's relation to reality is more seriously disturbed than is usually the case in experimentally induced psychotic states. (Despite all the hallucinations or delusions they may experience, participants in such experiments almost always manage to retain some awareness of the fact that they are taking part in a test, which can be broken off at any time or which will soon come to an end. Matussek has made the interesting observation that this is also usually true for delusions or hallucination experienced by people in complete isolation for long periods, such as polar explorers or sailors on solo ocean voyages.)[51]

One problem with these objections, however, is that they are based on rather naïvely reductionist ideas that do not take the interplay of biochemical and psychosocial factors sufficiently into account. This type of thinking tends to be found in the more exact experimental branches of science, which take a dim view of psychodynamic theories. It does not give enough consideration to the factor of time—drug-related psychoses last for hours or days, schizophrenic states for weeks or months—or to the influence of the altered psychosocial context in which schizophrenics find themselves. In "genuine" cases the appearance of psychotic symptoms goes hand in hand with a changed attitude toward the patient on the part of those around him; from the moment everything a person says, feels, thinks, or does is labeled "mental illness"—perhaps following a physician's diagnosis—it is devalued. Clearly this feedback will affect the patient's subjective experience, his self-confidence, and his sense of security; this can in turn influence the experience of psychosis and set a vicious circle going. Thus the only valid experimental strategy for comparing drug-induced psychoses and schizophrenia would be to give a subject a drug such as LSD for several weeks, *without his knowledge or the knowledge of anyone else around him, including all doctors and hospital staff;* but this would naturally be impossible for ethical reasons. In experiments that created quite a stir at the time, however, Rosenhan sent healthy test subjects to mental hospitals with complaints of hearing voices; despite otherwise perfectly normal behavior they were admitted and treated as schizophrenics for weeks. From these experiments we know that far less than a full-blown psychosis is sufficient to alter people's attitudes toward and perceptions of a person totally.[52] In such circumstances there can be no doubt that patients do not receive the type of normal feedback that constantly validates subjective experience. Yet according to my hypothesis of fragile systems of reference, this is precisely what persons at risk for schizophrenia need. Forms of genuine schizophrenia tend to develop in a pathological social milieu, in which autonomous thoughts, feelings, and behavior are not confirmed and esteemed but are instead devalued in a confusing and paradoxical manner. Thus chemical disorganizers very probably achieve their greatest pathogenic effect only in conjunction with a certain type of social context. Possibly further study of drug-induced psychoses will provide us with more information about the origin and subjective experience of schizophrenic states.

New insights into normal psychic functioning indicate that feedback mechanisms between the inner and outer worlds, and between feeling and thinking, operate in a complex manner. There is now some evidence that the altered perceptions of, for example, space and time caused by chemical disorganizers induce psychotic states mainly by interfering with and distorting this feedback. The effects of hallucinogenic drugs may thus be much closer to that of sensory deprivation that one might think at first. Experiments with radical exclusion of all sensory stimuli (in which subjects are kept immobile in total darkness, in soundproofed rooms, and in water maintained at body temperature, for example) achieve a cutoff of most of the environmental feedback (either positive or negative) that normally accompanies our perceptions, thoughts, and actions and provides a constant "commentary" on them. It has been known for a long time that perfectly healthy persons subjected to such deprivation will have distinct experiences of depersonalization, derealization, delusions, and visual and possibly auditory hallucinations after only a few hours. Such experiments may have real clinical significance, although when sensory deprivation occurs outside a laboratory other somatic, sociodynamic or psychodynamic factors (lack of communication, extreme conditions, hunger, thirst, or fever) will certainly be involved. The most spectacular example is prison psychosis after a long spell in solitary confinement, but similar states are known to occur among polar explorers, solo sailors, or people lost in deserts or the mountains. We also know from epidemiological studies and clinical observations that psychoses occur with statistically greater frequency in people who are socially isolated—such as immigrants, prisoners of war, and inmates of prison camps—if they have no contact with their own ethnic group or at least one significant other person. Certain near-psychotic or paranoid tendencies can be observed in many people who are hard of hearing, deaf-mute, or blind, and even after eye surgery, if the patient has had to spend several days immobilized in complete darkness. The most important type of feedback is the feeling—constantly provided by one's accustomed environment—of familiarity and "normality." This feeling usually accompanies all our perceptions without our being aware of it, and it is typically lost in the initial stages of psychosis. We can summarize these observations in terms fully consistent with the concepts of systems theory: *The psyche requires continual confirmation from without in order to maintain its normal structure and functions; in other words, the psyche represents an open, hierarchically structured system supported by numerous feedback mechanisms from its environment. The internalized functional processes of this system (affective-cognitive systems of reference) deteriorate rapidly if messages from the outside world fail to reach it or if they become radically different in character.*

Many authors have concluded from similar considerations that some psychotic symptoms such as hallucinations may be a kind of *compensation* for the lack of external stimuli. In the sensory-deprivation experiments mentioned above, for example, the participants were observed to develop a definite "craving for stimulation" after a time; if it remained unsatisfied, hallucinations took the place of the missing signals. Matussek reports on one experiment:

The subjects undressed and put a mask over their eyes; they then entered a pool that had water flowing through it at a constant temperature of 34.5° C. The only tactile stimuli were the mask itself and the bottom of the pool; all they could hear was their own breathing and the faint whirring of the water pump. Two subjects participated in the experiment and had received instructions to move about as little as possible. For the first three-quarters of an hour their thoughts were dominated by their daily concerns. Gradually the subjects began to feel peaceful and relaxed. During the following hour a "stimulus-action craving" slowly developed, and they made disguised attempts to provide their own stimulation by tensing muscles or making slight swimming motions. If the wish for more stimulation was not fulfilled, it began to seem impossible to continue with the experiment. Once they managed to get past this critical stage of intense longing for stimulation, the subjects suddenly became aware that thinking had given way to fantasies and dreams. Very personal images with a strong emotional coloring appeared. Two and a half hours into the experiment, one of the subjects noticed that the darkness had become three-dimensional and that strangely shaped objects with shining contours had gradually begun to appear in it. These bore a strong resemblance to the hallucinations that have been described in hypnagogic states.[53]

If experiments are continued for two or three days, the psychotic symptoms become more pronounced and less similar to normal experiences such as hypnagogic images. Schneider mentions, in a similar context, Platt's work on the role of "reafferent stimulation" in visual perception, which can function properly only via constant feedback between the inner and outer worlds.[54] Scheflen and other authors assume that certain regions of the brain, including the temporal lobe, are capable of developing autonomous activity in the absence of external stimuli; such messages are then transmitted to the cortex as if they were genuine external signals and create mistaken perceptions. Scheflen also refers to Jaynes's interesting speculations that hallucinations may have been normal occurrences in the prehistoric stages of human development, serving symbiotically functioning groups as a means of bridging the absences of their leaders, whose orders or instructions would be repeated in hallucinatory form.[55] He makes this point in connection with the observation that if schizophrenics are separated from another person with whom they have a symbiotic relationship, their hallucinations frequently increase.[56] Psychoanalysis assumes that a similar process occurs in "hallucinatory wish fulfillment," as when a small child sucks his thumb. Delusions or hallucinations also increase in the absence of activity or if activity is only routine; many patients will actually withdraw to a quiet place in order to experience them without being disturbed. It makes sense that such retreats into hallucination usually occur in situations of special stress—that is, they function as typical defense mechanisms; the more inconsistent and devaluing the echo from the outside world is, the more such withdrawal will lead to the construction of a compensatory inner world. Thus we may regard the tension-ridden and contradictory communication patterns discussed in the preceding chapter as a cause of particularly grave confusion in the harmonious interaction of a huge number of feedback mechanisms that are essential for normal psychic functioning.

Up to now we have gained a view of the psyche as a hierarchically ordered set of affective-cognitive systems of reference, which become equilibrated and structured over the course of development on the basis of experience, in a circular process of assimilation of and accommodation to the outside world. To this we may now add a view of the psyche as a highly complex set of interconnected feedback loops, by means of which the internalized systems receive constant reinforcement and are maintained in good working order, in a manner of speaking. Obviously such complicated "machinery," consisting as it does of somatic, organic, biochemical, sensory, affective, cognitive, and social components, can break down at many different points. Thus psychic disorganizers or "system alterers" can take many forms. Everything that disturbs the subtle interaction of intrapsychic mechanisms and the circular processes linking an individual with his environment can serve as a "disorganizer," producing such a state of tension within a system of reference that finding a new balance finally becomes imperative. In other words potential psychopathogenic mechanisms can cover a *whole spectrum, from organic, biochemical, and genetic influences to purely psychological and social influences. Such a broad spectrum not only appears plausible; we are virtually forced to postulate its existence.* What we have encountered here is a typical example of equifinality as it was defined in the discussion of systems theory in Chapter 1. It appears more and more likely that similar schizophrenic states can arise in a wide variety of ways. The old concept of a fixed disease entity with the same causes, symptoms, and progression in every case thus seems obsolete.

Ideas from systems theory and cybernetics also provide interesting insights concerning the energy involved in psychic "dis-orders." As was emphasized in Chapter 5, considerable amounts of energy are necessary to destabilize the carefully equilibrated states in which affective-logical systems of reference and behavior systems are maintained. According to his own account, Bateson became interested in the question of where this energy comes from when he was working as an anthropologist in New Guinea. To explain the escalation of certain social processes among groups there, he developed the concept of "runaway."[57] Bateson uses the example of a circular system of machinery similar to a steam engine: the faster the flywheel turns, the more fuel is provided, until the machine finally breaks down under the load. A good example of what is meant here is the fact—which we learned at school—that it is supposedly possible in theory to make a solid bridge collapse by applying the pressure of just one finger at the right place and at the right time, when it would increase an oscillation already present. Other examples from physics are avalanches, fires, and atomic reactions; in the area of human biology one instance would be sexual stimulation to the point of orgasm. Throughout his discussion Bateson emphasizes the importance of certain temporal rhythms, using the terms *oscillation* and *fluctuation*.

Schneider points out that Prigogine's "fluctuations" and "dissipative structures" are closely related to runaway and may also offer a possible explanation for the shift from one state of equilibrium to another. Both concepts are based on the principle of continuing positive feedback—of repeated reinforcement of certain reactions until a critical point is reached. This presupposes an open system with a constant energy supply. Prigogine consolidated such intuitive insights into an exact, scientifically verifiable theory after thirty years of research, for which he was awarded the Nobel Prize in 1977. Prigogine's theory offers the first generally applicable explanation for the way in which forms (or states of balance) in a lower order can naturally develop into forms of a higher order, in contradiction of the second law of thermodynamics, which predicts that disorder must inevitably increase (entropy). According to the excellent summary of this theory by Jantsch, this "order through fluctuation" works as follows: accidental fluctuations in open systems (which may be physical, chemical, biological, or social) are increased at one point by a continuing supply of energy until they cross a threshold of instability into a new dynamic regime, a new space-and-time structure.[58] Jantsch names as one of the simplest illustrations of this principle the "Bénard instability," which occurs when a thin layer of liquid is heated from a source underneath it:

The system moves further and further away from a state of equilibrium, that is, from a uniform temperature throughout. If the differences in temperature are small, the heat is transmitted by *conduction*. Beyond a critical difference, however, the heat is transmitted by *convection*. As a result convection cells of a regular shape, usually hexagonal, are formed. This structuring phenomenon corresponds to a *higher level of cooperation* between molecules. Before the onset of Bénard instability the energy of the system lies in the thermal energy of molecular motion; beyond the critical threshold, however, this energy takes in part the form of macroscopic currents containing a very large number of molecules.

Phenomena of this type, which occur far away from a state of equilibrium, have also been observed in the behavior of neuron groups and in the coding of sensory impressions. Jantsch continues:

If the imbalance between large, inactive neuron groups reaches a sufficient level, localized "active" states result. If further positive feedback occurs between the groups, these active states become unstable and can form dissipative structures, which can be registered in EEG patterns (of electrical brain waves). In particular a kind of limit-cycle behavior has been observed and associated with a decisive step in the coding of sensory impressions.

He then makes a point especially relevant to our topic: "If environmental impressions persist that *cannot be reconciled* with the dominant image, the dissipative structure can be forced through this instability into a new regime—*a new model of the situation*" (emphasis added throughout).[59]

It is certain that Prigogine discovered a general principle in these processes which is of the greatest significance for the evolution of life on earth, and which is also of interest in connection with my discussion of creativity in Chapters 3 and 5. Scholars in the social sciences and the humanities have recognized the usefulness of these ideas for their fields, and as far as I know Piaget was thoroughly familiar with them.

The cybernetic principles presented here as mechanistic for the sake of clarity are in reality principles of considerable complexity. Given this qualification, let us apply these notions to the dis-ordering of equilibrated affective-logical systems. Everyday experience teaches us that continued positive feedback can create a vicious circle in certain psychosocial processes until a breakdown is reached.[60] A simple example of this phenomenon, which Bateson calls "symmetrical escalation," is the way in which two people can escalate a disagreement until an actual fistfight occurs. Of course the destabilizing affective-cognitive "fluctuations" that may fuel psychotic disorders are not so simple; in addition they build up much more slowly and are not as visible as a brawl. Recent work in psychoanalysis and family dynamics has offered many suggestions about the specific phenomena which may be involved. Searles, in his famous 1959 essay, "The Effort to Drive the Other Person Crazy," described the disintegrating effect of rapid alternation between stimulation and frustration of sexual or other needs, constant shifts from one emotional "wave length" to another, and repeated jumps from one topic of conversation to another:

> For example, one deeply schizophrenic young man's mother, a very intense person who talked with machine-gun rapidity, poured out to me in an uninterrupted rush of words the following sentences, which were so full of *non sequiturs,* as regards emotional tone, that they left me momentarily quite dazed: "He was very happy. I can't imagine this thing coming over him. He never was down, ever. He loved his radio repair work at Mr. Mitchell's shop in Lewiston. Mr. Mitchell is a very perfectionistic person. I don't think any of the men at his shop before Edward lasted more than a few months. But Edward got along with him beautifully. He used to come home and say (the mother imitates an exhausted sigh), 'I can't stand it another minute!'"
>
> The now-deceased mother of another schizophrenic man was described by the patient's siblings as having been completely unpredictable in her emotional changeability; for instance, she would return from the synagogue with a beatific expression on her face, as though she were immersed in some joyous spiritual experience, and two minutes later would be throwing a kitchen-pot at one of the children. At times she was warm and tender to the patient, but would suddenly lash out at the child with virulent accusations or severe physical beatings. The patient, who at the time of my beginning therapy with him had been suffering from paranoid schizophrenia for some years, required more than three years of intensive psychotherapy to become free of the delusion that he had had not one mother but many different ones. He would object repeatedly to my reference to "your mother," protesting that he never had *one* mother; once he explained, seriously and utterly convincingly, "When you use the word 'mother,' I see a picture of a parade of women, each one representing a different point of view."[61]

Stierlin also points out the destructive effect of such phenomena. He describes typical escalating circles, both positive and negative, with reference to Wender's concept of "deviation-promoting feedback" and cites the case of a mother's abrupt shifts from excessive intimacy to hostile distance toward her seventeen-year-old daughter, who finally developed delusional psychotic symptoms.[62]

To summarize this discussion of acute psychosis I would like to report a case of my own that strikingly illustrates several of the mechanisms mentioned above.

Heinz was an unusually sensitive, imaginative, and artistically gifted boy of seventeen; his father was a scientist and his mother a musician. Partly because of his artistic interests he had always had a much closer relationship with his mother than his two brothers did. Now, however, the boy began to lead a more independent life; he ceased to appear punctually for meals and did not observe all the family rules. At a summer camp he showed an interest for the first time in a girl, a school classmate. When she rejected him, he discussed the situation with friends night after night, growing more and more upset and feeling misunderstood. In addition he began smoking hashish and horrified his family by striking up a friendship with a homosexual musician. At just this time he was on the point of finishing high school and needed to make some decisions about his future. He wavered between various scientific or technical alternatives, corresponding to his father's interests, and a career in music. On each of these subjects the whole family—but particularly the mother and son—developed conflicts with a typical double-bind structure, which were never openly discussed. (The boy was supposed to make his own decisions but still do exactly what his parents expected of him.) Heinz became increasingly tormented by an ambivalence that affected everything. He would approach first his mother, then the girl, then his homosexual friend; he was unable to decide on a future profession, began to skip school, stole money from home, and bought a set of drums. On one occasion, in an elevator, he embraced his mother with a vehemence that was partly erotic and partly aggressive. Then he climbed into his younger brother's bed several times and claimed that people were lying in wait for him in town and talking about him. He had the feeling that buildings were looking at him threateningly and began to hear voices, talk incoherently, and make geometric drawings in which he tried to symbolize his problems. In this state he was diagnosed as having a first schizophrenic episode and brought to me for treatment. I treated him for a number of years; in connection with choosing a profession and finding a girlfriend he suffered several similar psychotic episodes, each lasting several weeks. Finally, after family therapy, which concentrated on clarifying the conflicts *and* overcoming them, he was able to establish a stable relationship with a girl of about his own age, but who provided a kind of maternal support, and to begin a career as a musician. This stable condition has now been maintained for several years.

The most striking aspect of this case was Heinz's constant vacillation between a whole series of irreconcilable, contrary modes of experience. This vacillation increased during his psychotic phases and was also intensified by the efforts of his well-meaning but helpless parents. The most important of these opposing "worlds" or systems of reference were: infantile dependency versus adult independence, attachment to mother versus attachment to a sexual partner of his own age, identification with mother and an artistic profession versus identification with father and a scientific profession, and homosexuality versus heterosexuality. His situation was thus characterized above all by a pervasive ambivalence, associated with unsuccessful attempts to repress the one side or the other. (For example, Heinz kept his decision not to attend a technical school secret from everyone else for months, and to a certain degree even from himself.) As the preceding remarks suggest, the cardinal symptoms were his sensitive anxiety, tension, insecurity, and confusion; superimposed on them from time to time were acute psychotic manifestations such as experiences of being influenced, depersonalization, derealization, delusions, cognitive disturbances, and hallucinations; but these occurred only when he came under stress from several different sources at one time. Before his first acute episode these consisted of a first and unsuccessful romantic attachment, alienation from both parents and friends, contact with a homosexual, and an uncertain situation regarding his future combined with the pressure of final exams, lack of sleep, and the use of drugs. And despite the lack of a family history of schizophrenia, there was a definite fragility in the premorbid state of this sensitive young man, who possessed neither a robust constitution nor a firmly established identity. It seems likely that, in this case as in so many others, the fluctuations, which were both intrapsychic and interpersonal and kept in motion by family reactions and external events, affected the internalized self and object representations vital for maintaining a stable sense of identity and an adequate relationship to external reality. Searles provides drastic illustrations of what can happen when an insecure individual is confronted with contradictory communications and feedback from outside; in unfavorable circumstances these can lead in rapid succession to the activation and polarization of entirely contrary affects, thoughts, and ideas about oneself and others and about mutual relationships, tasks, and goals, which will veer back and forth between "all good" and "all bad." Massive disorganizers, both cognitive and affective, will "play off" against each other irreconcilable modes of thinking, feeling, perceiving, and behaving, destabilizing the "runaway" systems until both break down. Finally they are replaced by a new, psychotic system of reference and behavior system that can be regarded as analogous to Prigogine's "dissipative structures." It is possible that this new system of reference, the psychotic alternative, is unconsciously prepared or constructed bit by bit during the period when the extreme shifts from "all good" images to "all bad" are taking place. Once it has taken shape in the repeated extreme swings of the pendulum (borderline situations and states of mind), it can finally invade the sphere of consciousness and assume sole control of behavior. This would of course in no way exclude the possibility that, in addition to external, familial, or other psychosocial events, endogenous factors—either genetic, constitutional, or biochemical—are also involved in the process. One such factor could be a hereditary disposition toward abnormally strong psychophysiological reactions or emotions in one or more members of a family, as the results of some studies have suggested. For example, one particularly insightful schizophrenic patient writes of her situation:

> The largest problem I face—I think the basic one—is the intensity and variety of my feelings, and my low threshold for handling other people's intense feelings, especially negative ones. I have quite often experienced a euphoric "high" that is much like being in contact with some greater reality or meaning to life—accompanied by a kind of added brightness or extra dimension to everyday things around me. The other side of the coin, though, is a very intense anxiety from nowhere that typically hits me quite suddenly after a short period of time without medication. The two feelings are opposite, yet somehow connected.[63]

From the perspective of psychoanalytic ego psychology an abnormally low threshold at which agitation sets in represents one aspect of the specific ego weakness from which schizophrenics and those at risk for the disease suffer. Bellak and his associates have used ego-strength scales in careful comparative studies to determine other forms of ego function impairment, including disturbances in reality testing, forming judgments, drive control, cognitive functions, and the integration of complex information.[64] I have already mentioned the difficulties one patient had for months in certain situations in distinguishing hallucinations from reality, such as when she thought she heard someone in a café say, "She is a schizophrenic." If we recall the difficulties of reality testing for her, we can readily imagine how much more complicated the possibilities for escalation are when the attitude of the environment is confused, evasive, and contradictory *in actual fact.* If we add to this the fact that people in this environment may have good reason for covering up the realities of a situation (if a traumatic family event is not openly dealt with, for instance), then we can easily envision the likely results: a highly unstable, flickering state of shifting back and forth between different moods and thoughts, characterized above all by pervasive ambivalence. Such a situation must bring with it enormous *stress;* none of the available behavior systems provides relief; none reduces tension, and thus none can contribute to working through and coping with what has occurred. This "impossible" constellation is clearly the source of the energy that finally *compels* the person undergoing such stress to cross the threshold into a new system of behavior.

Here again we get a glimpse of the tremendous amount of energy that appears to lurk within paradoxes like a kind of "nuclear power." In this case it is negative, but we have already encountered its great *creative* potential if conditions are more favorable. The creative extraction of an invariance from two constructions that at first look very different not only reduces tension but also means that an optimizing "crossover" (Conrad) has occurred on a higher level of abstraction and development. One example of this would be the recognition that opposites such as good and evil, or love and hate, belong together and exist in feelings about oneself and others. This is exactly what the potential schizophrenic is not able to achieve, however, because of his fundamental ego weakness. Instead he evades "hard reality" (in Stierlin's phrase) in a manner that reduces tension but is at the same time a form of regression, a retreat into narcissistic, egocentric, magical, and animistic modes of perception and experience.

This brings us to the end of our exploration of acute psychosis and the mechanisms of disorganization that help to bring it about. Before we go on, I would like to add a few points that have interesting connections to an ongoing scientific debate.[65]

It is apparent that the source of energy that can destabilize an equilibrated physical or chemical system corresponds, on the psychic level, to the *information* (as defined in affective-logical terms) reaching the system of reference. This important insight could help us to recognize some illuminating parallels between biochemical and psychosocial processes. We can also see from our perspective—perhaps more clearly than from the perspective of the natural sciences—that *within* circumscribed systems of various hierarchical levels that arise contrary to a general tendency toward progressive disorganization, under certain conditions far from equilibrium, again homeostatic tendencies in the sense of the laws of entropy are at work to reduce tension and create more balance. In this "balance within imbalance" the irreconcilable opposition between entropic and antientropic forces which has often been postulated, and which poses so many riddles for modern science, appears to have been resolved in a strange manner: an increase in order (or tension, structure, or differentiation) at one point in the system appears to balance out general tendencies toward a decrease in order, so that on a higher plane paradoxical equilibrium is arrived at, namely an equilibrium between equilibrating and disequilibrating processes . . . Pursuing these ideas further would lead us too far afield, however.

The most important results of this discussion of acute schizophrenia can be summarized as follows:

Acute psychotic conditions may be regarded as disturbances and shifts of balance within large systems of reference; we may also view them as a sudden shift to differently structured affective-cognitive modes of functioning once a critical threshold has been crossed. In individuals at risk for schizophrenia this threshold is clearly much lower than in healthy individuals. Such shifts from one state of mind to another also occur in healthy persons, however, and the difference between such shifts and those of schizophrenics is only one of degree. Not only do many gradations exist, but there are also quite different stages or degrees of schizophrenic disorder, at least in the opinion of a number of authors. The stages display striking parallels, in phenomenological terms, to what occurs in an information-processing system of a given capacity, when progressive overloading will lead to a breakdown. From this perspective the central symptoms of psychosis are no longer indefinable primary or fundamental disturbances, but rather such common human reactions as tension, confusion, ambivalence, and anxiety, which have climbed to an abnormal level. Compared with the shifts from one state of mind to another in healthy individuals, the disorder of an acute schizophrenic psychosis is marked by a much higher degree of exclusion of other ways of feeling and thinking; it also lasts much longer, dissolves the normal boundaries between the inner and outer worlds, and reflects an expansion of an egocentric, autistic internal world at the cost of external reality. A further important aspect of psychosis appears to be a disturbance or distortion of the numerous mechanisms providing feedback from the environment, which are essential if the psychic apparatus is to function normally. It is precisely this set of feedback mechanisms that is affected by typical disorganizers so that it can no longer support and harmonize the interaction between internalized affective-cognitive systems of reference and the outside world, between feeling and thinking, body and mind. This makes the existence of a large number of potential disorganizers likely, extending from a psychosocial pole to a somatic and biochemical pole, but always producing similar symptoms. Among the possible disorganizers of unstable affective-logical systems of reference are stress resulting from ambiguous or paradoxical communication, excessive social demands, affective and cognitive imbalances of all kinds, and exogenous or possibly endogenous chemotoxic effects. These often occur in combination. Among the mechanisms in psychic disorganization that may play important roles are continued positive feedback and escalation processes between contrary modes of feeling, thinking, and behaving, analogous to Bateson's "runaway" principle or Prigogine's "fluctuations."

Chronic "Dis-Order"

We have now reached a point where we can ask some questions of great importance for the practice of psychiatry: How and why do some patients proceed to more or less rapid remission and cure, whereas others have frequent relapses or continue to suffer from residual effects of the disease? How and why does schizophrenia become chronic?

I mentioned earlier that only very few and unreliable criteria exist for predicting the long-term course or outcome of schizophrenia. The premorbid personality structure and a few characteristics of the early stage of the disease offer certain clues: the more stable the patient was before the outbreak of the psychosis, and the more acute and productive the initial symptoms, the better the prognosis as a rule. Other than that, however, we must watch as the disease runs its course in order to make a reasonably accurate judgment. Any type of pattern has a tendency to continue or to repeat itself; this holds true not only for the symptoms and course of single psychotic episodes but also for stabilized conditions and situations (such as social isolation or hospitalization) and for the long-term course, which may take the form of a persisting condition or of episodes occurring in waves, with strong or weak and regular or irregular fluctuations. One could speak in this connection, as I have suggested elsewhere, of a "principle of psychosocial inertia."[66] I have already noted that the predominant symptoms in chronic conditions are typically "negative" and "unproductive," that is, diametrically opposed to many symptoms of acute stages: the earlier tension, anxiety, and agitation give way to apathy and indifference. The former expansiveness has become narrow, strong affects grow blunted, the flow of words is replaced by silence, and the mood of anxiety or joyful exaltation is replaced by a nihilistic resignation. In the place of grandiose hopes we now find no expectations for the future at all.

Some authors of long-term studies, such as Huber and his colleagues, believe that the chronic conditions consist mainly in a "reduction of energy potential," reflecting a "basic process" of schizophrenia that they assume is a form of organic brain impairment. They are more and more inclined to view this loss of energy potential as a specific indicator of schizophrenia, citing the "basic symptoms" referred to above. Their arguments fall into three main groups. First, similar conditions can be observed in cases of cerebral injuries, in the form of a "post-traumatic reduction of brain activity," for example after injury to the skull. Second, in some cases they have found indications of brain atrophy in the form of pneumoencephalographically determined enlargement of the third brain ventricle. Third, they interpret the "thought disorders" of attention, focus, and so on, to which so much attention has been paid in recent years and which I discussed in Chapter 5, as evidence of organic disturbance.[67]

I have discussed this problem at length elsewhere and come to the conclusion that no convincing proofs exist for the organic origin of such chronic conditions, although we do have evidence suggesting that they must be viewed at least in part as the results of the acute psychosis, influenced by psychological and social factors. The findings on enlarged ventricles, for example, are irregular, restricted to a small subgroup, and still highly controversial.[69] As far as the thought disorders are concerned, they are more likely to be the expression and consequence of distorted forms of communication in the familial and social milieu of the patient than organic brain disorders in the usual sense. The system-of-reference hypothesis presented here suggests an interesting possibility for bridging the gap between the apparently irreconcilable somatogenic and psychogenic theories. According to the latest research, experiences of all sorts are registered and stored in the brain as specific dendritic and synaptic links. These experiences are also registered in internalized affective-logical systems of reference that, we have assumed, are confused in certain areas in individuals at risk for schizophrenia. Disturbed dendritic connections may thus be viewed as a form of "organic substrate." Findings in animals have shown that such connections are present in reduced number if external stimulation is withheld. It follows that even a certain amount of brain atrophy in chronic schizophrenics would not necessarily be evidence of an "organic process" in the traditional meaning of the term, but might be connected instead with a narrowing of their entire cognitive and affective field of experience, sometimes over a period of decades. It could also be the result of the tendencies to withdraw, the blunting of affect, and the psychosocial understimulation of which Wing speaks. Krüger develops exactly the same line of thought in his theory of "stimulation screening."[70] In any event we can hardly doubt that such connections will lead future researchers to regard the old and fruitless quarrel between proponents of "psychic" and "somatic" theories as unnecessary and out of date.

We have considerable positive evidence for the theory that important aspects of residual chronic conditions have a social origin; some of it is contained in Wing's work on "hospitalism," which I have already referred to.[71] These studies reveal losses of energy potential virtually identical with those of hospitalized schizophrenics in other long-term hospital patients (with the most varied and not necessarily psychiatric diagnoses), sanatorium patients, and prison inmates. In one of our own studies this condition was so prevalent among the patients who had been in institutions for many years that the original diagnoses of schizophrenia or other conditions, which had little to do with their behavior any more, had long since been forgotten by the hospital staff.[72] Ernst has also identified as "residual neurotic conditions" quite similar syndromes following severe cases of neurosis, physical illnesses, and stressful life events of all kinds.[73] Many authors very aptly refer to the typical and sometimes irreversible loss of vitality and elasticity that often occurs after particularly stressful experiences as the "broken spring syndrome," and a schizophrenic psychosis with all its consequences certainly represents one such experience. These authors usually associate the broken spring syndrome with organic causes, but those of us who have observed the humiliation and lack of understanding that people who have been labeled "schizophrenic" may encounter—not only in hopsitals but in society at large and sometimes even in their own families—are aware how resigned and demoralized some of them become. We have seen how many difficulties stand in the way of "rehabilitation," a term that has become standard usage for social reintegration, although the fact that it is borrowed from legal terminology speaks volumes. We have seen how so often, after several unsuccessful attempts, all those involved lose heart, not only the patient himself, but also his family, his doctor, and other mental health professionals. Whoever has observed this can have no doubt that the vital elastic spring of "energy potential" does not break solely as a result of organic processes in the brain. The undeniable fact that many of these residual chronic conditions do not improve even after a change of milieu or intensive social therapy is not a sufficient argument, in my view, for assuming the existence of a "basic disturbance" in the classical sense. For one thing we and all those involved in long-term studies can cite as counterevidence a certain number of cases of spectacular improvement even after decades of severe illness. On the other hand, we also know that psychological and social traumas can lead to irreversible damage, as the cases of former concentration camp victims demonstrate. Furthermore, an impoverishment of cerebral association networks, which may occur when the field of experience is severely constricted for decades, might not be reversible, especially in elderly patients, in the same way that inactive muscles atrophy. And last, the lack of energy evinced by patients who appear completely apathetic often proves to be merely a façade on certain occasions and may change with a change in their situation. It is a fatal effect of the principle of inertia that many patients with the typical signs of hospitalism protest vehemently against the slightest change in their surroundings, such as a different bed or room (not to mention larger changes such as a new kind of occupational therapy, a move to a new ward, or release from the hospital), even though it may appear advantageous to an outsider. As two of the case histories cited in the previous chapter illustrate, events of this kind can sometimes make it drastically clear that rigidity and apathy do not imply passivity, but instead represent a paradoxically active, powerful stance in a complex familial and social context in which circular communication prevails.

Additional but less obvious arguments for this point of view led me in a 1980 article to pose the challenging question: Is chronic schizophrenia perhaps not essentially a disease of the brain or any other organ, but in fact predominantly a psychosocial "artifact"? Not only has intense searching still not uncovered any organic substrate, but the role of hereditary factors (still the sole truly reliable indication of such a component) in chronic schizophrenia has been placed more and more in doubt by a number of recent findings. In long-term studies, including our own, little or no correspondence could be discovered between heredity and the actual course of the disease. Manfred Bleuler, whose work on schizophrenia in families uncovered only a few similarities in the *kind* of course the disease took, cites a large number of studies that arrived at much the same negative results.[74] In our own study a statistical comparison of the extreme groups—patients with three or more schizophrenics among their close relatives, as opposed to those with no history at all of schizophrenia or other mental illness in their families—revealed no significant differences in long-term course.[75] Although Kety and his associates found that secondary cases were more frequent among the relatives of chronic schizophrenics than in patients who suffered acute episodes of schizophrenia but recovered, the groups in this study were too small and were followed for too short a time to permit valid general conclusions.[76] In general we must regard the question of hereditary influence on chronic schizophrenia (in contrast to the outbreak of the disease) as still unanswered.

On the other hand, there is considerable evidence to suggest an influence of social factors. I shall mention only two, the familiar mechanism of the self-fulfilling prophecy and homeostatic family influences. The dynamic effect of future expectations probably contributed a great deal to what we observed in our study, and to other studies as well. The recovery of comparable chronic patients participating in rehabilitation programs was related to their own expectations and to those of their families and the mental health professionals looking after them. If these were all negative, recovery occurred much less often than if they were positive.[77] As far as family influences are concerned, as mentioned in the previous chapter statistical studies in Great Britain found that relapses occurred with significantly greater frequency in families whose partner relations were characterized by constant criticism and emotional overinvolvement ("high expressed emotions"). Recent research in family dynamics ranging from Searles, Bateson, and Laing to Boszormenyi-Nagy, Stierlin, and Selvini Palazzoli has also revealed that in many families there are (largely unconscious) mechanisms at work that tend to cement and perpetuate the dependent role of a family member as "patient" once he or she has fallen into it, and once it has been sanctioned by a professional diagnosis. The case histories of the two grown men still dependent on their mothers, cited in the previous chapter, provide striking illustrations of this phenomenon. Even if objective research on this latter concept is still insufficient, as critics correctly point out, clinical observation that takes events within the family into account reveals repeatedly that such mechanisms do exist and frequently play a fateful role.

The key question has been whether chronic schizophrenia is a "genuine" disease entity with an organic substrate or primarily (or entirely) a "social artifact," a pathological development arising from complex interaction between the patient and his environment. All in all I am of the opinion that we are not yet in a position to answer this question with scientific precision. Nevertheless, the indications that environmental influences play a decisive role so far outweigh the few and relatively hypothetical somatic factors that we should modify not only our view of the disease but also our therapeutic practices to take this into account. It used to be assumed that chronic schizophrenia resulted either completely or in the main from a basic organic process comparable to progressive syphilitic paralysis. If this is not the case, however, if chronicity on the contrary represents predominantly a reaction to ongoing life experience in vulnerable individuals (who have suffered one or more acute psychotic episodes and retain a disposition toward this form of decompensation throughout their lives), we must radically revise our view of schizophrenia: we must replace the idea of an all but inescapable fate with that of the interplay of virtually unlimited social, situative, and psychological influences, but also of somatic, constitutional, and genetic influences, both favorable and unfavorable. Not only does this open up almost as many possible avenues for therapy, but also it enables us better to understand the schizophrenic individual himself and a number of previously unexplained phenomena with which clinicians must contend daily. By this I mean the unpredictable variety of long-term developments, the surprising improvements that occasionally occur after long illness, the lack of reliable criteria for an individual prognosis, and the almost complete failure of somatic treatments, including neuroleptics, in chronic cases with unproductive symptoms. Here, taken from our long-term study, is one example of many indicating the difficulty of foreseeing how a patient will develop:

A tailor, born in 1879 into a family with a history of mental illness and character disorders, had an unstable work history and extreme inhibitions regarding contacts with women in the premorbid phase. He began to exhibit delusional tendencies in his late thirties, in the train of a broken engagement and work-related problems. Eventually he gradually developed extensive delusions of persecution and external influence, dominated by sexual themes. (He claimed that his neighbors were persecuting him after having used mirrors to observe him masturbating, and that poachers disturbed his sleep every night while gutting the animals they had caught, and so on.) He had auditory hallucinations of machines, of rapping on the walls, and later of voices that commented on his behavior and gave him orders. He broke into the apartment of a woman following these orders, and was admitted to our hospital in 1925 for the first time, at the age of 46. Later he was transferred to a clinic in his home town, from which he was not released until 1936 (at the age of 57), when his delusions, hallucinations, transient monomania, autistic and oppositional behavior, and sense of external influence had spontaneously subsided. He then moved in with his brother and took up work as a tailor again, showing no disruptive behavior apart from occasional quarrels with relatives.—When we visited him in the course of our follow-up study in 1967, 42 years after his first hospitalization, we encountered a physically and mentally active 88-year-old man, who had been living alone since his brother's death but maintained frequent contacts with nieces, nephews, and several friends. He had continued his work as a tailor until the age of 85 and was still taking care of his own household. He received us in a friendly manner, made good contact with the interviewer, and demonstrated excellent powers of memory for the distant past, although his short-term memory was slightly impaired. He referred to his past delusions as "things he had imagined while he was sick," and although he had some criticisms to make of his doctors and others in his environment at that time, he had clearly made his peace with them. He displayed no traces at all of his earlier psychosis, apart from a pedantic, almost obsessional love

of order and fairness and a certain rigidity and stereotypy in his thinking. Throughout his whole life he had never had any sexual contact
with women, but this had ceased to bother him many years ago.[78]

Our point of departure was the question: How are we to understand
such recoveries, or the acute relapses and chronic states that also occur, in the light of the previously described mechanisms of psychic
distortion that lead to the first outbreak of disease? We have assumed
that the different stages or degrees of psychic disorder represent altered affective-cognitive states of equilibrium, systems of behavior,
and modes of thought, achieved after phases of instability; these
might be compared to the different gears of an engine or the different
grids of an information-processing system. If this assumption is correct, then the "psychosocial principle of inertia" postulated above
would lead us to expect that a condition once reached will tend to
persist. Such a condition always represents a reduction of tension,
that is, the best and most energy-efficient way available for ordering
reality at any given moment (with a psychotic condition resulting if
reality has become unbearably contradictory, for example). For reasons of economy alone, and with a certain independence of reality, a
tendency will prevail for this condition to stabilize. Both clinical observation and modern crisis intervention theory confirm this. A certain amount of energy is necessary to dislodge a disordered system
and bring about the leap back into a normal mode of functioning; the
disordered system of reference must be destabilized again and reor-
dered, reversing the procedure of what happened before. One example of what this means in specific terms was illustrated in the
(highly unusual) case of the hebephrenic young man from our day
clinic who recovered to a surprising extent after being given a stern
talking-to. The following example, which anticipates some of the
ideas to be discussed in the next chapter, is taken from a short article
I published in 1979 on a "technique for provoking crises" in patients
whose chronic condition is so rigidified that no change by other
means appears possible:

> Mrs. X, a paranoid 51-year-old former schoolteacher, had spent years
> in a hospital ward for the chronically ill; she was withdrawn and anx-
> ious. She suffered from some residual symptoms but above all from a
> severe case of hospitalism. Through a tacit agreement with the staff and
> other patients she had acquired a monopoly on all "domestic chores"
> on the ward. Delusional fears of rain and snow prevented her from

leaving the hospital even in the nicest weather; she refused to travel by car or train or to let a dentist treat her badly decayed teeth. In general she resisted any slight change in her daily routine. After all other attempts had failed we intentionally provoked a severe anxious-depressive crisis by transferring her to a rehabilitation ward run on entirely different lines, withholding permission for her to perform her accustomed household tasks, and putting pressure on her to consent to dental treatment in which all her teeth were extracted. This crisis was a turning point, which was used by two staff members, a nurse and a social worker, to establish a strong supportive relationship with the patient. They initiated behavioral therapy with practical exercises that involved going outside the hospital, using public transportation, making small purchases, and so on. After a few months they were able to persuade Mrs. X to move into a family boardinghouse in the city, where she has since blossomed in an amazing fashion. She is now active and mobile and will soon begin working as an aide in a nursing home.[79]

Whether a destabilized schizophrenic system will in fact return to normal under pressure or whether, as Scheflen and Conrad suggest, it will progress to an even more pathological state probably depends on quite complicated factors. According to crisis-intervention theory the circumstances of the crisis itself and the influences to which the patient is exposed at this time are of considerable importance. Slight changes occurring at the right moment can have unexpected long-term effects. From a therapeutic point of view it is thus essential in destabilized situations to be able to polarize the entire psychosocial field with a particular goal in mind. It will also be important to determine if the change that this goal represents will reduce tension to a sufficient degree. Obviously if a previously confused or stress-ridden atmosphere in a patient's family or work environment, which contributed to the illness, is allowed to continue, it will make recovery more difficult; on the other hand, a new constellation can contribute to recovery. In addition, much depends on the nature of the relatively healthy systems of reference or behavior (both the patient's own and those of the people around him) that were constructed before his illness and continue to exist in latent form: What are they like? How long have they been out of use? How rigid or flexible, satisfying or unsatisfying was the patient's former state compared to his new (ill) one? The prognostic criteria mentioned above are in all likelihood connected with such factors. In our study of rehabilitation we observed that the patient's initial, subjective dissatisfaction with his social situation was a significant predictor: chronic patients who were content with their lot usually fared far worse in rehabilitation programs than did discontented patients.[80] The likelihood of a relapse after remission depends on corresponding factors: How solid is the foundation of the disturbed behavioral system, which also continues a latent existence during a period of remission? How long did it dominate the patient's behavior, and how much time has elapsed since? And how easy is it for the patient to fall back into such behavior? (We know that some former mental patients need only be stopped once by the police for some small incident of conspicuous behavior, for example, for them to require rehospitalization for months or even years. Once back in an institution, they revert to their previous form of disturbed behavior, just as if nothing had happened in the meantime.) In many cases the patient's whole familial and social constellation will be of crucial importance. All too frequently, unfortunately, we see that a certain patient's chronic condition (perhaps stabilized by long hospitalization) has been accepted by his entire social environment, until the two fit like hand and glove. Relatives and legal and social institutions may have grown used to the situation and even dependent on it, not the least for financial reasons involving insurance or retirement benefits.*

Any real change in such a constellation, which may have been functioning for years, would require immense effort and mean disruption in the lives of many people. It is thus not surprising that everyone involved—and not least the patient himself—often desires to maintain the status quo at any price.

I am aware that the ideas developed here do not offer a complete solution to the question of how schizophrenia progresses. In this area the reality is always more complex and variable than any schematic construct. Though provisional, however, what I have said here is consistent with the rest of the theory presented and can, as we shall see, be of use in practical therapy.

---

* *Translator's note:* In Switzerland and other European countries with well-developed health insurance and pension plans, families may have an economic incentive to keep an elderly relative in a mental hospital. An elderly person drawing a retirement pension would have to use that pension toward the expense of a normal nursing home, for example, whereas the cost of hospitalization in a mental institution would be covered by health insurance, leaving the patient's relatives free to collect his pension. Psychiatrists in such countries are not infrequently confronted by families seeking to institutionalize an elderly relative of perfectly sound mind, simply for the resulting financial advantage to themselves.

Summary: A New View of Schizophrenic Dis-Order

If we recall the three major stages of schizophrenic disorders—the premorbid phase, the phase(s) of acute psychosis, and the resulting chronic conditions—we arrive at the following general view: Certain individuals demonstrate a special type of vulnerability and sensitivity that is probably in part inborn and in part acquired. Like other members of their family they are often nervous, overreact in some situations with defensiveness and withdrawal, tend to feel insecure and inferior in dealing with others, and are frequently overdependent on a relationship with another person (symbiosis). Under stress they may easily become anxious and confused in interaction with the environment; they become distracted, disorganized, and fail to cope adequately with difficult situations. In particular, they become unable to focus attention, to think sequentially, and to construct correct categories. Under favorable conditions, however, some of these individuals may be more original, sensitive, and artistically creative than average.

If all goes well, many such people are able to lead normal lives, and sometimes even particularly rich and fruitful lives, despite—or just because of—these qualities, which also have *positive* aspects. Many others, however, spend their lives on the brink of collapse, seeking safety and grasping at straws; they retreat into a small, protected corner; their moods are unstable and they may show signs of psychotic reactions from time to time (variations of borderline personalities). They have great difficulty dealing with complex situations of stress (or complex information, in a wide sense) especially those requiring change and adaptability. They are particularly helpless when it comes to affective and cognitive contradictions in the area of interpersonal relations. Unable to see through them and to defend themselves, they often let themselves be manipulated by a stronger partner.

If a variable number of unfavorable factors comes together (personality structure, degree of vulnerability, general life situation, family constellation, special conditions at the time of the illness, a succession of stressful events, interaction with the environment), some of these people will experience a psychotic crisis; statistically they make up about one percent of the population. Even if the level of stress appears normal to others, for these individuals the state of tension will become unbearable and lead to progressive decompensation in the form of anxiety, ambivalence, and affective-cognitive confusion, finally reaching the point at which experiences of derealization and depersonalization, delusions, hallucinations, and other symptoms of psychosis occur. The energy necessary to produce such dis-order in the early precarious psychological equilibrium of individuals thus disposed appears to originate at least in part in positive feedback loops that escalate the tension between irreconcilable systems of thinking and feeling ("runaways," "fluctuations"). This imbalance is furthered by the vehemence of the individual's own affects and the contradictory reactions and injunctions reaching him from his environment. The altered modes of thinking, feeling, and behaving are to be understood as altered states of balance within comprehensive affective-cognitive systems of reference. They represent structures formed to decrease the tension that cannot be dealt with in any other way; these alternative structures have been gradually assembled as the individual is repeatedly pushed to the limits of what he can endure, and they finally take over his whole behavior, sometimes quite abruptly. Various stages of this dis-order exist, all characterized by a mounting degree of disturbance in the complex set of feedback reactions existing between the inner and outer worlds. From this perspective psychotic modes of behavior appear to be one aspect of a generally disturbed field of communication. Certain psychotic productions such as hallucinations or delusions may represent autistic substitutes for missing or distorted elements in a disordered global feedback system.

Such pathological modes of functioning have a certain inertia and obey their own laws; whether they become established, gradually disappear, or progress to even more psychotic conditions depends on a large number of factors, both internal and external. As I shall try to show in the next chapter, a great deal depends on how much understanding the schizophrenic receives from those around him and on the therapeutic steps taken; in other words, the social and psychological environment at this stage is decisive. In favorable circumstances a rapid and complete cure may be effected, although even at best the individual will remain fragile and vulnerable. In fact, since pathological patterns of behavior have become dominant on one occasion and will continue to exist in latent form, this vulnerability may even have increased. And we do know that several psychotic episodes may occur in succession with complete recovery after each one. If conditions are not favorable, however, the psychosis will become firmly established and chronic. Among such unfavorable circumstances are a long period of hospitalization, loss of social and professional contacts, several unsuccessful attempts to return to normal life, and an unsupportive family constellation. Residual conditions of varying degree will persist in these cases; pathological mechanisms from the acute phase will be carried over and become dominant or customary reactions, which can then be used to avoid meeting new demands if the level of stress should rise again. As the patient is demoralized by failed attempts to recover and by repeated setbacks, he develops more and more passivity, resignation, and listlessness, which also begin to affect those around him. His horizons narrow and he loses interest in things; future expectations give way to almost permanent indifference, interrupted by only brief flashes of attention. Such states can last for years or even decades and represent the fully developed "broken spring" or "clinical poverty syndrome." Whether organic factors are involved in such a condition must remain an open question for the time being. Recent research suggests that extreme impoverishment of the entire psychosocial field of experience in confined circumstances (chronic understimulation) might be reflected organically in an atrophy of cerebral association systems. Under certain conditions, however, which may be therapeutically induced or may occur spontaneously, surprising recoveries can occur even after years of stagnation. The loss of "energy potential" is reversed or disappears, and from behind the rigid, distorted façade of the chronic psychotic there emerges a sensitive, insecure human being, who in some cases has developed a characteristic form of ironic humor.

I postulated earlier that only the acute dis-order is actually specific to schizophrenia and the core of the disease, and everything else is only preparatory to or results from the acute phase(s). This claim should now appear in a clearer light. Of course other factors always play a role, which may be genetic and specific to the patient's personality or related to the dynamics of his family life. However, such factors are also present in cases in which no schizophrenia occurs. In other words, what some authors have described as a "basic disturbance" (Huber) or a "nonpsychotic schizophrenia" (Scheflen) does not seem to me to be a disease as such, but rather a possible variant of human modes of behavior that can range with gradual transitions from robust imperturbability at one end of the scale to a pronounced disposition toward psychotic reactions at the other end. Such reactions will occur when a person's tolerance threshold is exceeded, a point that varies considerably from individual to individual. In principle everyone is capable of psychotic behavior under the "right" conditions. Figure 8, adapted in part from the views of Manfred Bleuler, presents a schematic overview of these related factors.[81] This overview corresponds to the picture of schizophrenia that has been devel-

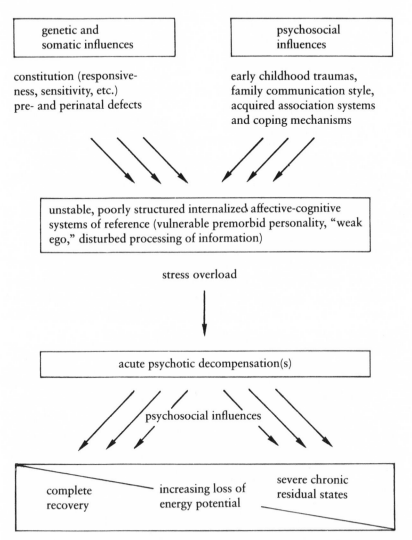

Figure 8.   A synoptic representation of the schizophrenias from the perspective of affect-logic (adapted in part from Manfred Bleuler, "Einzelkrankheiten in Her Schizophreniegruppe?" in *Schizophrenie: Stand und Entwicklungstendenzen der Forschung,* ed. G. Huber, Stuttgart and New York: Schattauer, 1981).

oped in several places with slight differences of emphasis on the basis of recent research, in particular the extremely systematic, pragmatic, and creative work of the London school. It thus participates in current attempts to categorize and summarize the enormous amount of detailed information available on schizophrenia under a more comprehensive perspective.

Before describing in detail the particular contribution that affect-logic can make to these efforts, I would like to summarize briefly one of the most comprehensive attempts at such a synthesis made in the last few years, that of Albert Scheflen in his book *Levels of Schizophrenia,* published posthumously in 1981. Using systems theory as a foundation, Scheflen examines the phenomenon of schizophrenia on eight different levels: society, institutions, the family, symbiosis and dyads, the individual, the central nervous system, metabolism and brain physiology, and neuronal and dendritic organization. On the first level schizophrenia appears to him as a form of social deviance that functions in a particular manner to bolster and equilibrate social norms. In order to deal with this deviance society uses a network of institutions on the second level (including the fields of medicine and psychiatry, hospitals, and support organizations), all of which serve to limit and stabilize the deviance and to keep it under control. On the third level of the family he views schizophrenia—much as I described it in the preceding chapter—in a context of relationships, dependency, coalitions, and oppositions between family members, with correspondingly complex and sometimes contradictory forms of communication. Scheflen also places special emphasis on the importance of the fourth level, a symbiotic dyadic relationship between the schizophrenic child (or the child at risk) and another family member, usually the mother. He makes the interesting point (which to my knowledge no one else has expressed so clearly) that it is often precisely when this symbiosis is disrupted that acute psychotic decompensation results. On the fifth, individual level Scheflen mentions the classic psychopathology and many accompanying somatic and psychomotor disturbances that are frequently overlooked; he also stresses the difficulty experienced by schizophrenics in performing sequential operations, in connecting these operations in a proper context, and in modulating affects in harmony with such a context. On the sixth level of the central nervous system, Scheflen discusses schizophrenia in terms of a disturbance in the integration of frontal, temporal, and limbic functions, whose interaction breaks down completely when florid psychotic decompensation occurs. On the seventh level, there are situated in the same regions the humoral disturbances that biochemists and brain physiologists today believe consist in dysfunction of the neurotransmitters dopamine and noradrenaline. On the last level of neurons and dendrites Scheflen emphasizes the significance of the recent discovery that experience can lead to the formation of new synaptic connections, a discovery that does away with the traditional distinction between "organic" brain disorders and those that are merely "functional": since in all probability every new acquisition of cognitive or affective experience leads to the formation of a corresponding dendritic network, the fine neuronal structure of the brain must necessarily vary according to individual experience, the way in which this knowledge is integrated, and the habits of thinking and feeling that are then established. This formulation of the situation represents only a slight extrapolation from Scheflen's ideas, and it should be obvious that it corresponds quite closely to the ideas presented in the previous chapters of this book. Of particular importance, in my opinion, is Scheflen's observation that establishing causal connections on one level (such as the genetic, biochemical, or other somatic level) by no means negates the significance of psychological or social factors. Only if we expand our view to include all these components can we avoid the error of monocausal reductionism, to which the narrow approach taken by specialists in one field or another has repeatedly led.

Scheflen's hypothesis of a four-stage development of schizophrenic psychoses maintains that on the basis of cognitive functioning and modulation of affects related to a symbiotic relationship, cortical and limbic functions grow more and more unstable or disintegrate as a result of continued positive feedback. As this process continues, a series of increasingly severe clinical states is reached that corresponds quite well to Kraepelin's subgroups of "simple," paranoid, hebephrenic, and catatonic schizophrenia. These successive stages would also reflect a progressive lack of functional differentiation. Conrad reached startlingly similar conclusions in many areas; he considered chronic states as being affected by a reduction of energy potential, which he saw as a loss of drive associated with the functions of the frontal lobe. Recent evidence from tests using PETT scans showing a reduced blood circulation in the frontal lobes of chronic schizophrenics appear to confirm this hypothesis.[82] If these preliminary findings, which are based on only a very small sample, should be substantiated, this certainly does not mean that we ought to neglect the psychological and social components of this loss of drive. As part of a circular process they contribute to a lasting reduction of cerebral functions, which can lead in turn to a lessening of general interest in the outside world.

Scheflen's survey is impressive and convincing on many points. However, large parts of it remain more of a synopsis than a true synthesis; the various aspects of the subject are juxtaposed but not really connected. A real synthesis would not only have to explain further the interplay of the different factors on all levels but also subsume them under one comprehensive theory. One such example of a comprehensive scientific theory today is Niels Bohr's unified theory of atomic structure and configurations, and the functional properties of atoms and molecules based on them, which has served to clarify the most varied micro- and macroscopic phenomena in the fields of biology, physiology, chemistry, and physics.

We remain far short of a comparable position of insight into psychological processes. Nevertheless, the current tendency to integrate the available information, including that assembled by Scheflen, into one general theory provides grounds for hope. The concept of affect-logic and the related systems-of-reference hypothesis represent a step toward this more comprehensive understanding and take us beyond Scheflen on some points. This step can be summarized as follows.

We have established the hypothesis that affective-cognitive systems of reference (or schemata, programs) are built up on an inborn substrate in the brain as a result of experience. Both biological (for example, genetic) and psychosocial factors can thus contribute to create a particular vulnerability. The human brain is extraordinarily "plastic"; that is, the path its development takes is affected to a large degree by external influences. In certain areas of their total experience (presumably mainly in the field of interpersonal relations), individuals at risk for schizophrenia seem to have formed unstable and confused systems of reference, which become destabilized under stress and establish a new equilibrium, the "dis-order" of acute psychosis. This model seems to me to integrate more hard evidence and plausible surmises about the nature of schizophrenia than any other I have encountered: it contains ample room for hereditary, constitutional, biochemical, physiological, and somatic influences as well as psychogenic and sociogenic factors of all kinds. It thus appears to mesh with the latest findings of all the above-mentioned disciplines and to conform to the multicausal thinking now so prominent in much of modern science. We have further formulated the theory of the psyche as an equilibrated, hierarchically structured affective and cognitive double system; in this view the psyche develops and acquires differentiation through a process of abstraction, the extraction of invariances, which are then stored in corresponding cerebral association networks. One advantage of this approach is the possibility it offers to narrow the gap between the material substrate (physical or chemical processes in the brain) and intellectual or psychological phenomena. In addition this model is fully consistent with the principles of systems theory. In combination with psychoanalytic insights, the dynamics of affective as well as cognitive and psychosocial phenomena can be included in the theory to the full. We have also created a plausible link between individual, intrapsychic events and interpersonal, familial processes.

This same theory also integrates a great many psychopathological clinical observations. It subsumes all the facts (known to me) concerning the various stages of development of schizophrenia (or the schizophrenias) under one unified heading, thus offering an explanation for their enormous variety while still leaving room for new findings.

And finally—what is perhaps most important—this model, though highly theoretical in part, brings us closer to understanding the individual schizophrenic human being, by replacing the long-prevailing view of his disturbance as something utterly strange and remote with a concept of the disease as a peculiarly intensified and distorted form of normal, (almost) everyday experience. I shall try to show in the final chapter that this opens new avenues for practical therapeutic activity.

Before going on to this subject, however, I would like to add one important qualification to the summary above. Many parts of this theory are nothing more than an outline or sketch: I have endeavored to take the realities of scientific research into account, but I have also filled in gaps in our knowledge with speculations about how things might be. Much of what I have said still lacks firm evidence to back it up; some of the ideas presented here may turn out to be correct, and others will prove false. I do believe that one aspect of my approach that will remain valid is its general direction, which understands human beings, whether healthy or sick, always as both body *and* mind, individuals *and* social beings and at the same time places the human psyche—that is, our feelings, thoughts, and actions, including all technology, civilization, and culture—once again in its proper framework: the framework of *nature* and its fundamental laws, even though much of their beauty still remains hidden to our eyes.

7 Consequences for Therapy

With what do we actually live,
Where do we experience life,
If not with our feelings?

—Hermann Hesse,
Nuremberg Journey

This chapter will show what bearing the ideas discussed up to now can have on the practice of therapy. This discussion will be far from comprehensive, since my goal has not been primarily to develop new procedures and techniques, but rather to strive for a better understanding of certain aspects of the human mind. Nevertheless, some practical consequences have emerged from the theoretical discussion; and in fact some conclusions appear compulsory, even if this result was not my main intention. The resemblance of some of these conclusions to recent trends in quite different schools of thought is an interesting, and certainly not coincidental, phenomenon.

General Therapeutic Principles

What follows is designed, like the rest of this book, to refer mainly but not exclusively to the treatment of schizophrenic and other related disorders. If it has a more general application, then this is connected with the fact, which Manfred Bleuler has repeatedly emphasized, that no form of treatment for schizophrenia alone can exist: whatever is favorable for the psychological growth and maturity of human beings in general will also help schizophrenics, and vice versa.[1] The preceding chapters should have made it clear that schizophrenics do not "have" a disease in the way that we can (supposedly) "have" the flu, or rheumatism, or even an organic cerebral problem such as progressive syphilitic paralysis, some of the symptoms of which are not dissimilar to schizophrenia. Schizophrenics and people at risk for schizophrenia are first and foremost vulnerable individuals who in certain circumstances become tense and confused more easily than others and, as a result of many interacting forces, finally develop the symptoms of psychosis. They do not differ from "healthy" or "normal" people in any fundamental respect, and thus it follows that whatever is "good for" or "not good for" others in principle will have a similar effect on schizophrenics.

We should also keep in mind that we are dealing in the main not with a *disease*, but rather with a particular *person* in a *situation* that is contributing to his illness. The strong links between the psyche (or psychosis) and the environment that have become apparent in these chapters are probably the most important result of this study, both theoretically and practically. All the pieces of information collected here point to the conclusion that we cannot begin to understand—let alone treat—either the healthy or the unhealthy psyche apart from a social context. The psyche is formed from the very beginning in close interaction with a particular milieu; depending on what it encounters, it acquires a clear or confused structure. As the discovery of the significance of feedback mechanisms has shown, the psyche relies at every moment on what is occurring in the world around it, to a much greater degree than we had assumed before. The dynamic effect of expectations generally held about a person shows further that even his future development is determined to a large extent by his interaction with his surroundings ("self-fulfilling prophecies"). It should be obvious that these circumstances contain, in addition to the possibility for pathological developments, great therapeutic potential as well. Yet to realize this potential represents an incomparably larger task than the prescription of medication or individual psychotherapy. The first general conclusion we must draw is that such procedures have a relatively small chance of success if used alone, since they disregard many of the most important factors. This conclusion is supported not only by everyday clinical observations but also by many statistical findings.[2]

A number of further consequences arise as a result. One key question is how the patient's *social milieu* should be constituted so as to have a healing instead of a pathogenic effect. It is far easier to answer this question in theory than in practice. In theory, as we have seen, many things can lead to psychotic confusion: ambiguity and contradictions of all kinds, particularly in existentially crucial areas such as the family situation, relationships with parents, strivings for autonomy, the choices of a profession and a life partner. It then follows that creating clarity in the same areas ought to reduce confusion and tension. Some central goals in establishing this clarity are (1) to draw unequivocal lines between the generations in the family and to break up any dysfunctional alliances, such as a symbiotic relationship between one parent and a child directed against the other parent; (2) to promote the children's growth toward independence and emancipation, to establish any explicit arrangements that may be necessary to achieve this, and to see that all family members consent to abide by them; (3) to discuss and expose conflicts existing in this regard, if necessary, and to seek constructive solutions; and (4) to strive for the gradual transference to the children of responsibility for themselves. These goals are recognized by most schools of family therapy and are based on a view of fundamental stages of development in the human life cycle as understood by Erik Erikson and others.[3] They consist of basic affective-cognitive tasks in childhood and puberty, choosing a profession and spouse, establishing a family, raising children, middle age, the roles of parent-in-law and grandparent, old age, and death. Authors such as Minuchin and Haley have given us superb descriptions of how such developmental problems can be dealt with in practice, and I shall return to several specific aspects of this therapeutic approach as we go on.

To be successful, however, the aim of therapists to establish unambiguous situations will need to include far more than the patient's immediate family. The entire field of social experience is important, including the work sphere and significant personal relationships outside the family. As I will try to show later, the therapeutic setting—meaning both the institutional infrastructure and the creation of integrated programs of treatment—is also a key area. When the latter exist at all, they usually lack a clear framework and continuity, a point I have discussed elsewhere.[4] Only by keeping the institutional structure as uncomplicated as possible—such as personnel, administration, finances, use of space—and striving for clarity in the other essential areas mentioned above can we effectively counterbalance the confusion in which many schizophrenics operate and which they bring with them to the therapeutic situation. This confusion arises partly as a result of their pathological family dynamics and partly from their reduced capacity to deal with complex information. The professional team treating such patients represents a central element in their social milieu and can have an enormous influence, either positive or negative. To be able to work effectively, this team has an urgent need for institutional continuity and clarity. Their ability to go about their job in a secure and goal-oriented atmosphere will awaken a corresponding confidence in patients and their families, allowing them to develop the realistic positive expectations that recent research has shown to be so important.

In the best of cases the social field of the schizophrenic patient will be poorly structured and confusing; in the worst it will be rigidified and severely counterproductive. In all cases, we might compare effective therapy to the action of a magnet on a field of scattered iron shavings: the entire field must be polarized so that a clear pattern and lines of orientation are created along which, in the end, all the participants will be able to proceed. In other words, the primary aim of therapy must be to establish *explicit and specific common goals* for the patient, such as moving into a halfway house or his own apartment, beginning a training program, or finding a job. The goals must be worked out among the patient, his family, the therapeutic team, and any other people involved in the patient's care; an essential part of the therapy will be devoted to negotiating a commonly accepted *therapeutic contract*. It is not easy to achieve such an ideal in practice, of course, and innumerable difficulties will be encountered along the way. I shall return later to measures that can help to reduce problems of an organizational nature.

Some further general principles of treatment can be derived from the view of acute psychosis as what occurs when particularly sensitive individuals with a reduced capacity to process information are *overstimulated,* and from the related view of chronic conditions as the result of understimulation. According to this, treatment should consist in finding the *optimal level of stimulation:* When acute productive symptoms (tension, anxiety, confusion, agitation, experiences of depersonalization and derealization, thought disorders, delusions, and hallucinations) appear or increase, the main aim should be systematically to reduce psychosocial demands on the patient. Such demands may stem from his work situation, contacts with other people, other sources of excitation and change, amount of information to be absorbed, and so on. What we have learned about the effects of feedback mechanisms and other environmental influences makes it clear that for the confused and hypersensitive psychotic the physical and social character of his surroundings and the way in which people deal with him will have great significance: ideally they should all provide a sense of relaxation and tranquillity. This is a far cry from the usual atmosphere in the emergency rooms of large hospitals and mental institutions where acute psychotics are normally seen first. Unfortunately, high doses of tranquilizing medication are often seen as the only way to prevent a vicious circle of escalation between psychotic agitation and the restraining measures necessary to control it (see the case histories in the next section).

In the case of chronic, unproductive symptoms (blunted affects, withdrawal, apathy, indifference, and resignation; "loss of energy potential"), opposite measures are called for: carefully calculated amounts of social activation and increased stimulation and demands on the patient. For long-term patients in mental institutions, where such symptoms are frequently met with, this could mean transfer to a smaller, more personal and active ward, encouragement to make contacts outside the hospital, starting a rehabilitation program, and preparations for moving to a more independent form of housing. If the patient is already living outside an institution, the goal would be to make similar changes toward more stimulating or demanding conditions in his living or work situation, social contacts, leisure activities, and so on. Often the patient, his family, *and* those taking care of him will cling to medication like a crutch, even though it is no longer really necessary; and reducing it can have a positive effect. Usually it is advisable to proceed through these steps in gradual stages, but occasionally the technique of intentionally provoking a crisis can be successful, as the example in the last chapter showed. Every experienced clinician will be aware, however, that all efforts to raise the level of demands on the patient will often be initially opposed by a united front of family members, guardians, caretakers, *and* the patient himself. The homeostatic tendencies, the "principle of psychosocial inertia," will operate in such situations in many ways, both open and hidden, the worst of which is disguised as overprotection against all kinds of responsibility for the patient. Yet the results of rehabilitation programs show that equally determined efforts to bring about real change *in the long run* can lead to extraordinarily positive developments (see the case history below).

At the same time we must not lose sight of the realistic *limits* of endeavors of this kind. The maneuvering room between understimulation and overstimulation, between resignation and overeagerness on the therapist's part, is often very small. The reactivation of psychotic productions can also be used as a weapon in the battle against any change, whether by the patient himself or by people in his surroundings who unconsciously provoke it. In many cases hopes for full reintegration and complete disappearance of residual conditions are illusory. Furthermore, although the concepts of "productive" and "unproductive" symptoms can be a barometer for the type of treatment indicated, they are hardly a panacea, nor are they the only factors to be considered. Finally, some aspects of the situation are not yet entirely clear, such as the way in which different forms of treatment (rehabilitation programs, family therapy, group therapy) affect each other and the best way to combine them.

Since any real change is likely to encounter the kind of resistance just described, the question arises again and again as to just what kind of goal it is reasonable to strive for. Is it reintegration into society and the work force at any price? The best possible state of subjective well-being for the patient? The greatest benefit to the patient's family as a whole or to society? In some cases the last-named goal may not be identical with the patient's own contentment. Should the aim be for the patient to lead the richest possible life—one that involves taking risks—or the most "normal" and safest? Questions such as these have endless implications and cannot be given general answers, important though they may be for the practice of therapy. Subjective well-being and contentment are not only hard to define; they are also highly relative; they change; they have conscious and unconscious elements; and so on. In our own study of rehabilitation programs we found that after one year there was no correlation at all between the degree of contentment chronic patients expressed with their overall situation and the extent of their social reintegration in terms of jobs or housing.[5] However, those who expressed discontent with their situation at the start of the program had clearly better chances of success. This study was based on observations in the rehabilitation ward of a psychiatric hospital over several years, after which we could report that a number of anxious and rigidified long-term patients with severe cases of hospitalism began by furiously resisting any change, as did their families. Yet once they had finally taken the major step of moving out into a halfway house, a therapeutic community, or their own apartment, they often blossomed amazingly and refused even to consider a return to the hospital. If the move had been prepared carefully enough, patients almost never wanted to be rehospitalized. Consider the following case.

There were three completely passive, obese, chronic schizophrenics, all middle-aged, in the special rehabilitation ward; two of them had extensive delusions and one was more or less "stuck" in a depression. All of them had spent between five and fifteen years in the hospital, and they had all fought tooth and nail against being transferred to this ward. Once there, they sat together in a corner, refusing to participate in group discussions and always voting in a block against every suggested activity, whether it was a dance or an excursion. (At least their casting a vote was progress of a kind!) They took no part in social programs. After about six months, however, one of them visited a residence for former patients in the city, where he encountered some people he had known in the hospital and enjoyed a good meal. This experience appeared to make the first dent in his resistance. About the same time I gave a talk in the ward on the subject of hospitalism. Even though I had purposely kept its tone quite neutral, it proved surprisingly effective: along with other patients, these three began to accuse each other of showing symptoms of this so-called hospitalism. After a few more months two of them moved to the residence, finally followed by the third. One of them remained there for years, another found an apartment to share after some time, and the third rented a room of his own. Twice the trio took an Easter trip to Paris together, and one later began a relationship with a woman. At first all three worked in our hospital workshop and at the rehabilitation center; later one found a relatively undemanding job with the city's public transportation system. As time passed they lost contact with one another and we with them.

These and many similar experiences have convinced me that the most "normal" possible environment is better in the long run than the best and most progressive psychiatric hospital, even in cases in which everything, including the patient's own attitude, seems to argue against such a move. Of course enormous differences exist among individual cases, and it has already been noted that criteria for prognosis are hard to come by, so that generalizations would be out of place here. Nonetheless this point of view does suggest general guidelines on which to base decisions: the chances are good that patient and persistent attempts to relieve at least the *social* isolation of the "mentally ill" will be worth it in the end. On the other hand, the danger is great that passivity and resignation, the easiest solution for everyone involved to start with, will result in those tragic caricatures of human existence that can be met with in all kinds of psychiatric institutions.

Other general principles of therapy can be derived from the view of psychic and psychotic structures presented here; those that can be categorized as *techniques for altering systems of reference* will be discussed in a later section. But every effective form of psychotherapy can be regarded as measures standing in a reciprocal relationship to the disordering and disorganizing mechanisms discussed in Chapter 6. What these measures achieve is a reordering of pathological systems of reference. Such systems must first be destabilized, and to do so it is necessary to introduce a quantity of new and "unsettling" information (in the affective-logical sense).

A final general principle that emerges clearly from the concepts presented above is that *the accent must be placed on the healthy side of the disturbed individual*. There has been a great deal of justified criticism of prevailing methods in psychiatry and psychotherapy in recent years, which argues that they borrow too much from models of somatic medicine. These methods concentrate on what is diseased, first "exposing" it in order to treat it. In contrast, the view of psychosis taken here emphasizes what is still healthy or intact that remains behind the disorder of the psychotic or individual at risk for psychosis. The sensitivity and "thin skin" of schizophrenics has a *positive* as well as a negative side; the same is true of their remarkable powers of intuition and observation (resulting from the unstable boundaries of their egos), their genuineness, unconventionality, and potential for creativity (associated with the typical "loosening of associations"). All of these qualities should appear as possible variations of the normal, at *one* extreme of a scale that runs all the way to the other extreme of too "healthy" and rigid insensitivity and callousness. The therapeutic approach that results concentrates on treating such patients with respect for these qualities and on making the most of the possibilities for development contained in them. It is clear that therapists need to have a certain sensitivity themselves for this task, as well as sufficient ego strength.[6] Expecting people who are entirely unsuited for the job to take care of schizophrenics—something that still happens too often—is like asking a person with hands rough from hard manual labor to play the harp. People with an intuitive gift for working with schizophrenics, by which I do not mean gushing sentimentality but rather sincerity and directness, are able to elicit sympathetic vibrations in them, can get them to laugh and sparkle. Every human being is born with the laws for healthy growth implanted in him, like a tree; if conditions are unfavorable and cripple the tree, the law is still in effect, and many parts of the tree will still be healthy. One must just know how to find and recognize them, be able to uncover, to discover, the mischievous girl in the wrinkled face of an old woman, or the brash twelve-year-old in the stony features of an embittered old man.

Now that we have discussed a few general principles, let us take a closer look at some important specific problems in practicing therapy with schizophrenics.

The Therapeutic Setting

Just as my primary aim in this book has been to reach a better understanding of psychosis and psychotics, and the therapeutic measures suggested by this line of inquiry have therefore been of secondary concern, I would like to consider the ideal setting for therapy first, without reference to existing institutional limitations, although these will of course have to be taken into account afterward.

From what has already been said about the structure of psychosis it should be clear what kind of setting is best suited for treating schizophrenics: in *acute phases,* when they are confused, hypersensitive, unable to cope with anything unfamiliar or to process complex information, and likely to misinterpret events in a delusional manner, what is needed above all is a quiet, relaxed, and natural atmosphere, a relatively small space in which they can feel protected. Hectic goings-on should be avoided, and the people dealing with them should be few in number, calm, reliable, understanding, and, above all, healthy themselves.

Patients whose affects are supposedly blunted, but whose reactions are still quite vehement under the surface, need a similar milieu. However, for these *chronic patients*—insecure, devalued, withdrawn, with rigid defenses—the setting should ideally be more open and spacious, more stimulating and in certain ways more demanding; it should promote gradual development and positive change, activating healthy forces in the patient but without urgency or stress. It should also convey respect for individual differences, be flexible and lively, and work against all tendencies toward apathy and robotlike stereotypy.

New research findings indicate that beyond these fundamental considerations the ideal therapeutic setting could be even further specialized and differentiated, depending on which psychopathological condition and stage of disease was being treated. Thus Maxwell Jones's

"therapeutic community" (emphasizing partnership between therapists and clients, working out solutions of conflicts in cooperation,
sharing responsibility, cotherapy, and the like) can be a very beneficial
milieu for certain kinds of psychiatric patients. For schizophrenics,
however, it turned out to be quite often overtaxing.[7] Heim and his
colleagues showed that only an outgoing and active "type A" schizophrenic is likely to profit from such a community, whereas the more
withdrawn "type B" feels even less secure.[8] Passive, regressed long-
term patients with unproductive symptoms appear to react very positively to highly structured programs with a behavioral or family-
therapy orientation of the kind developed in the United States in
recent years by Robert Liberman or Carl Anderson.[9] Efforts to create
different therapeutic settings for various stages of illness have only
just begun, but we can already recognize a certain contrast between
two types. In the former, which we might call "maternal," acutely
anxious patients are calmed and soothed in an indulgent but protective atmosphere; in the latter, more "paternal" type, limits are set and
demands imposed in a kind but respectful way, so as to stimulate
chronic patients and gradually draw them out of their shell. Many
intermediate types can be imagined, including the type of therapeutic
community in which the patient is urged to take first active steps in a
positive direction. Clearly, a great deal of research remains to be done
in this field, but everything suggests that not only the intellectual and
structural qualities of the therapeutic setting deserve attention, but
also their *affective* qualities. I shall return to this point in my discussion of dealings with patients and questions of organization.

The requirements for an appropriate therapeutic setting as set out
above are not new; they are largely a matter of common sense, and
they are brought forward again and again by those who have not
become "case-hardened" in their contacts with the mentally ill. Family members voice such concerns when inquiring about the best possibilities for treatment; nursing students mention them after seeing
chronic wards in old-fashioned institutions for the first time; and
medical students challenge their professors with them when cases are
presented.

Nevertheless, despite the familiarity of these calls for reform, it cannot be disputed that the institutional settings in which schizophrenics
are treated do not generally conform to this ideal picture at all. Someone suffering an acute schizophrenic episode is usually taken to the
emergency room of a general or psychiatric hospital; often family
members, a doctor, or the police have intervened in a way that is

unclear and more upsetting to him. He may then be sent to a ward full of other confused and agitated patients, where there is frequent coming and going. In this totally unfamiliar atmosphere he is subjected to incomprehensible procedures by a swift succession of different people; his personal belongings, clothes, and valuables will be taken from him; he may be washed, restrained, given injections and possibly shock treatment, and in the meantime there will be forms to be filled out and administrative matters to be taken care of. Finally, depending on his condition, he may be transferred to another ward within a few days or weeks, where there will be different patients, a different staff, perhaps even different doctors, and new rules and regulations. Even in places where these conditions have been improved,[10] from the point of view of the patient, who was confused to begin with, this "treatment" will resemble a trip to an inferno. It would be difficult enough for a healthy person to endure, and it must of necessity worsen the state of someone who is already acutely psychotic. For this reason large doses of neuroleptics and sometimes further measures (isolation, restraint) have to be taken, which may inhibit the pathological symptoms but also suppress healthy forces at work within the patient.

The atmosphere is usually just as stifling, though in a different way, in many wards for the chronically ill, where the patients' own tendencies, staff attitudes, and administrative convenience contribute to a rigid, monotonous, and enormously inflexible climate. The rules and regulations, supported by force of habit, tend to promote rather than deter the development of the "clinical poverty syndrome." The following example from my own experience can stand for many.

On a visit to a "sheltered" apartment shared by four former mental patients we were astonished to learn that months after their release from the hospital they were still going to bed regularly before seven o'clock! The reason for this was habit; after years spent in institutions they had completely forgotten how to fill their evenings. In the hospital the lengthy procedures of serving and clearing away dinner, undressing the patients, and getting them ready for bed had to begin at five, since after six or seven no kitchen or regular nursing staff were available.

In all fairness, however, it must be admitted that much has gone on in the last ten or fifteen years to change the practice of psychiatry not only outside but also inside mental hospitals. New ideas, people, and schools of thought have begun to make themselves felt, including the ideological criticism of the "antipsychiatry" movement and also the British school of social psychiatry (including Wing, Brown, Bennet, and Leff) already mentioned frequently earlier. We have started to chip away at the worst abuses within rigidified institutional structures. But old habits die hard; they crop up in the most unexpected places even in progressive institutions, partly because it is so hard to change cumbersome, unwieldy bureaucracies.

> In the closed admission ward for agitated men that it was my duty to supervise about fifteen years ago in a university psychiatric hospital with 300 beds and a deservedly high reputation, it took *months* of persistent negotiations with the nurses, orderlies, doctors, and the administrative hierarchy before the patients there were finally allowed to have knives at meals like all the other patients in the hospital. Once the change had been made, however, there was never the slightest incident, and after a while it would never have occurred to anyone to stop giving out the knives at mealtimes again.

Such experiences, viewed in conjunction with the points discussed above concerning an ideal therapeutic setting, strongly suggest that the whole idea of a mental *hospital*—which has been taken over from somatic medicine—is not really suited to the treatment of schizophrenics. At the very least it appears that institutions above a certain size are not advantageous. It would seem much more appropriate to have small, flexible, familylike groups of understanding and healthy people, each of whom would look after one or a small number of schizophrenic patients over a longer period in the most normal atmosphere possible.

Even better would probably be the treatment of a schizophrenic directly *in* and *with* his customary environment, at home, at work, and in his neighborhood, as far as humanly possible. This is the aim of much community psychiatry, family therapy, and *network therapy*, and experiments along these lines have been undertaken since the 1970s with good results in Italy, Great Britain, and the United States. Further research in this area is needed, however. Another alternative is to set up small psychiatric units within general hospitals, in combination with centrally located patient day centers, halfway houses, therapeutic residences, workshops, and other part-time care arrangements, such as are now being established in many places. If we keep in mind the needs of the patients themselves, leaving aside the question of existing pressures and limitations, then the widespread development of these new, comprehensive care systems appears as much more important than the bare modernization of the traditional mental hospital.

These proposals will sound unrealistic in the light of conditions actually prevailing in many places. If at all, they can be realized only through long and difficult processes of transformation. Nearly everywhere in the world, the treatment of schizophrenics is still concentrated in large hospital units that must treat many other conditions, some of them extremely difficult, such as depression, addiction, senility, personality disorders, epilepsy, and mental deficiency. In view of their often deplorable state and as a result of public pressure, high priority is currently being given in many places to renovating old mental hospitals and increasing personnel. In addition, some transitional facilities designed for small numbers of patients are being established where budgets permit. The creation of mobile units consisting of a social worker, nurse, and physician is still rare and in many places faces almost insurmountable administrative difficulties. For this reason, among others, a radical attempt has been made in Italy, where institutions in many parts of the country were extremely antiquated, to abolish mental hospitals altogether. In some areas day clinics are being set up and in others small psychiatric units established in general hospitals; in a few places mobile crisis-intervention units of the type just described are already doing superb work. However, in many cases the results of abolishing mental hospitals without replacing them with something else indicate that great caution is necessary. Some years ago in California, where the then Governor Reagan closed many state mental hospitals (for far different ideological reasons), the lack of alternative arrangements for treating schizophrenics meant that many of them simply landed in the street or became the victims of unscrupulous operators of nursing homes, some of which had no medical supervision. There conditions developed that were even worse than in the old mental institutions.

All of this does not mean that the formulation of ideal conditions as a long-term goal is irrelevant; on the contrary, we must make attempts to approach them as closely as possible in the practice of therapy, starting from whatever conditions may currently exist. It is too seldom recognized that schizophrenia is one of the greatest unsolved problems of modern medicine next to cancer; its cost, in both economic and human terms, is enormous. *Every* possibility of alleviating it therefore deserves the most serious attention of professionals and the general public. Recently it has come to seem as if we were focusing on the luxury of psychologizing every phase from the cradle to the grave in the lives of relatively healthy people,[11] when our first priority ought to be to expend our limited resources on better treatment for the very seriously ill, many of whom are still being shamefully neglected. There is all the more reason to do this since recent developments have brought new life and hope to a once stagnant field.

Several models show that the proposals discussed here *can* be implemented, at least in part. One of these, of great interest for the treatment of acute psychotics, is the Soteria Project, an extensive experimental program begun in the 1970s by Loren Mosher for the National Institute of Mental Health in the United States. Mosher and his associates, intrigued by the work of Ronald Laing and other unconventional approaches to treatment, created several small groups located in houses in ordinary residential neighborhoods. There the groups looked after a small number of acute schizophrenics, up to six per house, who received therapy there instead of in hospitals. The patients spent several months living with the healthy group members, who had been very carefully selected on the basis of their personalities and general experience. These helpers spent two to three days a week living in the group; spending the rest of the week in a completely nonpsychiatric milieu was regarded as an important counterbalance to their experiences in the group. In case of need they could call on a medical team from a nearby community mental health center (a type of institution created by the Kennedy Act of 1963, in which physicians, psychotherapists, and social workers take care of patients in their own neighborhoods as far as possible). The condition, psychopathological and social progress, and subjective experience of the patients were followed over several years in a careful comparative study using control groups of patients undergoing standard treatment in mental hospitals. In the program the treatment consisted primarily of the group living experience; medication was used only rarely. If patients were agitated, staff members would remain with them constantly, for two or three days if necessary, in a stripped-down quiet room furnished with cushions and shatterproof glass. A striking result of this approach was that patients almost always calmed down during this period without medication. Difficulties with neighbors remained within reasonable limits. The results, published in more than twenty articles, showed that the patients' progress was just as good as or in some cases better than the progress of those in the control groups (especially in social development and subjective experience), even though total costs in the experimental program tended to be lower.[12] When I visited one of these projects I had the impression that almost all the criteria mentioned above for an ideal therapeutic setting were met. Since then more has been published on similar projects in various parts of the world, where positive results have been reported.[13] One of them is currently working successfully under my direction in Bern, Switzerland.

Another project of the 1970s that is of great interest in this context is the attempt of Paul Polak in Denver to revive the old idea of *family care*. Polak succeeded in finding suitable families willing to take on the care of psychiatric patients, among them not a few acute schizophrenics, for a limited time during a phase of crisis. He developed possibilities for accompanying mobile crisis intervention and organized many volunteer helpers in the community. Here, too, a team of psychiatrists was always on call, in particular to supervise the high doses of medication often required at the beginning. Using these methods, Polak was able within a few years to reduce the annual number of hospitalizations in one section of the city from several hundred to less than thirty.[14]

The main drawback of these unconventional treatment centers is clearly their small capacity, but at the same time this represents one of their greatest strengths: they are more flexible and open than large institutions. Once a start has been made, they can be expanded to deal with patients in significant numbers. In one town in Switzerland with a population of less than 20,000, more than twenty "sheltered" apartments, each housing four or five long-term schizophrenic patients, were opened within a few years.

The same flexiblity exists in other types of social-psychiatric institutions designed to help patients make the transition from hospital to normal life: day clinics, night clinics, crisis-intervention centers, residences, social centers, and workshops. Of course, like all the other types of treatment centers mentioned, they can develop their full therapeutic potential only if they are located close to the patients' homes and places of work, that is, if they are *decentralized* and geographically distributed in autonomous districts with a population of 100,000 to 250,000. Our current experience suggests that a network of six to eight such centers, caring for a maximum of 15 patients at one time (with the exception of outpatient clinics), will require a total staff of about 50. Together they can treat up to 1,500 psychiatric patients a year, most of them moderately severe cases of schizophrenia, on a very flexible and largely outpatient basis—in other words, just as many as a medium-sized mental hospital can treat. Where the potential of such treatment centers has been fully developed, as in one region of Switzerland that has been organized in this way for more than fifteen years, a study showed that the number of patients requiring long-term hospitalization was correspondingly reduced: from a total population of 280,000 only 40 psychiatric patients remained in the hospital for longer than a year (excluding 136 cases of senile dementia and oligophrenia). Although the number of beds in the local mental hospital was reduced in the same period from more than 400 to less than 200, many more inpatients could be treated per year.[15] Social-psychiatric institutions provide transitional services bridging the gap between full hospitalization and full social reintegration on *two* "axes," as the table below shows.

Housing axis	*Work axis*
1. Full hospitalization	1. Full hospitalization
2. Crisis-intervention center, day clinic, or night clinic	2. Therapeutic workshop
3. Quarterway or halfway house	3. Rehabilitation center
4. Therapeutic apartments	4. Supervised workshops for former patients
5. Partially supervised special living arrangements (in families, boardinghouses, etc.)	5. Partially supervised workplace (special arrangements in normal jobs)
6. Autonomous housing situation	6. Autonomous work situation

One of our studies followed a group of eighty-one long-term, mainly schizophrenic patients who were receiving treatment in one or the other form of transitional or outpatient centers in this same region of Switzerland on a chosen day. One year later 72 percent had either reached or were maintaining levels 4 to 6 on the housing axis, and 36 percent were at levels 5 or 6 of the work axis.[16]

A network of such small autonomous clinics and centers has a great deal of potential for meeting the criteria for treatment described above. Not only does it provide a therapeutic setting with a relaxed, personal, and noninstitutional atmosphere, but it also allows for many flexible and individual combinations: a patient may live in a small therapeutic community and slowly attain more independence on the work axis, or he may work in a rehabilitation center and make progress toward a more independent living situation. This permits a progressive (or, if necessary, regressive) degree of "social stimulation" to meet the changing needs of each patient, in accordance with the general theory of schizophrenia therapy outlined before. In addition, these two axes allow us to replace vague goals (such as "better adjustment," "personality development," "improved psychological state") with concrete steps that can be easily understood and agreed on by all concerned—patients, their families, and staff members. As a result the specific content of therapeutic programs can be worked out at each stage.

The following basic social skills are essential for life in normal society; in some cases schizophrenic patients will need help and guidance in practicing them if the specific goal of independent living arrangements is to be reached. They must be able to:

Look after their own food and clothing
Take care of their own bed, room, or apartment
Use telephones and public transportation
Deal adequately with money
Take care of their own personal hygiene; use medicines properly;
    keep doctor's appointments
Deal with agencies and institutions (banks, post office, etc.), legal
    guardians

Similarly, if the goal is autonomous employment, in addition to specific job skills and the work performance itself the following minimal abilities must be realistically taken into account:

Regular and punctual attendance
Work speed
Concentration
Neatness
Ability to get along with others
General behavior
Independence

Using graded scales developed to evaluate these abilities as they are acquired, we have found that they develop best in a program of useful jobs at the patients' level of competence and at *realistic pay rates*.[17] This approach is far more constructive in the long run than keeping chronic schizophrenics endlessly occupied with pseudo-creative leisure-time hobbies or "occupational therapy," which at bottom carries the unspoken message, "You aren't fit to do anything really useful." Again, it is not a question of just forcing these goals on the patient, but rather of *negotiating* them with him—as the person most concerned—in discussion with his family, guardians, and staff members as necessary helpers. It is precisely through these concrete clarifications and *actions,* directed at visible and definable goals, and not through mere words, that a schizophrenic can stabilize (often not without real conflicts) the boundaries of his own self. With the development of goal-directed wishes and desires, feelings and thoughts, roles and responsibilities, his sense of identity becomes firmer. At the same time he will be able to experience a variety of interpersonal relations and, in short, to acquire that degree of internal and external autonomy and maturity that must be the true aim of all psychotherapy. Without this link to concrete reality, the danger exists for schizophrenics in particular that psychotherapeutic work will remain too theoretical and constantly be contradicted by unfavorable feedback from the outside world. As we have already seen, there is a direct path from (appropriate) action to an internalized image or system, and from there to clearer, healthier thinking and feeling. That certain more "verbal" therapies can also be quite useful will be made clear below.

The idea of a number of small, largely autonomous but complementary social-psychiatric units presents one particularly thorny problem: *How to provide for continuity* in the long run? Nothing is more confusing to patients and their families than to be confronted again and again with new personnel, new programs, and new expectations. A certain amount of changing from one unit to another is inevitable in this type of social psychiatry, however, and it is not a bad idea for each local team of mental health professionals to feel that they have some degree of independent authority. This problem, which is analogous to the problems of large hospitals with many different departments and concerns both personnel and programs of treatment, becomes especially acute when continuity should be maintained as a patient moves repeatedly from full hospitalization to intermediate care (day or night clinic, halfway house) and to outpatient status (family physician, outpatient clinic, rehabilitation program). To my knowledge, no entirely satisfactory solutions have yet been found. Two radically different approaches have been tried. One is to combine all the different phases of treatment under one team, so that the same people divide their time between hospital, intermediate, and outpatient care. A prerequisite for this approach is the division of health care into very clearly defined geographic sectors.[18] The other is to concentrate all (or almost all) aspects of treatment in one location, in very small, familylike communities.

One manageable compromise that we have been exploring in our own region is to establish central but mobile teams (physician, nurse, and social worker) to "accompany" a patient through all the stages of a long-term rehabilitation program. This team formulates the long-range goals and coordinates the work of all the different professionals involved. Of particular importance is a conclusion which may sound self-evident but which is often neglected in practice, namely that the long-range programs should always be hierarchically superior to short-term treatments in different institutions (day clinics, crisis-intervention centers). The latter must adapt to the former rather than vice versa.

A final question remains: What consequences does the view of psychosis presented here have for traditional *mental hospitals?* They are likely to remain as the main centers of treatment in many areas for a long time, particularly for the more severe and acute cases, if only for reasons of their large capacities. In principle the consequences are the same as for the less conventional small institutions just described. First and foremost, instead of large, noisy wards, which can only increase psychotic confusion, schizophrenics need small and quiet departments with specially selected personnel. Examples from progressive mental hospitals show that a great deal can be done to implement the proposals outlined here (with the limitations already mentioned) even in large institutions. New construction and remodeling can facilitate the creation of small departments; the emphasis can be placed on social reintegration and prevention of long stays in the hospital; hospitals can be made more open and can work toward systematic cooperation with external services. In addition, innovations in some hospitals have led to the dismantling of overly rigid structures and measures inconsistent with psychotherapeutic goals, such as the separation of the sexes in different wards, institutional clothing, excessive limitations on free-time activities, inflexible hierarchies, and strict bureaucratic regimens for both patients and staff. All these changes represent steps toward the realization of the therapeutic ideals I have mentioned. However, the most important consequence of a new understanding of schizophrenia has no connection with a particular type of institution. Rather, it is an attitude toward patients and therapy that can make itself felt in any contact between individuals, no matter where it occurs. It is behind the oppressive walls of old-fashioned mental institutions, in the worst and most backward surroundings, that one understanding person, who knows how to react sensibly and how to talk sense with "crazy" people, can do the most good. It makes an enormous difference whether someone has at least *one* friend in need, or no one at all!

Dealing with Schizophrenics

Various subjects discussed in the preceding chapters contain a wealth of suggestions for how to deal with schizophrenics. These subjects included the interaction between individuals and their environments, especially the role of feedback mechanisms and the effects of a contradictory style of communication; the concept of internalized affective-logical systems of reference; and the theory that in schizophrenics these systems are unclear and poorly structured. Many of the recommendations that follow lie between two poles that may at first seem irreconcilable but are in fact complementary.

As a general rule we can say that every kind of communication that contributes to clarity and avoids misunderstandings is good for therapy, and everything that does the opposite is bad. Social roles and functions, goals, agreements, tasks, and expectations should be explicit for *all* participants, including the patient, his family, and therapists. Policies, procedures, appointments, and financial arrangements should be made equally clear.[19] If something *must* be left indefinite (such as the length of treatment or date of release from the hospital), then this fact should be explained. Schizophrenics should know where they stand with their therapist, be aware of what he is or is not, wants or does not want, what he is or is not thinking and feeling. The therapist has his own role and identity, just as the patient has his: the therapist is a member of a helping profession and is paid for his work; the patient pays and receives help in return. The one has responsibility (perhaps for a group); the other has none, or less responsibility; the one is healthy, the other is ill. Each is also clearly male or female, young or old, fat or thin; they come from this place or that;[20] they are not all "equal."

At the same time, however, the opposite of all this is also true, and should be made unmistakably clear to patients in what is said and done: They are *not* (just) ill, *not* fundamentally different, *not* less good, less responsible, less mature, less worthy than I am as their therapist! What they think, feel, say, and do is just as true and correct as what I think. They may come from a different background, be a different gender, have different education and experience, but that does not matter in the least—in every essential respect we are like each other.

Dealing with schizophrenics (as with all patients and in fact with every partner) teaches us to deal with two counterparts: our own self-assertion and that of the other person. Anything that tends to cover up this situation, such as seeking to avoid conflict at all costs, is bad for therapy, but it is also bad to *seek* conflict at all costs. Everything is bad which puts *me* and my identity before the other's, which puts me above him, does not show respect for him, does not let him respond calmly to my own calmness. However, it is also bad if I do not let him know in some way if I happen to be frightened, nervous, or impatient, so that he can *understand* why I am acting as I am, why I will not let him leave at the moment, or why I have no time for a long conversation. He should be aware that at times I am unsure of myself—though not in any fundamental sense—that I may not know this or that, and that I may make mistakes. But in spite of that, I am still someone, not nothing, as his destructive nihilism will sometimes lead him to believe, about himself as well as about me.

The opposite of this approach, however, is also necessary at times: *not* always to say what one is thinking, *not* always to show one's feelings, *not* always to be forthright and direct, but sometimes to be *indirect,* in subtle ways involving suggestions, metaphors, or paradoxes.

An additional polarity (expressed in the work of Heinz Kohut and Carl Rogers) is to accept the patient completely as he is (to be a mirror, a support) and yet to *refuse* to "let him be," to let him remain as he is—regressed, stunted, distorted, "insane"—and to manipulate him into making progress. In a similar way in the world of nature a cat or fox mother will nurture her young according to their own rhythms and needs, but when the time comes she will throw them out of the nest, brutally if necessary, and *force* them to become independent. Too often we forget that the goal of therapy is not to create the closest possible bond between therapist and patient. In some cases (but not all) this bond is merely a useful aid in achieving the actual goal, which is to make the bond itself, and the therapist, *superfluous*.

A final important but confusing polarity exists between actions and words, between preverbal and verbal communication, between thinking and feeling. As we have seen, often the nonverbal is much more important than the verbal; "actions speak louder than words." We should not preach to patients, but instead *do something* for and with them. Yet it is also important—when they are agitated, anxious, confused—to be able *to do nothing at all,* to sit with them in silence, to let them make the first move. Words, too, however, can be very important; sometimes they convey more information than actions; they can "say" more. But at the same time, in talking with schizophrenics we should above all *keep still and listen;* we should not *lead* discussions but *follow* them, although this does not mean that a therapist can never be the one to break the silence or take the initiative. Here is one example of how this can work in practice.

The day clinic regularly begins with a forty-five-minute group discussion in the morning. All the patients (among them several schizophrenics) and staff, about fifteen people altogether, are sitting around a large table drinking coffee or tea. There is *no* set plan or topic for discussion. At the start there is an embarrassed silence or an exchange of trivial remarks ("Nice weather today," or "Did you sleep well?"). But *always,* without fail, something important will come up . . . but one must be very alert not to miss it. Someone will make a face or whisper something to his neighbor; that may be the significant event. Yesterday two of the patients were in the midst of a quarrel, and the whole group was affected by the atmosphere. Then someone makes a "trivial" remark about a train trip, about how slippery the platform is in wintertime, about the sudden drafts, about how you have to be careful not to get sucked under the train . . . He is expressing his own suicidal fears and fantasies. Someone else says that you just need to get a good foothold and not stand too close to the edge; a staff member (a nurse, social worker, psychologist, or doctor) may repeat this remark and praise the man's good, sturdy legs. He looks down at them in astonishment, and relaxes. The group, now in the grip of

a peculiar excitement, talks about nothing but this station platform for five minutes—how the wind almost seems to pull you
down when the train comes in, how it is worst in the morning,
and so forth. No one has offered an "interpretation," but everyone senses what is being talked about; everyone feels included and
addressed—if only the therapists are observant enough and react
correctly, following on the same wavelength and not interrupting
because *they* haven't been able to keep up, or because *they* can't
bear the silence.

Then nothing much happens for a while; people are silent, star-
ing off into space or passing the tea and sugar around the table,
until someone mentions that he still has not succeeded in finding a
job. Or one of the therapists may start up a conversation with a
patient who has not said a word for weeks, a sullen Italian who is
ignored because his foreign accent is hard to understand and because nobody likes him. The therapist starts to ask all about
him—where does he come from? Precisely from *which* little village near Venice? He comes from a large family, from a farm; it's a
little remote . . . *How many* cows do they have? How many pigs?
What brought him to Switzerland? Soon he has livened up, started
talking; it turns out that one of the other patients once spent a
vacation in that part of Italy. All at once the Italian is "somebody"
in the group, although for weeks he has been a nobody . . .

In this kind of approach everyone is important. No distinction exists
between the doctor who can "treat" patients and the new student
nurse who "can't." This does not mean that a person with years of
psychoanalysis and training behind him should not make this competence available to the group: Everyone should be and is permitted
to be himself, including the trainee who is there for the first time and
who will therefore see, sense, and authentically *know* what is happening differently than we do. Most important of all, the patient is permitted to be himself. We are "whole"—that is, "therapeutic" in our
effect—only when we communicate in an "entire" (or "holistic")
way, with harmony between words and actions, mind and body,
thoughts and feelings, verbally and nonverbally. We can thus communicate and pass on to the patient something whole—that is to say,
just what he is lacking and what will "do him good": an affective-
cognitive or affective-logical unity.

It is possible to establish a connection between the unfavorable influences in a schizophrenic's family milieu and communication style, about which much has been said earlier, and the specific symptoms of his disease. There will be parallels between the two, from which favorable therapeutic approaches and influences can be deduced. The results are striking. Such a list (see table) shows almost the complete psychopathology of schizophrenic conditions, providing further evidence that many symptoms and aspects of schizophrenics' behavior are determined by their milieu (or, at the very least, induced and amplified by environmental influences).

The table indicates very clearly what kind of setting and approach toward patients appear therapeutically beneficial for each category of symptoms.[21] It is not different from the atmosphere and behavior that have a favorable influence on human development in general: quiet, calmness, simplicity and lack of ambiguity, dependability and continuity, trust, tolerance, directness, and authenticity. All these qualities should be associated with the main goal of demarcating the boundaries between myself and the other person, between *my* feelings and *his* feelings, between my thoughts, wishes, strivings, and his; the aim is to validate *his* identity without giving up my own. According to everything we have learned from psychopathology, psychoanalysis, and systems and communications theory, this list says something about the basic structure of psychosis, the structure of the intrapsychic and interpersonal spaces associated with psychosis, and the dynamics of their interaction. The only surprise is how simple and plausible the connections seem to be.

That matters are not quite so simple in reality, however, is suggested by the polarities implicit in the therapeutic approaches discussed above. These will take on an even more complex character as we come to some technical aspects of altering systems of reference, including such sophisticated methods as the therapeutic double bind and paradoxical prescriptions.

Techniques for Altering Systems of Reference

If we regard schizophrenic psychosis—and in a broader sense every severe psychic disturbance—as a leap into "dis-ordered" or pathological states of equilibrium and systems of reference, then the goal of all therapy must be to "re-order" these systems. A technique for altering systems of reference would thus have to make use of the same mechanisms that led to the disorder, but in the reverse direction.

Pathological versus therapeutic influences in the environment of schizophrenics

Pathological milieu (e.g., family, institution)	Psychopathological disorders in the patient	Optimal therapeutic setting
Tension, anxiety, friction, too many stimuli	Tension, anxiety, agitation, productive psychotic symptoms	Security, serenity, reduction of stimuli
Complex, unclear, confusing environment	Derealization	Simple, clear, well-arranged environment
Anonymity, too much change, large group	Confusion	Personal atmosphere, little change, small group
Instability, discontinuity, unpredictability	Instability, erratic behavior, inconsistency	Stability, continuity, dependability
Inability to share focus of attention	Inattentiveness, absent-mindedness	Clear focusing of of attention
Distrust, devaluation, intolerance	Distrust, tension, anger, rage, low self-esteem	Trust; validation of perceptions, thoughts, and feelings; tolerance
Lack of understanding, coldness, indifference, lack of involvement	Disappointment, dysphoria, withdrawal and blunting of affect	Understanding, warmth, encouragement, dialogue, explanations
Symbiotic, narcissistic relationships; forced consensus; denial of differences, "pseudo-mutuality"	Unclear ego, boundaries, oversensitivity, inability to deal with conflict, negation, denial	Clear demarcation of persons; recognition of differences in opinions, feelings, and behavior
Irrationality, mystification, ambiguity, lack of clarity	Irrationality, lack of clarity, distortion	Rationality, clarity, no ambiguity
Contradictory instructions and injunctions (double bind) "impossible mission," contradictory implied expectations	Ambivalence, thought disorders, affective disorders, incoherence, delusions, hallucinations	No ambiguity in instructions and injunctions; realistic, clear, explicit instructions
Infantilization, dependency, lack of responsibility	Regression, infantilism, dependency, incompetence	Autonomy, responsibility, trust
Rigidity, stereotyped roles	Rigidity, stereotyped behavior, mannerisms	Mobility, flexibility in roles
Impoverished stimulation, lack of openness, intellectual and affective construction	Indifference, passivity, withdrawal and blunting of affect, narrowness	Intellectual and affective stimulation, openness, space

Source: Based on L. R. Mosher and A. Z. Menn, "The Surrogate Family: An Alternative to Hospitalization," in *Schizophrenia: Science and Practice,* ed. J. C. Shershow (Cambridge, Mass.: Harvard University Press, 1978), pp. 223–239.

The internalized programs for thinking, feeling, and behaving are a condensation of all the significant experiences of a person from childhood on; they are reactivated again and again, for instance in the phenomenon of transference. Until recently, a real and lasting, and especially a rapid, alteration of these programs has been regarded as difficult if not impossible, largely under the influence of psychoanalysis. All of psychoanalytic practice seemed to indicate that such change could be expected, if at all, only though complicated therapeutic procedures requiring years of interpretative exploration and revision of the patient's past. Quick cures of symptoms, though observable now and again, were considered superficial and, because of the supposedly inevitable appearance of new symptoms to replace the old, practically useless.

However, findings during the last two or three decades force us to revise these views at least in part. Among these findings are Sargant's observations on brainwashing and similar techniques, as well as some results of crisis-intervention research and behavior therapy. In many cases the cure of specific symptoms did not lead to the production of substitute symptoms, but on the contrary to an observable general improvement in the patient's whole condition. In one case of a traveling salesman, who had become socially devalued and a complete invalid and got into severe financial difficulties, the treatment concentrated on curing his long-standing phobia about traveling by train; the disappearance of this phobia brought about sweeping improvements in his professional and family life, his self-esteem, and his relations with others. But above all it is our new experience with the methods derived from systems and communications theory that has shown that, under special conditions, internalized systems of reference and behavior can be more easily destabilized than we used to assume. Particularly challenging examples of this are provided by the unconventional techniques of Milton H. Erickson based on hypnotherapy.

Before analyzing some of these techniques in detail, let us consider a few everyday instances of how systems of reference are altered:

When a child burns its fingers on a hot stove for the first time, or is stung by a wasp, or slapped hard by a neighbor who had always been friendly before, the child revises its internalized system of reference for this context, at once, for good, *and* independently of past experience.

Similarly, an adult will thoroughly revise his corresponding system of reference if he visits a country whose inhabitants he had always idealized as "friendly" and "sincere" and there becomes the victim of an aggressive attack.

The same applies to *every kind* of severely traumatic experience, that is, every negative experience that makes a very strong impression. But in certain circumstances positive events can also leave an ineradicable impression, one that will have a lasting influence on feeling, thinking, and behavior no matter what may have gone before. Someone who has been lost in the mountains and given up hope will never forget the sight of his rescuer; someone who has ever been desperately thirsty is unlikely to forget the face of the stranger who offered him a cold glass of water. They will remain present below the surface levels of the mind; they have been added, as relevant information, to the related systems of association and will be reactivated from then on in similar situations (for example, as persistent hope or, perhaps, as increased fear and caution in potentially dangerous situations). Pre-existing systems of reference can thus be altered by particularly intense emotional experiences in the present.

Such observations, in full agreement with the previous description of how affective-cognitive schemata are formed, allow us to deduce for therapy *a certain primacy of the present, the here and now, over the past, and a primacy of concrete action (carefully polarized in a specific direction) over thinking and speaking.* This corresponds to the fact— the implications of which have not been sufficiently grasped up to now—that it is not primarily a way of thinking that is to be changed, but ways of acting and feeling. The *affective*-cognitive concept of information is central in this context. It becomes increasingly clear that, as new information from experience is added to existing systems of feeling and thinking, condensation into images and other intermediate stages between external action and internalized "intellect" (such as symbolic acts, rituals, metaphors) plays a pivotal role, in much the same way that consciousness was assumed to develop in Chapter 4.[22]

Two little illustrations of therapeutic alteration of a system of reference were included in the description of the morning conversations at our day clinic. As an antidote to the latent suicidal fantasies of one patient who was anxious and unsure of himself, the therapists tried to suggest in an indirect manner a quite different self-image and body image, namely that of a robust person able to stand firmly on two strong legs on the slippery platform (that is, in life) and to resist the dangerous draft from the train (his suicidal impulses). This suggestion was successful at the moment and later led, in connection with other influences, to a general improvement in his condition. In the other case a "faceless" patient without an identity, completely devalued both by himself (on an intrapsychic level) and by his environment (on an interpersonal level), was retrieved from this obscurity and provided with qualities, warmth, color, and outline (in the form of a place of birth, a family, a biography, and so on). For a moment, at least, he was transformed in his own eyes and those of others; his own and their systems of reference were altered, and a therapeutic breach in his defenses was opened, which could be widened with more of the appropriate treatment (although in this instance our efforts met with only partial success).

Both of these examples contain many of the elements known to be significant in dealing with schizophrenics. The distinct actualization of events is important, as are the intentional use of metaphors and symbols and an "unconscious" level of therapeutic communication, which is largely one of action. (Addressing and turning the spotlight on a previously overlooked member of a group is at least as much an action, an event, as it is a matter of words.) Another equally important element—which may not have emerged clearly enough from the description, but which is essential for every alteration in a system of reference—is *emotional intensity*. The use of symbolic language in these examples reflects a psychoanalytic approach and method, while the inclusion or polarization of the patient's social field is inspired by systems theory.

The long-term effects of metaphors, used at the right moment to inform an existing system of reference, can sometimes be surprisingly strong, as the following case reveals:

> I recently happened to meet a thirty-year-old woman who is now flourishing and full of energy, but to whom I had once spoken years earlier when she was very ill and being treated in our crisis-intervention center. Severe family problems had led to a suicide attempt; the patient was feeling completely devalued, disheartened, and exhausted. She reminded me during our chance encounter that at that time I had compared her in a conversation to a "wilted flower," which "only needed water to come back to life."

She had never forgotten that image, she said, and for months afterward the idea that despite her pitiful state she still had something of a flower in her had strengthened her desire to regain her health.

Comparisons having to do with a person's body image—which psychoanalysis teaches us is a central aspect of self representation—can make an indelible impression, positive as well as negative ("old goat," "cow," "witch"). Metaphors can occasionally be useful in the cognitive field, too. Another patient, who tended to be highly erratic and disorganized, profited greatly from a group discussion around a large table piled high with objects of all different kinds. She was shown very graphically how important it is to "start with what is nearest at hand and then go on to what is further away." Later she was able to use this metaphor as a way of orienting herself in many different situations.

The purpose of symbolic actions and rituals is to "brand" or "print" such information on existing systems of reference. The more intense their affective stamp, the more effective they will be. The apple that Mme. Sechehaye gave to her schizophrenic patient at a highly emotional point in her psychotherapy as a symbol of her (Mme. Sechehaye's) breast is a well-known example of the enormous effect of such procedures at the "καιρός," the right and—in the original sense of the word—critical moment.[23] This is also the underlying meaning of social ceremonies such as puberty and initiation rites, weddings, and funerals. They represent a visible "sign" to all the participants, an emotionally effective enacted metaphor that helps them adjust their affective and cognitive systems of reference to the altered reality. Clearly a direct path to internalization must exist from normal activity through ritual and metaphor to fixed mental images. Psychodrama and the technique of guided affective imagery both make use of this path.[24] Milton Erickson was a master in the use of such metaphorical language, and Mara Selvini Palazzoli reports on the use of therapeutic family rituals that can simultaneously represent paradoxical "prescriptions of the pathology":

The four-member nuclear family of a patriarchically organized Italian clan of peasant origin came to us for treatment of the psychotic 15-year-old daughter. We prescribed the following paradoxical antidote to the family myth of unconditional loyalty to the clan, which was stifling all conflict. Without any further explanation we instructed them to perform a ritual: "Every other night the family was to lock and bolt the door and sit around the dining room table, which would be cleared of all objects except an alarm clock. Each member of the family, starting with the eldest, would have fifteen minutes to talk [without interruption], expressing his own feelings, impressions, and observations regarding the behavior of other members of the clan . . . As for relations with members of the clan, a doubling of courtesy and helpfulness was prescribed." The goals of this ritual, which led rapidly to a therapeutic breakthrough which had long been sought in vain, were complex: Among other things its aim was to isolate and demarcate the family group undergoing this treatment from the rest of the clan precisely by "prescribing the pathology" (that is, the emphasis of taboo and myth) and to change the family structure by establishing equal rights for all members.[25]

Another method for bringing about therapeutic change in affective-cognitive systems of reference consists in selectively redistributing single elements in a system (in a reversal of the disorganizing mechanisms), either by attaching a different value to them or by changing the "punctuation" (division into sequences, classification, taxonomy).[26] An amusing example of the former technique can be found in Mark Twain's *Tom Sawyer:*

Tom has been given the unpleasant job of painting a garden fence one afternoon, to his dismay, and the other boys make fun of him, since they are free to play and amuse themselves. But Tom suggests to them that the job is so demanding that only he could be trusted with it, thereby achieving his purpose: the whole gang of boys competes for the honor of being able to pay him for a chance to paint the fence under his supervision.

One could say that *whoever establishes the system of reference has the power,* or at least a very decided advantage. This person creates the framework of the "field" in which all succeeding transactions must take place, and he determines what these transactions will be as if they were self-evident, that is, without the others noticing and thus all the more effectively, according to his own convenience and values. Paul Watzlawick means much the same thing when he speaks of "defining a relationship": every interpersonal relationship exists within a shared system of reference that must first be "defined" and established.[27] This occurs to a great extent through nonverbal and unconscious channels. Among other things it establishes who "leads" and who "follows" in a relationship. Here is a nice example:

> As I was talking to a woman I didn't know who had struck up a conversation with me at a crowded conference center, I suddenly became aware that she was constantly shifting the angle at which she faced me, forcing me to perform a little dance around her and follow her slowly in a certain direction through the mass of people. As soon as I stopped playing along and remained in one position, her flirtatious behavior changed abruptly. She lost all interest in our conversation and turned to talk to someone else.

Definitions of relationships, which establish fundamental dependencies and complementary or rival symmetries (Bateson), play a decisive role not merely in such fleeting encounters but also in longlasting relationships, where they can develop into typical double-bind constellations. These definitions are highly significant in therapy, since the therapist must be in a position of *leadership* if he is to make any headway against the pathological homeostasis of disturbed individuals and groups, although he may sometimes have to adapt his movements to those of his "opponent," like a judo wrestler. The following case history from one of the great modern "magicians" of psychotherapy illustrates this point strikingly, as well as several further elements in the altering of a system of reference.

> At a seminar[28] Salvador Minuchin showed a video tape of the first and only family therapy session with a working-class family. The family consisted of an overworked, inflexible, and dominating mother; the weak, evasive, and shadowy figure of the father; and a fifteen-year-old son bound up in a symbiotic relationship with his mother. The son, the "designated patient," displayed an attitude of indifference and created a more or less hebephrenic impression; for months he had been incapable of getting out of bed before noon or pursuing any useful activity. Within one hour Minuchin succeeded in altering the systems of reference of this depressed group so thoroughly that in the end the father appeared as an energetic authority figure, the mother was both relieved of her

burden and neutralized, and the son abandoned his passive attitude. How did this "miracle" come about? Minuchin, presenting himself in the role of "expert," began by rapidly establishing a very warm and genuine contact, particularly with the parents; he accomplished this in a kind of opening "dance"—as he very aptly calls this procedure—in which he asked a number of seemingly harmless questions about their names, background, occupations, and so on. Then, unexpectedly, he seized on something which had been mentioned only in passing and to which no one had attached any particular importance, the fact that the father had worked as a pipe fitter for the same company for thirty years and got up every morning at five to go to work. He built this up as a tremendous achievement, feigned disbelief, congratulated the man, and got him to describe his work day and several episodes in his life in exact detail. In so doing Minuchin conjured up a picture for all present of a tough, solitary, struggling but unappreciated fighter who never gave up no matter how badly things might be going against him. At the same time he subtly began to draw the son into the conversation, spoke of how he would gradually loosen the "lines of communication" to his mother and of how he had the chance, now that he was growing up, to "tap the potent energy source" of his father. Minuchin then opened up the perspective of a "breaking of the connection" that would occur later of its own accord, praised the young man's height, and predicted that he would grow even taller. Finally he let everything that had been said taper off into ordinary social conversation, with a clear drop in the level of emotional intensity, and took his leave of them in a relaxed atmosphere, wishing them well like a friend who had dropped by.

This session initiated a decisive turn for the better: the son became active and finally entered a vocational training program. The whole regressed and blocked family began to develop in a healthy direction again.

This kind of approach to therapy is highly interesting from a number of different perspectives. A "structural systems therapist," which is how Minuchin describes himself, will place the greatest emphasis on changes in the family constellation—which in this case are indeed impressive. A psychoanalyst, on the other hand, will focus on the weakening of the symbiotic ties between mother and son and the opening up of the possibility for a constructive identification with the father, and will of course also note the obvious transference phenomena. New shifts in accent, new "punctuation," and new, consolidated metaphors all play a large role, supported by a pleasurable atmosphere of understanding and emotional intensity. Other striking elements of this session are the manner in which attention is focused on the present or future, while all discussion of the past history of family conflicts is avoided; the subtle but total domination of the situation by the therapist; and the deliberate avoidance of conscious insight.

The most surprising aspect of the session is surely that it was at all effective, and that this effect was lasting. This can be explained in part by the extremely clear, even stark polarization and restructuring of the entire field of force within the family, in both cognitive and affective terms. In favorable circumstances this can lead to a corresponding repolarization of internalized self and object representations, which will then receive continued support in the form of altered feedback from other family members. If the constituent elements of the external field—in this case father, mother, and son—are shifted by effective action to their correct positions, then, we must assume, their internal representations will undergo a corresponding shift. If this does not occur, then intrapsychic changes will remain ineffective, since they will be denied and contradicted by discordant feedback from external reality. In my view there is yet another side to this approach, but it is one that Minuchin avoids mentioning as he explains his techniques. This is the induction, unnoticed by the participating family, of a "common everyday trance," to use Milton Erickson's phrase. A case history reported by this even more fascinating "magician" illustrates what this phenomenon is.

A 26-year-old man with an M.A. degree in psychology came reluctantly to the writer for hypnotherapy at his father's dictatorial demand. His problem was fingernail biting, begun at the age of four as a measure of escaping four hours' daily practice at the piano. He had bitten his fingernails to the quick until they bled, but his mother was unmoved by the bloodstains on the keys. He continued the piano and the fingernail biting until the latter had become an uncontrollable habit. He resented greatly being sent for hypnotherapy and freely stated so. I began by assuring him that he was justified in his resentment, but I was amused that he had allowed himself to participate in self-frustration for 22 long years. He looked at me in a puzzled way, so the explanation was given,

"To get out of playing the piano you bit your fingernails to the quick until it became an unbreakable habit despite the fact you have wanted long fingernails. In other words, for 22 years you have literally deprived yourself of the privilege of biting off a good-sized piece of fingernail, one that you could really set your teeth on satisfyingly."

The young man laughed and said, "I see exactly what you are doing to me. You are putting me in the position of growing fingernails long enough to give me some genuine satisfaction in biting them off and making the futile nibbling I'm doing even more frustrating." After further semi-humorous discussion he acknowledged that he was not sure he really wanted to experience a formal hypnosis. I accepted this by adamantly refusing to make any formal effort. This constituted a reverse set double bind: He asked for something he was not sure he really wanted. It was refused. Therefore, he was bound to want it, since he could now do so safely. In the ensuing conversation, however, *his interest was maintained at a high pitch and his attention was rigidly fixated,* as he was told earnestly and intently that he could grow one long fingernail. He could take infinite pride in getting it long enough to constitute a satisfying bite. At the same time he could frustrate himself thoroughly by nibbling futilely at the tiny bits of nail on the other nine digits. Although no formal trance was induced, his high response attentiveness indicated he was in what we might call "the common everyday trance" that is brought on by any absorbing activity or conversation.

This light trance suggestion was reinforced by the measure of arousing him with casually irrelevant remarks and then repeating the instructions. What is the purpose of this measure? When you casually repeat suggestions in the awake state right after he heard them in trance the *patient says to himself,* "Oh, yes, I know that already, it's okay." In saying something of this sort to himself the patient is actually taking the first important step toward internalizing and reinforcing the suggestion as an aspect of his own inner world. It is this internalization of the suggestion that makes it an effective agent in behavior change.

Many months later the patient returned to display normal fingernails on each hand. His explanation, while uncertain and groping, is adequately descriptive of the effect of the double bind. He explained, "At first I thought the whole thing hilariously funny, even though you were serious in your attitude. Then I felt myself being pulled two ways. I wanted 10 long fingernails. You said I could have one only and I had to end up by biting it off and getting a "real mouthful of fingernail." That displeased me but I felt compelled to do it and to keep gnawing at my other fingernails. That frustrated me painfully. When the one fingernail started growing out I felt pleased and happy, I was more resentful than ever at the thought of biting it off but I knew I had agreed to do so. I eventually got around that by growing a second nail—that left eight fingers to gnaw on and I wouldn't have to bite the second long one off. I won't bore you with the details. Things just got more confusing and frustrating. I just keep on growing more nails and nibbling on fewer fingers, until I just said "to hell with it!" That compulsion to grow nails and nibble nails and to feel more frustrated all the time was just unbearable. Just what were the motivations you put to work in me and how did it work?"

Now, more than eight years later, he is well-advanced in his profession, he is well-adjusted, a personal friend, and he has normal fingernails. He is convinced that the writer used hypnosis on him to some degree because he still remembers a "peculiar feeling as if I couldn't move when you were talking to me."[29]

Even though the problem in this case history is much less severe than a psychosis, it still contains instructive elements for our topic. First of all, Erickson mentions the "common everyday trance," which, in my opinion, must be a part of *every* therapeutic influence of any intensity and of course represents, in psychoanalytic terms, a powerful force in transference. Apart from this, the report shows very clearly how the internalization of "disturbing" new information can destabilize old systems of reference. And finally, it illustrates the *technique of the therapeutic double bind.* Experiences with this new method during the last decade have revealed it to be one of the most effective means of shaking up rigid systems of reference or behavior. We are only now beginning, in the wake of Bateson, Erickson, Haley, Watzlawick, Selvini Palazzoli and others, to grasp the mechanisms at work in this procedure and to learn how to apply them.

Erickson defines the therapeutic double bind as a situation in which the patient is offered an illusory freedom of choice between two possibilities, neither of which really appeals to him, but both of which are expressed in positive terms. To make his point Erickson cites his father, who used to ask him if he would rather feed the chickens or the pigs first, and whether he would prefer to go to bed at eight o'clock or stay up until eight fifteen. Every time he would be surprised at himself for agreeing to one of the two alternatives, although he really wanted to do something quite different. The two possibilities offered appear to exist within a frame of reference on an implied higher plane of logic that is immutable and inescapable. Analogies to the pathological form of the double bind are evident, and they also include one point that does not emerge so clearly from the simple examples given, namely that in Erickson's method not just one, but in fact a whole complicated series of double binds is offered. The key difference between pathological and therapeutic double binds is that the latter contains a *positive* situation and relationship. The "fundamental message" is that whatever the therapist may do or suggest is done for the patient's benefit, to serve his health, his growth, and his autonomy, and not to serve the therapist's own needs. In other words, a positive basic transference is an essential prerequisite for this kind of prescription to be effective: the patient swallows the bitter pill because he is convinced that it will do him good. Double binds that are not in the patient's real interest fortunately do not succeed, as Erickson emphasizes, nor do hypnotic procedures; like a pathological double bind, they evoke only deep-seated tension and rage.

A further decisive difference between the two kinds of double bind lies in the fact that the therapeutic situation contains (and must necessarily contain) an element of genuine freedom: the patient comes for treatment of his own free will, and he is free to stop coming. The same applies to psychoanalysis, which in some ways resembles a double-bind situation. The fundamental rule, which the patient must accept, *demands* that he associate *freely*. This very aspect of both methods makes it apparent that any form of treatment involving coercion, no matter how skillful, will inevitably have a negative, paradoxical character. Not only the receiver but also the sender of therapeutic double-bind messages must alter his system of reference to a certain extent: he must keep an open mind, be flexible, and contemplate *several* possible solutions instead of just one, at least on a superficial level; he must be sure to keep a second, deeper level of treatment and his "fundamental message" extremely stable.

Erickson's own writings and the many books that have now been written about him, such as Jay Haley's *Uncommon Therapy* and E. L. Rossi's *Nature of Hypnosis and Suggestions,* give many striking examples of how therapeutic double binds can alter systems of reference.[30] Similarly unconventional methods with much the same structure have been devloped by Selvini Palazzoli and her colleagues; they use sophisticated counterparadoxes, such as the "prescription of pathology" in the case of the taboo ritual cited above. Her "golden rule" belongs in the same context: avoiding all criticism of patients' behavior, however pathological it may be, and so creating the basis for a positive therapeutic relationship and alliance.

In general all these approaches represent forms of psychotherapy that combine familiar methods from psychodynamics, psychoanalysis, and hypnotherapy with newer ones developed by communications and systems theory. The resulting new techniques for altering systems of reference force us to reconsider the merits of the more traditional therapies, including psychoanalysis. An example from my own experience illustrates this point.

An unmarried woman of over fifty who had been diagnosed elsewhere as having a "personality structure with severe narcissistic defects" was brought in as an emergency case in a state of suicidal depression and despair. This occurred two years after her psychoanalyst had broken off her treatment against her wishes. The analysis had begun well and continued for several years, but toward the end had clearly taken a most unfortunate course. The entire past of this woman was characterized by traumatic losses and frustrations. Her parents had been involved in long and bitter divorce proceedings throughout her childhood; one brother had committed suicide, and several relationships with men, though initially promising, had not lasted. She had always had depressive tendencies and strong feelings of her own worthlessness. She felt ugly, old, incompetent; the people around her appeared unreliable and bad. It was apparent at first glance that her central problem was the theme of separation, represented at the moment by the unresolved and highly ambivalent transference relationship with her (male) psychoanalyst. The patient demanded that I take over her interrupted analysis and unconsciously expected me to provide reparation for all the disappointments she had suffered.

I offered her a total of ten hours of treatment, no more and no less, leaving the choice of when they were to take place up to her. She could decide whether they should all take place immediately, in a few weeks, in a year, or in ten years. At first she "needed" several hours in quick succession. Although a distinctly positive relationship developed, she used these sessions to give vent to her frustrations, both past and present, and to try to make me change my mind and consent to psychoanalysis, or at least to a few more hours of treatment. I remained adamant as I offered direct interpretations of a negative transference. Gradually, with the aid of techniques like those described above, I succeeded in contributing more positive elements to her images of herself and her body; I saw and emphasized not her weaknesses and insecurities but rather her tremendous hidden strength in the face of all the blows of fate she had suffered: her ability to be by herself, her powers of observation, and—a "legacy" from her father—her creative and very characteristic sense of humor. This last quality had long been buried but began slowly to reemerge. After six sessions she began to introduce longer and longer breaks; the last one, before the ninth hour, lasted exactly one year. Her depression improved at about the same rate, except for minor ups and downs, giving way to a degree of efficiency and enjoyment of her work that she had never experienced before. Both her appearance and her self-image underwent striking changes. In the eighth and especially the ninth hours I set up the following multilayered therapeutic double bind: She could decide to keep the tenth hour in reserve for an unspecified length of time, or she could use it up at some point and thus bring the therapy to a conclusion. In both cases she would become capable of living her life with her own resources. Since then three years have gone by with, as I once heard, more very positive developments. The tenth hour is still "up in the air."

Why is such a situation thoroughly therapeutic, meaning constructive instead of destructive? The main reason is probably that the "fundamental message" containing and continually communicating the therapeutic double bind is based on a positive relationship and expresses a genuine and unshakable confidence in the hidden strengths of this devalued and careworn woman. The same holds true for all the arrangements with regard to her therapy, which contain a recognition of the need for limits and separation as well as the element of "attachment," that is, a (paradoxical) recognition of her need for long-term support.

The danger exists that the few examples and case histories offered here, which are intended to illustrate the positive possibilities in new techniques for altering systems of reference, may create the false impression that they are always crowned with rapid success. Nothing could be further from the truth. For one thing, even with these methods some cases can still require years of treatment, comparable to intensive psychoanalysis (such as Erickson's patient "Harold," discussed later), and for another even the most skilled therapists report instances of errors and failure.[31] For the achievement of spectacular successes, years of practice and preparation are usually necessary as in the case of the Japanese calligraphers who work with lightning speed. The use of the new methods in psychotherapy is still by and large a learning process, although it is going on in many different places, and as yet neither their possibilities nor their limits are fully apparent. Their status in relation to older, traditional procedures such as psychoanalysis, cognitive methods, and drug therapies is just as open a question.

As far as psychoanalysis is concerned, the success of the new techniques has forced us to reconsider many theoretical as well as practical elements. In the light of these modern procedures classical analysis begins to appear more and more as an instrument for fine adjustments, comparable perhaps to surgical techniques using microscopes, and suited as therapy only in very special and exceptional cases. Most of the time the experienced general surgeon will give preference to less fine but faster and more efficient procedures. Whoever desires to study the fine details of intrapsychic workings, however, like the psychotherapy specialist, will not be able to do without the knowledge of their fine structure that only the "microscope" of psychoanalysis can provide, just as the physician cannot do without the basic disciplines of histology and physiology, even though in practice he may make very little direct use of them himself. Freud seems to have anticipated such a development when he wrote in 1926: "The future will probably attribute far greater importance to psycho-analysis as the science of the unconscious than as a therapeutic procedure."[32]

This view of the matter reflects the fact—which has become an open secret—that many psychoanalysts now seldom treat anyone except other members of their own profession, that is, future psychoanalysts, psychiatrists, and psychotherapists. It applies even more to the immensely difficult and time-consuming attempts to treat schizophrenics in individual psychoanalysis, undertaken twenty or thirty years ago (with some success) by pioneers such as Rosen, Fromm-Reichmann, Sechehaye, C. Müller, Benedetti, Stierlin, and Selvini Palazzoli. It is striking that most of the pioneers of modern family and systems therapy have a firm grounding in psychoanalysis, a training that leaves its stamp everywhere in their work. Mara Selvini Palazzoli, for example, by no means rejects a psychoanalytic understanding of intrapsychic and interpersonal processes, despite her considerably different methods of therapy. Explaining why she makes no attempt to determine the causes of problems in family therapy sessions, she writes: "Causes, reasons, and feelings should all remain in Pandora's box, as it were. This does not mean that we therapists, having a psychoanalytic formation as we do, do not regularly discuss the session using the linear and psychoanalytic model."[33]

Erickson's intuitive grasp of situations also appears specifically psychoanalytic in case after case, in contrast to his techniques; his therapy sessions often strike one as "actualized" or "performed" psychoanalysis, projected into the present and future instead of the past. The goals of "structural family therapy" as practiced by Minuchin are to create clear lines of demarcation between generations and family members, to break up dysfunctional alliances, and so on; the methods used are intended to achieve these goals by influencing the external social field, and thus run parallel to the goals of psychoanalysis with respect to intrapsychic processes.

One aspect of this general problem that will perhaps require particular study is the *dimension of time*. A firm grasp of the ways in which we experience time and their fundamental significance to us—and we have a long way to go in this respect—would probably provide important evidence on the formation and structure of the psyche. The theoretical foundations and therapeutic methods of the systemic and structuralist schools are strongly present-oriented; systems therapists (appear to) work only in a synchronic system and to neglect diachrony, whereas Freud's key discovery and the main field of psychoanalytic work (appear to) lie exclusively in the patient's past history. If we look closely, however, both observations must be qualified. Systems therapists do explore and employ important elements from the past; Selvini Palazzoli, for example, uses them to construct highly effective counterparadoxes.[34] And it is a well-known fact that if psychoanalysis does not succeed in reawakening the emotions of the past in the here and now of the transference, it remains ineffective. As we saw in Chapter 3, there exist in the mind both a synchronic system of the present and a past-future system along a longitudinal time axis; the two are connected in an intricate manner, interacting and influencing each other in ways that are not yet well understood.[35] This function represents a fundamental unsolved problem. A similar problem exists in many disciplines—biology, linguistics, political science, and economics—and would certainly suggest interesting new insights and possibilities for a number of them. All of this indicates that it would be a serious error simply to jettison psychoanalysis, as some extreme systems theorists have proposed; we would do far better to endure the tension inherent in the opposition between the two approaches, so that in the end the congruent elements in both can be applied to further creative development. Of course such a process would require psychoanalysis to come to grips with a whole range of new facts and questions, including the following.

Experiences in the present, if they possess enough affective intensity, can in special circumstances restructure affective-cognitive systems of reference internalized in the past, including even the crucial systems of self and object representations. This restructuring can be accomplished with amazing rapidity and lasting effectiveness if it is later confirmed by feedback from a correspondingly restructured social field. Such experience raises the question of whether the arduous detour via the systematic reactivation of the past should ever be taken. Both psychology and learning theory have shown that affective-logical systems of reference become extended and strengthened through use. Therefore, old and possibly already partly inactive ways of thinking, feeling, and behaving—such as regressive, aggressive, or depressive modes that may have been experienced and established during phases of severe frustration in early childhood—would necessarily be first *reinforced* through long and frequent actualization in the therapeutic process, creating the need for dismantling them later with great effort and some risk. Similar doubts have recently become apparent in the psychoanalytic profession itself, quite apart from any influence of systems theory. Benedetti, for instance, places the main emphasis on the present in his treatment of schizophrenics.[36] In the cases of neurotic patients the goal of systematically investigating the past is also often modified. Short-term therapy based on psychoanalytic principles but with a specific focus is one example;[37] the work of the French analyst Serge Viderman is another. Viderman uses the interpretation of "analytic material" primarily as a means to constructing entirely in the present an "analytic space"—that is, to creating a common language for the dialogue between patient and therapist.[38] In principle, this amounts to the same thing as polarizing the social field by constructing a shared system of reference. In this case it is limited to the analytic relationship between only two people, but it thereby acquires the enormous emotional weight it must have to alter behavior. This is of course exactly what classical analysis strives to achieve by concentrating all essential problems in the "transference neurosis."

The role of transference in modern techniques for altering systems of reference is very apparent from a psychoanalytic point of view;

their successful use is regarded in some quarters as merely a superficial sort of "transference cure." On the other hand, it is well known that in (either short- or long-term) psychoanalysis regression to an intensive transference is considered to be the essential therapeutic force; the only difference is that in the new techniques it is directly focused. Many of the new forms of therapy certainly make use of the transference as a vehicle for change. This is done implicitly instead of explicitly, but it can still reach depths far beyond the effects of a superficial transference reaction. The internalized affective-logical schemata affecting behavior and the transference, such as those connected with self and object representations, could be compared to acquired, intrapsychic "matrices" or "genes," which produce the same response to fundamentally similar situations. To the extent that radically innovative techniques such as the therapeutic double bind or paradoxical prescriptions can effectively modify such central structures, they may perhaps represent a new kind of "psychological gene manipulation"—with, it must be repeated, both possibilities and limits that have not yet fully emerged.

Important questions also exist regarding the significance of awareness and insight as the ultimate goals of successful psychotherapy. New methods of altering systems of reference suggest they might have a different value. Erickson, Minuchin, Selvini Palazzoli, and others appear to make an intentional effort to avoid conscious insight in the traditional sense on the patient's part; and we know from Piaget that conscious attention focused on the actualization of internalized cognitive schemata can be more of a hindrance than a help. Even in the hypnotic techniques of Milton Erickson, however, we always observe at least a temporary concentration of conscious attention, accompanied by intense feelings, on the area to be changed.[39] This phenomenon tends to confirm the assumption that a reshaping of affective-logical systems of reference cannot be accomplished without direct affective and cognitive focus on them. Clearly, the concentration of attention and intensity of affect necessary to achieve this can be developed in a strong transference. After the new information has been integrated and the reshaped system practiced, however, such a focus and the consequent "conscious insight" are probably superfluous and may even be counterproductive. (Naturally I do not mean to imply that Freud's famous therapeutic fiat, "Where id was, there ego shall be,"[40] is no longer valid, but this "ego" might consist of *unconscious* components to a much greater extent than has been assumed until now.)

Clearly the few points mentioned here suggest a wealth of complex theoretical questions that go far beyond the scope of this book. We are still in the early stages of finding possible answers, especially as regards a revision of psychoanalytic thinking. Erickson's techniques and also those of Selvini Palazzoli (with their blend of intuitive psychoanalytic understanding and quite different practical methods) show that somewhere must lie a fascinating and fruitful synthesis of the two approaches, which may lead to the psychotherapy of the future. An important case of Erickson's, presented at some length by Jay Haley, provides one more example of how profound and effectual the alteration of a system of reference can be with these new procedures.

"Harold" was a migratory laborer with homosexual leanings and an extremely hostile attitude toward women. Lonely and often desperate, he was treated at long intervals over a period of several years by Erickson, who employed the seemingly inexhaustible arsenal of his techniques—some hypnotic and concentrating on the individual, and some which effectively involved the social field. Harold changed almost beyond recognition during this period; he acquired a radically new and positive self-image and view of the world, went back and finished high school, successfully found work as a private secretary, made friends, and finally began a sexual relationship with a woman, an older, motherly person, for the first time in his life. He was able to end this relationship and then experienced, toward the end of his therapy, the following:

"Monday morning I got up early and left for work, not knowing why I went early. It didn't take long to find out. I was driving down the street when it happened. A girl came along towards me on the pavement and I was so startled I had to pull up at the curb and watch her out of the corner of my eye until she got past. That girl was beautiful—the first beautiful girl I had ever seen. Two blocks further on, the same thing happened again. Only this time it was two absolutely beautiful girls. I had a hard time getting to work. I wanted to stop and look at things. Everything was so changed. The grass was green, the trees were beautiful, the houses looked freshly painted, the cars on the street looked new, the men looked like me, and the streets of Phoenix are lousy, just absolutely lousy with pretty girls. It's been that way ever since Monday. The world is changed."[42]

An experience of this kind is a striking counterpart to the experiences of psychotic disorder presented in the previous chapter, such as Conrad's patient, Corporal K., or the young woman who heard voices in the rain. It is a joyful experience of "re-ordering," of things being back in their proper place, of openness and harmony. It is an experience of the law of growth and development that is innate in every human being.

The fact that most of the examples of dramatic cures or improvements presented in this chapter do not involve schizophrenic patients may give rise to a question, however: Are these techniques for altering systems of reference in fact suited to cases of severe psychosis? The answer is that many of these methods were actually developed in the treatment of schizophrenics. In their book *Paradox and Counterparadox* Selvini Palazzoli and her colleagues report on nothing but cases of psychosis, although they concentrate on instances of children and teenagers who were not hospitalized during therapy. Erickson also treated schizophrenics, sometimes with amazing success. Bandler and Grinder report in detail on the case of a hospitalized catatonic patient who had spoken only an incomprehensible private language for five years and was otherwise completely mute; Erickson was able to cure him within a year by inventing an analogous language of his own. In this language he succeeded in making contact with the man, gradually carrying on more and more lively "conversations" with him until the patient finally began to speak intelligibly and to move and act as well.[43] The following case from my own experience shows that interesting possibilities exist even with chronic schizophrenics, or perhaps *especially* with them.

In our day clinic we attempted for fourteen months in individual therapy to improve the condition of a twenty-nine-year-old patient, but we met with the same lack of success as his previous therapists. He had formerly attended a commercial training course and had studied music, but in the preceding ten years he had had to be hospitalized several times for episodes of schizophrenia with delusions and hallucinations. In between hospitalizations he had tried to carry out highly unrealistic plans for a career as a painter or pianist. We wanted to "bring him back down to earth" and encourage him to organize his life more constructively, but whenever he was presented with any specific changes, his hallucinations and delusional fears increased to such an extent that all plans had to be abandoned. Finally we sent him back home, to a well-known therapist (Gottlieb Guntern) who began sessions with the patient and his family. He concentrated at once on the patient's positive creative and human qualities, and redefined all the schizo-

phrenic symptoms as a form of "private entertainment" designed
to help the young man pass the time and avoid adult responsibilities. Simultaneously the therapist worked at establishing a closer
relationship between the "designated patient" and his younger
brother and at improving the lines of demarcation between the
parents and the younger generation by giving them a heightened
sense of self-worth. Then, once he had created a relationship of
genuine trust with all participants, they worked out a plan in minute detail together, containing clear rules of behavior for every
member of the family. The first step toward the final goal of autonomy for the patient was for him to find a part-time job at
once. Influences running counter to this goal (from a physician
and other sources) were tactfully but systematically neutralized by
the therapist. He worked to repolarize a number of affective-
cognitive systems of reference (goals, values, future expectations,
ideas about the nature of the patient's current difficulties and the
prognosis) for all family members, altering them in the direction
of health, strength, and independence. The immediate result was
that, with the consistent support of his brother and parents, the
patient's attitude underwent a dramatic change, and after only
one week he took on a strenuous job as a dishwasher. As time
passed his characteristic attitude of evasive, anxious nervousness
gave way to a clear decisiveness even in moments of conflict; his
hallucinations and delusions receded. Two years later, with the aid
of one family session per month, not only the patient himself but
also his brother and parents continue to develop in a positive direction, despite a number of complications that have had to be
faced.

The decisive factor in this case was undoubtedly the skillful and in-
formed redefinition of the general situation and the goal to be worked
for. These were no longer defined as the treatment of a disease, but as
a united effort to encourage a natural, healthy development that had
failed to take place before.

Besides the methods already discussed, many more techniques for
therapeutically altering systems of reference must surely exist; like the
variety of "disorganizers," these could cover the whole spectrum from
social and interpersonal influences to biochemical ones. In a broader
sense we may also reckon various rehabilitative procedures among

these techniques, including new and sophisticated methods of cognitive behavior therapy, assertiveness training, role playing, and formalized work and behavior therapy. Even some effects of medication, such as the striking changes sometimes observed with antidepressants or antianxiety drugs, can be regarded as typical alterations of a system of reference. From the perspective of affect-logic the effectiveness of all the factors named will depend on how clearly and consistently the various therapeutic steps are combined, and on how well the social field can be involved in support. This is exactly what one of the most thorough American studies of recent years has shown. The variables listed below are in complete agreement with the general principles of treatment proposed in this chapter; in this study, which followed two groups for five years, they proved to be decisive in the successful treatment of chronic mental patients (mainly schizophrenics). One group underwent routine treatment; the other received intensive milieu therapy in a therapeutic community and in structured social learning programs.[44]

1. Treatment as a "client" and not as a "patient"
2. Induction of specific positive expectations
3. Structured activities with progressive increases of responsibility
4. Concentration on action (not on explanations)
5. Organized, structured programs
6. A stable, predictable environment
7. Emphasis on individually selected skills necessary for living in society (jobs, housework, etc.)
8. Creation of social contacts
9. Supportive and educational follow-up care after return to the community

As for medication, and the neuroleptics in particular, the view developed here does not question their potential usefulness, either in acute conditions or as preventive measures against relapses. Their ability to reduce sensitivity to stress and the vehemence of emotions, and thus to act as an effective "brake" in cases of psychotic "runaway," suggests that their main function is as general buffers. Although this function may certainly be advantageous in some situations, it may be superfluous or even harmful in others. Well-known studies by Vaughn, Leff, and others have shown that neuroleptics can contribute a great deal to preventing relapses, especially when patients live in close contact with emotionally overinvolved families.[45] If there is a less strained situation or no contact, however, then negative pharmacological and social side effects (such as blunting of affect and personality, loss of energy potential, tiredness, sluggishness, ocular disturbances, infantilization, social labeling, and irreversible motor disturbances) tend to prevail, particularly if high doses are being given. Medication represents a potentially useful tool that is best employed only when a patient's total social and personal situation is taken into account. The results from the Soteria Project indicate that drug therapy can become unnecessary even for acute schizophrenics if other conditions for therapy are particularly favorable. In our follow-up studies of former patients with severe chronic schizophrenia, we found a large number who had been living without medication or relapses for years or even decades.

Conclusion

I would like to close this chapter and the book with two thoughts; one is connected with questions of therapy and the other with the general subject of affect-logic.

The few points I have touched on with regard to therapy are *elementary* in the double sense of being both "simple" and "basic." The ideas I have tried to formulate, apart from the sophisticated techniques for altering systems of reference referred to at the end, are mostly a matter of common sense. Possibly they have become forgotten "secrets" for that very reason. Again and again they threaten to be swept away by a flood of subtle and hyperintellectual theories. But the ideas on therapy described here are simple enough to be understood by everyone, and this, I believe, is their main virtue: they are accessible not merely to specialists of various schools (psychoanalysis, family dynamics, systems theory, or behavior therapy) but should also appear down-to-earth and sensible to family physicians, to the nurses and support staff who play a far more important role than doctors do in the everyday experience of mental patients, to social workers, to directors of rehabilitation programs, to relatives, and last but not least to those people for whom all these efforts are undertaken, the patients themselves. Everyone should be able to form a picture of the specific goals, programs, and methods I have mentioned; one can discuss them, accept or reject them—in short, work with them in a constructive way. To this extent they represent, mainly for schizophrenics but certainly also for many other mental patients, a kind of solid foundation upon which more differentiated special techniques can be based. In the extreme situation of schizophrenic psychosis something becomes recognizable that we have difficulty perceiving in the more subtle disturbances of neurosis, perhaps because we are too close to the latter. Thus, from a pedagogical point of view, the basic principles of psychotherapeutic treatment for schizophrenics should not necessarily be regarded as the culmination of the therapist's art, to be reached by only a small elite; on the contrary, and in contrast to current notions, we ought to see these principles as a possible *starting point:* whoever has acquired a real grasp of them will profit greatly in the treatment of all other, milder disorders.

I would like to emphasize again, however, that much remains to be learned about the newer methods of therapy; we must bring some order to their confusing variety and assign the correct weight to each. We must learn what the best combinations are and distinguish more clearly between what is specifically effective and what is not. On the other hand, the approach taken here certainly suggests more than I have been able to cover explicitly. One subject that received too little mention is the physical aspect, *the therapeutic approach to the affective-cognitive double system of the psyche by way of the body.* In practice there are almost endless fruitful possibilities for approaching a patient's problems from the physical, nonverbal side; in combination with verbal therapy (groups, ergotherapy, social therapy, rehabilitation programs, and individual or family psychotherapy), we can use pictorial, symbolic, and ritual experiences that as forms of action can strongly affect emotions. Of course this can be achieved only by fully integrating physical therapists in the therapeutic team. Specialists such as dance and exercise therapists and gymnastics teachers would have to participate in other therapeutic activities, group discussions, and staff meetings to design and evaluate programs, and not merely in occasional exchanges of information. The same applies to music and art therapy. As I have said before, the goal is to create the fullest possible sense of harmony in body and mind, feelings and thinking, verbal and nonverbal modes of expression and communication.

Further important but often neglected therapeutic possibilities exist in personal contact with animals and plants, in "communication" with the fundamental and marvelously clear laws of nature, especially for schizophrenic patients. Whoever has tried, literally, to *talk* to animals or even to plants, knows that subtle answers are quick to come.

Another aspect that has received little attention in this book is *prevention*. The straightforward and low-tension forms of communication that have been mentioned as essential parts of good therapy naturally have a prophylactic effect as well. In addition, we could establish as a sensible goal of *primary prevention* (that is, preventing a first outbreak of disease) teaching children *how to deal with complex affective-cognitive information*. Montessori kindergartens, some Piagetian concepts concerning the cognitive field, and ideas developed by the anthroposophs (disciples of Rudolf Steiner) in their work with children concerning the emotions all suggest what form such primary preventive care might take. In the area of *secondary prevention* (preventing relapses) we have already noted the proven efficacy of medication in stress situations, and we could also envisage the development of improved methods for dealing with difficult family or work environments. One simple approach would be to teach patients how to set up a better hierarchy of internalized coping mechanisms, as in the case of the woman who learned to deal first with immediate problems and then with more distant ones. An analogous general motto might be: Tackle the simple problems first and then the more complicated ones! Another possibility of social learning is currently being explored by British research teams: families who are fairly successful in dealing with a mentally ill relative can teach a great deal to more seriously disturbed families. Methods of *tertiary prevention* (preventing disease from becoming chronic) are implied in much of what was said above about avoiding full hospitalization, especially for longer periods, and about developing alternate forms of treatment, stimulation, and social reintegration.

At the same time everything I have said here about therapy for schizophrenics needs to be understood in its proper context. Affect-logic contains hints and suggestions; it sets new accents and poses many questions, some of them new, but it does not offer guarantees or prescriptions for success. We are still searching, especially in our everyday work as members of a therapeutic team; we are learning and developing new ideas in a process of trial and error. Like other therapists, we have encouraging achievements, but also our share of only partial successes and outright failures. And much research remains to be done; in particular, the claim that treatment programs combining several of the approaches mentioned here are more effective must be carefully studied and verified.

This leads to the second question that I want to discuss briefly: After traveling all this way, how far have we come in our search for a logic of affects and the affects of logic, for a more holistic understanding of the interaction between feeling and thinking in the healthy mind and in psychosis?

Certainly we have made progress in clarifying one possible view of things. We have established a sort of comprehensive system of reference in which many disparate observations have found a place with some consistent order. But several gaps remain. As this final chapter in particular has shown, this system of reference can function as a basis for action; that is, it can be used as a way of dealing with the daily reality that we encounter. This does not mean that it is the whole truth; like every other "truth," every "right answer" or synthesis that reduces an area of tension, it is merely *one* perspective, *one* fragment of a still unknown whole.

But let us consider, for a moment, how we usually answer questions of the type: Is affect-logic actually one "truth," or at least one "right answer?" Putting the question this way produces several interesting points: We cannot answer it with thinking alone, with cognitive observation and measurement, no matter how objective; we must consult our feelings at the same time. In other words, the instrument we use to tell whether something is "right" or not is not solely logical thought, nor is it only a feeling, an uncontrolled emotion. It is *both*, feeling and thinking in a specific economical *equilibrium*—and not only in this case, but *always*, I am convinced, even when the simple "truth" of reciprocal relationships such as $2 \times 2 = 4$ and $4 \div 2 = 2$ dawns on us for the first time. This state of equilibrium represents a harmonious resonance, a minimum of cognitive-affective tension and a maximum of structuring at once, both "release" and "constructive achievement." It is such a balance between feeling and thinking that we constantly strive to reach, and when we do, it is not a Nirvana, a state of complete release from tension—as Freud thought for a while that it might be—but a pleasurable experience of greater harmony. *This kind of pleasure thus appears to be the driving force behind all mental and intellectual development.* I am further convinced that what we have in this particular case is only one instance of a very general tendency in nature for things to reach a state of equilibrium. If the often-postulated hypothesis is correct that everything that exists has a dual structure of part and counterpart, then this striving for harmony is an interesting reformulation of the fundamental natural principle known as the second law of thermodynamics: the ubiquitous tendency toward a maximum reduction of tension. In any event our psyche, with its affective and cognitive "poles," clearly is able to register this special balance or "rightness" as we feel-think-know things; we carry it with us everywhere as a kind of compass. It must certainly have something to do with "the evidence of our senses" on which all axioms are founded. This form of experience is suspect to philosophers, but it is also one they have never been able to do without. In the last analysis we use just such experience to decide whether an explanation, a situation, a scientific hypothesis is "right" or not, whether it is economical and harmonious or lopsided, either a sterile intellectual theory or an emotional flight of fancy.

As theories go, this is not an easy one to swallow; it gives the emotions a weight equal to (though not greater than) intellect as a way of knowing. We are accustomed, in the sciences at least, to regard logic alone as valid—and have for this reason developed a civilization that is, all in all, insanely one-sided, rational, cold, technological, and efficient . . . I would claim that we misinterpret the emotional component of great scientific theories—for Copernicus when he began to discover the "true" relationship between the sun and the planets, for Kekule when he discovered the ring structure of benzene, for Watson and Crick when they grasped the double-helix structure of DNA. Blind to reality, we persist in repressing and denying this component. The feelings of these scientists were not merely pleasure as a *reaction* to a successful discovery, however. Instead, a striving for pleasure, for a feeling of harmony and "rightness" was itself an instrument of discovery, just as a persistent feeling of disharmony tells us that something is *not* right, despite all superficial appearances to the contrary.

The following thought may help to place much of the fragmentary evidence of earlier chapters in a large context and make its significance clearer: If it is in fact true that emotions represent invariance and the intellect variance in our affective-logical systems of reference, then both feeling and thinking *together* are necessary to grasp structure as we have defined it. What we call "feeling," that is, what we mainly perceive through the instrument of the body as a whole, grasps primarily entities and similarities; as we have seen, these holistic perceptions probably are closely related to the right hemisphere of the brain. The analytic, abstract, "left-brained" intellect then fills in the details in these "intuitive" basic perceptions and "modulates" them. Just as in binocular vision, not until both aspects are *combined* do our perceptions become sharp and accurate; each in isolation leads to its own kind of flatness and distortion.

To return to our question: Is the theory of affect-logic "true"? My own "feeling" is that the answer is not yet entirely clear; my pleasure is mixed, although as I wrote I always strived to let my compass lead me in the "right" direction. I have a sense that the *direction* is the good one, but we are still a long way from our goal. In our search for "reality" we can rely only on our instrument of perception, which is both cognitive and affective; we must think sharply and logically, observing, measuring, and drawing conclusions at times. But at other times we must also depend on our feelings and our intuition in order to perceive the "true" state of things. We *must* do this, for to act in this way reflects a natural movement toward equilibrium between the two poles of the psyche, which cannot be evaded and which continuously regulates the workings of our mind. But this back-and-forth, these "fluctuations," we suddenly come to realize at the end of our reflection, constitute a special kind of "runaway," namely a *creative process!* They draw us on inevitably, just as the pheromones carried by the wind attract the moth from one "right" place to the next. We have no choice but to stagger on together toward a larger truth.

Notes

Index

Notes

1. Psychoanalysis and Systems Theory

An earlier version of this chapter was published in *Psyche*, 35 (1981).

1. T. S. Kuhn, *The Structure of Scientific Revolutions* (Chicago: University of Chicago Press, 1970).
2. Ludwig von Bertalanffy, *Modern Theories of Development* (1928; reprint, New York: Harper Torchbooks, 1962). See also idem, "An Outline of General Systems Theory," *British Journal of Philosophical Science*, 1 (1950), 134–165.
3. J. G. Miller, "General Systems Theory," in *Comprehensive Textbook of Psychiatry*, ed. A. M. Freedman, H. J. Kaplan, and B. J. Sadock (Baltimore: William and Wilkins, 1975), pp. 98–114.
4. M. Zahn, "System," in *Handbuch philosophischer Grundbegriffe*, ed. H. Krings, H. M. Baumgartner, and C. Wild, 3 vols. (Munich: Kösel, 1974), III, 1458–75.
5. Jean Piaget, *Structuralism*, trans. Chaninah Maschler (New York: Harper & Row, 1970); first published as *Le structuralisme* (Paris: Presses Universitaires de France, 1968).
6. Gottlieb Guntern, "Die kopernikanische Wende in der Psychotherapie: Der Wandel vom psychoanalytischen zum systemischen Denken," *Familiendynamik*, 5 (1980), 4 and 7.
7. I have ignored here the various stages of development of this doctrine before the 1920s. I refer to the fully developed theory, including aspects of economy and dynamics ("psychoanalytic metapsychology").
8. Sigmund Freud, *Beyond the Pleasure Principle* (1920), *The Standard Edition of the Complete Works of Sigmund Freud*, ed. James Strachey, 24 vols. (London: Hogarth Press and Institute of Psycho-Analysis, 1953–74), XVIII, 1–

64; "The Economic Problem of Masochism" (1924), *Standard Edition*, XIX, 155–170.

9. Anna Freud, *The Ego and the Mechanisms of Defense,* trans. Cecil Baines (New York: International Universities Press, 1946; 1st German ed. 1936).

10. Karl Menninger, *The Vital Balance: The Life Process in Mental Health and Illness* (New York: Viking Press, 1963), pp. 102 and 104.

11. Heinz Hartmann, *Ego-Psychology and the Problem of Adaptation* (New York: International Universities Press, 1939).

12. Otto Kernberg, "Psychoanalytic Object-Relations Theory, Group Processes and Administration: Toward an Integrative Theory of Hospital Treatment," *Annals of Psychoanalysis,* 1 (1973), 363–388.

13. Murray Bowen, "Schizophrenia as a Multi-Generational Phenomenon," in *Beyond the Double Bind,* ed. M. M. Berger (New York: Brunner and Mazel, 1978), pp. 101–123; Ivan Boszormenyi-Nagy and G. Spark, *Invisible Loyalties* (New York: Harper & Row, 1973).

14. Salvador Minuchin, *Families and Family Therapy* (Cambridge, Mass.: Harvard University Press, 1974).

15. Mara Selvini Palazzoli et al., *Paradox and Counterparadox: A New Model in the Therapy of the Family in Schizophrenic Transaction,* trans. Elisabeth V. Burt (New York: Jason Aronson, 1978); first published as *Paradosso e controparadosso* (Milan: Feltrinelli, 1975).

16. L. C. Wynne, I. M. Ryckoff, J. Dave, and S. J. Hirsch, "Pseudomutuality in the Family Relations of Schizophrenics," *Psychiatry,* 21 (1958), 205–220.

17. Michael Balint, *The Basic Fault* (London: Tavistock, 1968).

18. H. F. Searles, "The Effort to Drive the Other Person Crazy," *British Journal of Medical Psychology,* 32 (1959), 1–19.

19. Gregory Bateson, D. Jackson, Jay Haley, and J. W. Weakland, "Towards a Theory of Schizophrenia," *Behavioral Science,* 1 (1956), 251–264.

20. Boszormenyi-Nagy and Spark, *Invisible Loyalties;* see also Helm Stierlin, *Von der Psychoanalyse zur Familientherapie* (Stuttgart: Klett-Cotta, 1975), pp. 182–183.

21. See the concept of delegation in Helm Stierlin, *Delegation und Familie* (Frankfurt: Suhrkamp, 1978).

2. On Affect-Logic

An earlier version of this chapter was published in *Psyche,* 36 (1982).

1. Sigmund Freud, "Project for a Scientific Psychology" (1895), *Standard Edition,* I, 281–293; idem, *The Interpretation of Dreams* (1900), ibid., IV and V.

2. Ferdinand de Saussure, "Psychologie génétique et psychanalyse," *Revue Française de Psychanalyse,* 6 (1933), 364–403; David Rapaport, "On the Psychoanalytic Theory of Thinking," *International Journal of Psycho-Analysis,* 31 (1950), 161–170; Michel Gressot, "Psychanalyse et connaissance" (1955), in *Le royaume intermédiaire* (Paris: Presses Universitaires de France, 1979); Thérèse Gouin-Décarie, *Intelligence and Affectivity in Early Childhood,* trans. E. P. Brandt and L. W. Brandt (New York: International

Universities Press, 1965); S. K. Escalona, "Patterns of Infantile Experience and the Developmental Process," *Psychoanalytic Study of the Child,* 18 (1963), 197–224; André Haynal, "Parallelen und Differenzen zweier Entwicklungspsychologien," *Psyche,* 29 (1975), 242–272.

3. Henri Schneider, *Die Theorie Piagets: Ein Paradigma für die Psychoanalyse?* (Bern: Huber, 1981). Although Schneider's book did not appear until after my own manuscript was completed, I have been able to incorporate some of his findings.

4. Jean Piaget, "La pensée symbolique et la pensée de l'enfant," *Archives de Psychologie,* 18 (1923), 273–304; idem, "La psychanalyse et le développement intellectuel," *Revue Française de Psychanalyse,* 6 (1933), 404–408; idem, "The Affective Unconscious and the Cognitive Unconscious," in *Piaget and His School,* ed. Bärbel Inhelder and H. H. Chipman (New York and Berlin: Springer, 1976), pp. 63–71.

5. Piaget's notes for a lecture series at the Sorbonne at 1953–54, titled "Intelligence and Affectivity: Their Relationship during Child Development," were published posthumously in 1981 in T. A. Brown and C. E. Kaegi, eds., *Annual Reviews Monograph* (Berkeley and Los Angeles: University of California Press), after my own manuscript had been completed. This is by far the most detailed discussion of the connections between affectivity and intelligence in Piaget's work, but curiously it is a subject to which he hardly ever returned. I have presented my own views on these lectures in a recent article, "Zur Integration von Fühlen und Denken im Licht der Affektlogik: Die Psyche als Teil eines autopoetischen Systems," in *Psychiatrie der Gegenwart,* ed. K. P. Kisker, H. Lauter, J. E. Meyer, C. Müller, and E. Strömgren, I (Berlin and Heidelberg: Springer, 1986), 373–409. Piaget's lectures contain many highly interesting details but present no fundamental contradictions to the hypotheses developed here.

6. Jean Piaget and Bärbel Inhelder, *The Psychology of the Child,* trans. Helen Weaver (New York: Basic Books, 1969; 1st French ed. 1966), p. 158.

7. Otto Kernberg, *Object Relations Theory and Clinical Psychoanalysis* (New York: Aronson, 1976).

8. See Rapaport, "Psychoanalytic Theory of Thinking"; Gressot, "Psychanalyse et connaissance."

9. Hartmann, *Ego-Psychology and the Problem of Adaptation.*

10. Piaget, "Affective Unconscious and Cognitive Unconscious," pp. 63–64.

11. See Jean Piaget, *The Psychology of Intelligence* (New York: Harcourt Brace, 1967).

12. Ibid., pp. 129–131.

13. Jean Piaget, *The Equilibration of Cognitive Structures: The Central Problem of Intellectual Development,* trans. Terrance Brown and K. J. Thampy (Chicago and London: University of Chicago Press, 1985; 1st French ed. 1975).

14. In his autobiography Piaget connects his interest in intellectual functions with the "unpredictability of the unconscious" ("la malice de l'inconscient") and also with his mother, who was emotionally unstable. His father, by contrast, became a model of seriousness for him early in life. This may be the most important source of Piaget's lifelong rejection of the importance of af-

fect. See *Jean Piaget et les sciences sociales: Autobiographie* (Geneva: Droz, 1966), pp. 129–159.

15. Inhelder and Chipman, *Piaget and His School*, p. 155.
16. Jean Piaget, *The Moral Judgment of the Child*, trans. Marjorie Gabain (New York: Free Press, 1965; 1st French ed. 1954). But see note 5 above.
17. Piaget and Inhelder, *The Psychology of the Child*, p. 21. See also René Spitz, *The First Year of Life: A Psychoanalytic Study of Normal and Deviant Development of Object Relations* (New York: International Universities Press, 1965); Gouin-Décarie, *Intelligence and Affectivity*; Escalona, "Patterns of Infantile Process."
18. Escalona, "Patterns of Infantile Process."
19. Piaget and Inhelder, *The Psychology of the Child*, pp. 114–115.
20. Ibid. This corresponds closely to D. W. Winnicott's psychoanalytic concept of the "transitional object."
21. Jean Piaget and Bärbel Inhelder, "The Gaps in Empiricism," in Inelder and Chipman, *Piaget and His School*, p. 32.
22. Gouin-Décarie, *Intelligence and Affectivity*, cited in Piaget, "Affective Unconscious and Cognitive Unconscious," p. 71.
23. H. C. Shands, "Structuralism and Genetic Epistemology" (Paper presented at the Sixth International Interdisciplinary Seminar on Piagetian Theory, University of Southern California, Los Angeles, January 1976).
24. Piaget, "Affective Unconscious and Cognitive Unconscious," p. 64.
25. Jacques Lacan, *The Four Fundamental Concepts of Psychoanalysis*, trans. Alan Sheridan (New York: Norton, 1978; 1st French ed. 1964), p. 20.
26. Piaget, "Affective Unconscious and Cognitive Unconscious," p. 71.
27. Piaget, "La pensée symbolique."
28. On the basis of the same passages Schneider arrives at a quite similar conclusion, namely that Piaget's theories imply "structural isomorphs" in the cognitive and affective areas and consequently imply the necessity of reflective abstractions for the latter as well; *Die Theorie Piagets*, p. 73.
29. Piaget, "Affective Unconscious and Cognitive Unconscious," p. 68.
30. Sigmund Freud, "Formulations Regarding the Two Principles in Mental Functioning" (1911), cited in Gressot, "Psychanalyse et connaissance," p. 89.
31. Jean Piaget, *Mes idées: Propos recueillis par Richard I. Evans-Denoel* (Paris: Gouthier, 1977), p. 58; cited in Schneider, *Die Theorie Piagets*, p. 147.
32. G. A. Miller, E. Galanter, and K. H. Pribram, *Plans and the Structure of Behavior* (New York: H. Holt, 1960).
33. Karl Popper and John Eccles, *The Self and Its Brain* (Berlin and London: Springer, 1977), p. 273.
34. Kernberg, *Object Relations Theory*, pp. 62–63.
35. Cited in M. B. Arnold, "Perennial Problems in the Field of Emotion," in *Feelings and Emotions* (New York: Academic Press, 1970), pp. 169–185.
36. Schneider, *Die Theorie Piagets*, p. 142.
37. J. D. Watson, *The Double Helix* (London: Weidenfeld & Nicholson, 1968).
38. Gressot, "Psychanalyse et connaissance," p. 187.
39. Cited in Haynal, "Parallelen und Differenzen," p. 249.

40. The fact that feelings also affect the body via the peripheral nervous system (the autonomic nervous system in particular) adds another dimension to the circumstances described here but does not fundamentally alter them.

41. See K. D. Hoppe, "Die Trennung der Gehirnhälften: Ihre Bedeutung für die Psychoanalyse," *Psyche*, 29 (1975), 919–940; B. E. Wexler, "Cerebral Laterality and Psychiatry: A Review of the Literature," *American Journal of Psychiatry*, 137 (1980), 279–291.

42. It is doubtful, however, that the psychoanalytic constructs of the ego, id, and superego can be understood on this basis. These hypothetical structural elements cannot simply be equated with Piaget's operational schemata.

43. P. Marty, "Sur la pensée opératoire," *Revue Française de Psychanalyse*, 36 (1972), 805–816; J. C. Nemiah, "Alexithymia: Theoretical Considerations," in *Toward a Theory of Psychosomatic Disorders,* ed. W. Brautigan and M. von Rad (Basle: Kastle, 1977).

44. Piaget, *Mes idées,* p. 58; cited in Schneider, *Die Theorie Piagets,* p. 147.

45. See Chapter 4, note 39.

46. Quite strikingly similar lines of thought to those pursued in this chapter have since been presented by Fritz B. Simon in *Der Prozess der Individuation. Über den Zusammenhang von Vernunft und Gefühlen* (Göttingen: Vanderhoeck & Ruprecht, 1984). In particular, his concepts of coenaesthetic perception (Spitz) and diacritical perception correspond to my use of "affect" and "cognition."

3. Differentiation, Structure, Systems, and Systems of Reference

1. Gregory Bateson, *Mind and Nature: A Necessary Unity* (New York: Dutton, 1979), p. 68.

2. Claude Lévi-Strauss, *Structural Anthropology* (1963; reprint, New York: Basic Books, 1976); first published as *Anthropologie structurale* (Paris: Plon, 1958).

3. Roger Bastide, ed., *Senses et usages du terme "structure"* (The Hague: Mouton, 1962).

4. Ibid., pp. 23–28.

5. Ibid., p. 14.

6. Ibid., p. 16.

7. Piaget, *Structuralism,* p. 5.

8. Ibid., pp. 19–20.

9. In Bastide, *Senses et usages du terme "structure,"* pp. 82–83.

10. J. Platt, "The Two Faces of Expression," in *Perception and Change* (Ann Arbor: University of Michigan Press, 1970), p. 38; cited in Schneider, *Die Theorie Piagets,* p. 29.

11. See R. W. Sperry, "Cerebral Dominance in Perception," in *Early Experience in Visual Information Processing in Perceptual and Reading Disorders,* ed. F. A. Young and D. B. Lindsley (Washington, D.C.: National Academy of Science, 1970), pp. 167–178.

12. Popper and Eccles, *The Self and Its Brain,* pp. 352, 335, and 462.

13. In Bastide, *Senses et usages du terme "structure,"* p. 32.

14. "Language is a system; all its parts can and must be regarded in their synchronic solidarity"; Ferdinand de Saussure, *Cours de linguistique* (Lausanne and Paris, 1916).

15. J. G. Miller, "Living Systems: Basic Concepts," in *General Systems Theory and Psychiatry*, ed. W. Gray, F. J. Dual, and N. D. Rizzo (Boston: Little, Brown, 1969).

16. See Piaget, *Structuralism*, pp. 7 and 17.

17. One can probably also put it in the following terms: *structure* refers more to certain realities of a differentiation, whereas *system* refers more to the potentialities of a differentiation.

18. Boszormenyi-Nagy and Spark, *Invisible Loyalties*.

19. C. Dorazé, "Les structures temporelles" in Bastide, *Senses et usages du terme "structure,"* p. 120.

20. Gregory Bateson, in Berger, *Beyond the Double Bind* (New York: Brunner and Mazel, 1978), p. 211.

21. In this context, every relevant bit of "information" must be regarded as "experience" in the sense of affect-logic.

22. Bateson, *Mind and Nature*, p. 132.

4. On Language and Consciousness

1. Noam Chomsky, *Language and Mind* (New York: Harcourt, Brace, and World, 1968); M. Bierwisch, "Strukturalismus: Geschichte, Probleme und Methoden," *Kursbuch*, 5 (1966), 77–152.

2. Henri Ey, *Consciousness: A Phenomenological Study of Being Conscious and Becoming Conscious,* trans. John J. Flodstrom (Bloomington: Indiana University Press, 1978; 1st French ed. 1963). See also H. Heimann, "Bewusstseinsstörungen," in *Lexikon der Psychiatrie*, ed. C. Müller (Berlin and New York: Springer, 1973), pp. 61–69.

3. Popper and Eccles, *The Self and Its Brain*, p. 375.

4. Ibid., pp. 355–356.

5. See C. Haring and K. H. Leickert, *Wörterbuch der Psychiatrie und ihrer Grenzgebiete* (Stuttgart and New York: Schattauer, 1968), p. 108. Freud expressed a similar view when he spoke of "a fact without parallel, which defies all explanation or description—the fact of consciousness. Nevertheless, if anyone speaks of consciousness we know immediately and from our most personal experience what is meant by it"; *An Outline of Psycho-Analysis* (1940), *Standard Edition*, XXIII, 157.

6. Karl Jaspers, *General Psychopathology*, trans. J. Hoenig and Marian W. Hamilton (Manchester: Manchester University Press, 1963; 1st German ed. 1953), p. 9.

7. Ludwig Pongratz, *Lexikon der Psychologie,* I (Fribourg, Basel, and Vienna: Herder, 1971), 266.

8. Ey, *Consciousness*.

9. Christian Scharfetter, *Allgemeine Psychopathologie* (Stuttgart: Thieme, 1976), p. 25.

10. Of course even the best-informed person has access to only a tiny portion of

total consciousness. Each individual is, so to speak, the *place* where consciousness occurs—that is, where it is actualized and perhaps developed a tiny step further. But the whole of human knowledge and awareness, the tradition handed down from generation to generation, is constantly developing and is beyond the realization of an individual.

11. Scharfetter, *Allgemeine Psychopathologie,* p. 25.

12. It becomes evident here that the attempts of perceptual psychology to make sharp distinctions between general feelings, physical feelings, and sensory impressions do not make much sense from this perspective. In a manner of speaking, the whole body is a single sensory organ, registering continually whatever affects it. The total of the information received is then centrally processed and becomes a gradually more differentiated "world view."

13. Lévi-Strauss, *Structural Anthropology.*

14. Bierwisch, "Strukturalismus," pp. 92–97 and 104–120.

15. Chomsky, *Language and Mind,* p. 63.

16. Massimo Piatelli-Palmarini, ed., *Language and Learning: The Debate between Jean Piaget and Noam Chomsky* (Cambridge, Mass.: Harvard University Press, 1980).

17. *Signals* in de Saussure's terminology (French: *indices*) are a part of what is signalized, such as the smell of a particular food, the smoke of a fire, the visible part of a mostly invisible object. *Symbols* (French: *symboles*) still have a certain resemblance to what they symbolize, for example, gestures that represent a situation or a person. *Signs* (French: *signes*) are conventions completely removed from any resemblance to the things they represent, such as words, numbers, and algebraic signs.

18. Hermine Sinclair, "Developmental Psycholinguistics" and "Epistemology and the Study of Language," in Inhelder and Chipman, *Piaget and His School,* pp. 189–204 and 205–218.

19. Freud, *Beyond the Pleasure Principle,* pp. 14–15.

20. Claude Lévi-Strauss, *The Savage Mind* (London: Weidenfeld and Nicholson, 1966), p. 131; first published as *La pensée sauvage* (Paris: Plon, 1962).

21. Ibid., pp. 159 and 161.

22. Ibid., p. 143.

23. It is most noteworthy that in the view of genetic epistemology the first "object" whose permanence is grasped is a person, generally the mother. Clearly, this corresponds to the psychoanalytic view.

24. Sinclair, "Developmental Psycholinguistics," p. 197.

25. Bärbel Inhelder, "The Sensorimotor Origins of Knowledge," in Inhelder and Chipman, *Piaget and His School,* p. 158.

26. Ibid., p. 159.

27. Heinrich von Kleist, "On the Gradual Fabrication of Thoughts While Speaking," in *An Abyss Deep Enough: Letters of Heinrich von Kleist with a Selection of Essays and Anecdotes,* trans. Philip B. Miller (New York: E. P. Dutton, 1982), p. 218.

28. Cited in Arthur Koestler, *The Act of Creation* (1964; reprint, London: Pan Books, 1975), p. 118.

29. Koestler, *The Act of Creation.*

30. Schneider, *Die Theorie Piagets*, p. 143.

31. René Spitz, *No and Yes: On the Genesis of Human Communication* (New York: International Universities Press, 1957).

32. Popper and Eccles, *The Self and Its Brain*, pp. 235–236.

33. Ibid., pp. 261–262.

34. Ibid., p. 386.

35. See J. C. Eccles, *The Understanding of the Brain* (New York: McGraw-Hill, 1973). See also C. W. Cotman, *Neuronal Plasticity* (New York: Raven, 1978); K. Alert, "Morphologische Vielfalt und Komplexität vor Synapsen und Mikroschaltungen," *Schweizer Archiv der Neurologie, Neurochirurgie und Psychiatrie*, 125 (1979), 217–229.

36. See Hoppe, "Die Trennung der Gehirnhälften"; B. E. Wexler, "Cerebral Laterality and Psychiatry."

37. Popper and Eccles, *The Self and Its Brain*, chap. P1, P3, P4, P5.

38. Psychoanalysis assumes the existence of a primary unconscious, which is never capable of becoming conscious.

39. Schneider (*Die Theorie Piagets*) appears to arrive at quite a similar conclusion when he emphasizes the importance of making something conscious (in psychoanalysis) for "the formation of structures." However, the conclusion he draws from this—with reference to a remark of Piaget's—that the unconscious must therefore be understood as that which is not (or not yet) structured does not seem to me to be admissible. If the unconscious were actually characterized merely by the fact that something was lacking or nonexistent, then certain central unconscious phenomena such as psychoanalysis understands them would become inexplicable—such as the compulsion to repeat actions, transference, and, more generally, the determination of unconscious processes. These phenomena suggest to me that, on the contrary, the unconscious must be understood as something structured, namely as a *system of rules*, some of which are innate and some of which are acquired. This system of rules determines a large proportion of our behavior. If something is not (yet) structured, it cannot have any effect on behavior.

40. By "new and unusual" I mean "unusually difficult"; this applies to any task that has not become so automatic that we can perform it without having to think consciously about it.

41. C. A. Shannon and W. Weaver, *The Mathematic Theory of Communication* (Urbana: University of Illinois Press, 1949).

42. Bärbel Inhelder, "Memory and Intelligence in the Child," in Inhelder and Chipman, *Piaget and His School*, pp. 100–120.

5. Contradictions, Paradoxes, and the Double Bind

1. Bateson et al., "Towards a Theory of Schizophrenia."

2. E. Ringuette and T. Kennedy, "An Experimental Study of the Double Bind Hypothesis," *Journal of Abnormal Psychology*, 71 (1966), 136–141.

3. Berger, *Beyond the Double Bind*.

4. See Bateson, *Mind and Nature*.

5. See S. R. Hirsch and J. P. Leff, *Abnormalities in Parents of Schizophrenics* (London: London University Press, 1975).

6. Minuchin, *Families and Family Therapy.*

7. See G. W. Brown, I. L. T. Birley, and J. K. Wing, "Influences of Family Life on the Course of Schizophrenic Disorders," *British Journal of Psychiatry,* 121 (1972), 241–258.

8. See L. Chapman, "Recent Advances in the Study of Schizophrenic Cognition," *Schizophrenia Bulletin,* 5 (1979), 568–580.

9. Stierlin, *Delegation und Familie.*

10. Selvini Palazzoli et al., *Paradox and Counterparadox.*

11. Otto Kernberg, *Object Relations Theory and Clinical Psychoanalysis; idem, Borderline Conditions and Pathological Narcissism* (New York: Aronson, 1975); idem, *Internal World and External Reality* (New York and London: Aronson, 1980).

12. R. R. Fairbairn, *An Object Relations Theory of the Personality* (New York: Basic Books, 1952); E. D. Jacobson, *The Self and the Object World* (New York: International Universities Press, 1964); Margaret Mahler, *On Human Symbiosis and the Vicissitudes of Individuation* (New York: International Universities Press, 1968); Kernberg, *Object Relations Theory* and *Borderline Conditions.*

13. I am grateful to Dr. Dieter Signer, Bern, Switzerland, for making this diagram available to me and for his summary of Kernberg's concepts in an unpublished lecture.

14. Krings, Baumgartner, and Wild, *Handbuch philosophischer Grundbegriffe,* III, 1164–65.

15. Paul Watzlawick, J. H. Beavin, and D. D. Jackson, *Pragmatics of Human Communication* (New York: Norton, 1967), p. 191.

16. Gregory Bateson, "The Cybernetics of 'Self': A Theory of Alcoholism," *Psychiatry,* 34 (1971), 1–18.

17. Jean-Paul Sartre, *Questions de méthode* (Paris: Gallimard, 1960), pp. 6, 9, 10.

18. Arthur Koestler, *The Sleepwalkers: A History of Man's Changing Vision of the Universe* (New York: Macmillan, 1959), pp. 193–194.

19. Bateson, *Mind and Nature,* p. 79.

20. Watzlawick, Beavin, and Jackson, *Pragmatics of Human Communication,* p. 188.

21. In Krings, Baumgartner, and Wild, *Handbuch philosophischer Grundbegriffe,* II, 1051–59.

22. Ibid., p. 1159.

23. As I observed in Chapter 2, even such a seemingly emotion-free field as mathematics definitely has its own affective component. This consists, in part at least, of the pleasure felt about a harmonious relationship of parts; later, the particular affective sign may consist of just that typical "coolness" between pleasure and unpleasure that appears to be characteristic of mathematics.

24. Bateson, *Mind and Nature,* pp. 122–123.

25. Of course—precisely in the double bind—a pathogenic relationship can be

maintained by constant "proofs of affection." However, as we shall see, this is an instance of a form of love that prevents development rather than encouraging it.

26. See Berger, *Beyond the Double Bind,* pp. 72 and 129.

27. S. R. Hirsch, "Eltern als Verursacher der Schizophrenie: Der wissenschaftliche Stand einer Theorie," *Nervenarzt,* 50 (1979), 337–345.

28. Bateson et al., "Towards a Theory of Schizophrenia," p. 259.

29. Berger, *Beyond the Double Bind,* pp. 242–243.

30. See J. H. Weakland, "The Double Bind Hypothesis of Schizophrenia and Three-Party Interaction," in *The Etiology of Schizophrenia,* ed. D. D. Jackson (New York: Basic Books, 1960).

31. M. T. Singer, L. C. Wynne, and B. A. Toohey, "Communication Disorders in the Families of Schizophrenics," in *The Nature of Schizophrenia,* ed. L. C. Wynne, S. Cromwell, and S. Matthysse (New York: Wiley, 1978).

32. J. S. Kafka, "Ambiguity for Individuation: A Critique and Reformulation of the Double-Bind Theory," *Archives of General Psychiatry,* 25 (1971), 233.

33. Lilo Süllwold, *Symptome schizophrener Erkrankungen* (Berlin and New York: Springer, 1977).

34. Gottlieb Guntern, ed., *First International ISO Symposium on the Transformation of Human Systems* (Brig, 1981).

35. Piaget, "La pensée symbolique."

36. Frieda Fromm-Reichmann, "Notes on the Development of Schizophrenia by Psychoanalytic Psychotherapy," *Psychiatry,* 2 (1948), 263–273.

37. Jay Haley, "Ideas Which Handicap Therapists," in Berger, *Beyond the Double Bind,* pp. 67–82.

38. Kernberg, *Borderline Conditions,* pp. 315–316.

39. A. E. Scheflen, "Communicational Concepts of Schizophrenia," in Berger, *Beyond the Double Bind,* p. 142.

40. Helm Stierlin, "Die 'Beziehungsrealität' Schizophrener," *Psyche,* 35 (1981), 49–65.

41. Marianne Krüll, *Freud and His Father,* trans. A. J. Pomerans (New York: Norton, 1986).

42. See Jacques Lacan, "Le stade du miroir comme formateur de la fonction du Je," in *Ecrits,* I (Paris: Seuil, 1966).

43. Helm Stierlin, *Von der Psychoanalyse zur Familientherapie* (Stuttgart: Klett, 1975), p. 136.

44. See Watzlawick, Beavin, and Jackson, *Pragmatics of Human Communication,* pp. 51–52.

45. Balint, *The Basic Fault.*

46. Selvini Palazzoli et al., *Paradox and Counterparadox,* p. 36.

47. Bowen, "Schizophrenia as a Multi-Generational Phenomenon," pp. 101–123; Boszormenyi-Nagy and Spark, *Invisible Loyalties.*

48. Weakland, "Double Bind Hypothesis."

49. Scheflen, "Communicational Concepts of Schizophrenia," pp. 125–150.

50. See Singer, Wynne, and Toohey, "Communication Disorders."

51. Süllwold, *Symptome schizophrener Erkrankungen.*

52. See P. Hartwich, *Schizophrenie und Aufmerksamkeitsstörungen* (Berlin and New York: Springer, 1980).

53. R. W. Payne, "Cognitive Defects in Schizophrenics: Overinclusive Thinking," in *Deficits in Cognition*, ed. J. Hellmut (New York: Brunner and Mazel, 1971); J. Poljakov, *Schizophrenie und Erkenntnistätigkeit* (Stuttgart: Thieme, 1973).

54. Theodore Lidz, "Egocentric Cognitive Regression and Family Setting of Schizophrenic Disorders," in Wynne, Cromwell, and Matthysse, *The Nature of Schizophrenia*.

55. E. Schmid-Kitsikis, A. M. Zutter, Y. Burnand, J. J. Burgermeister, R. Tissot, and J. de Ajuriaguerra, "Quelques aspects des activités cognitives du schizophrène," *Annales médico-psychologiques*, 133 (1975), 197–235.

56. Leopold Bellak, M. Hurvich, and H. K. Gedimann, *Ego Functions in Schizophrenics, Neurotics, and Normals: Ego Strength Rating Scales* (New York: Wiley, 1973).

6. On Schizophrenia

1. L. C. Morey and R. K. Blashfield, "A Symptom Analysis of the DSM-III Definition of Schizophrenia," *Schizophrenia Bulletin*, 7 (1981), 258–268; J. H. Stephens, G. O'Connor, and G. Wiener, "Long-Term Prognosis in Schizophrenia," *American Journal of Psychiatry*, 126 (1969), 498–504.

2. See G. Huber, G. Gross, and R. Schüttler, *Schizophrenie: Eine Verlaufs- und sozialpsychiatrische Studie* (Berlin and New York: Springer, 1979). See also Albert Scheflen, *Levels of Schizophrenia* (New York: Brunner and Mazel, 1981); Klaus Conrad, *Die beginnende Schizophrenie* (Stuttgart: Thieme, 1958); W. Janzarik, *Dynamische Grundkonstellationen in endogenen Psychosen* (Berlin: Springer, 1959).

3. Manfred Bleuler, *The Schizophrenic Disorders: Long-Term Patient and Family Studies*, trans. S. M. Clemens (New Haven: Yale University Press, 1978); first published as *Die schizophrenen Geistesstörungen im Lichte langjähriger Kranken- und Familiengeschichten* (Stuttgart: Thieme, 1972); Huber, Gross, and Schüttler, *Schizophrenie;* Luc Ciompi and Christian Müller, *Lebenslauf und Alter der Schizophrenen: Eine katamnestische Langzeitstudie bis ins Senium* (Berlin and New York: Springer, 1976) (in this study 289 former schizophrenic mental patients were followed up an average of 36.9 years after their first hospitalization).

4. Ciompi and Müller, *Lebenslauf und Alter der Schizophrenen*.

5. Careful studies conducted in Germany over more than a decade have shown that schizophrenics commit neither more nor fewer acts of violence than the general population, namely in about 1 case in 2,000! See W. Böker and H. Häfner, *Gewalttaten Geistesgestörter: Eine epidemiologische Studie auf Bundesebene* (Berlin and New York: Springer, 1973).

6. Luc Ciompi, "Ist die chronische Schiziophrenie ein Artefakt? Argumente und Gegenargumente," *Fortschritte in Neurologie und Psychiatrie*, 48 (1980), 237–248.

7. S. S. Kety, D. Rosenthal, P. H. Wender, and F. Schulsinger, "Studies Based on a Total Sample of Adopted Individuals and Their Relatives: Why They Were Necessary, What They Demonstrated and Failed to Demonstrate," *Schizophrenia Bulletin*, 2 (1976), 413–428.

8. See H. E. Spohn and T. Patterson, "Recent Studies of Psychophysiology in Schizophrenia," *Schizophrenia Bulletin*, 5 (1979), 581–610; L. Erlenmeyer-Kimling, B. Cornblatt, D. Friedman, Y. Marcuse, J. Rutschmann, S. Simmens, and S. Davi, "Neurological, Electrophysiological, and Attentional Deviations in Children at Risk for Schizophrenia," in *Schizophrenia as a Brain Disease*, ed. F. A. Henn and H. A. Nasrallah (New York: Oxford University Press, 1982), pp. 61–98.

9. Luc Ciompi, "The Natural History of Schizophrenia in the Long Term" *British Journal of Psychiatry*, 136 (1980), 413–420.

10. J. K. Wing, "Clinical Concepts of Schizophrenia," in *Schizophrenia: Toward a New Synthesis* (London: Brunner and Mazel; New York: Academic Press, 1978), p. 29.

11. With positron emission transaxial tomography (PETT) it has become possible through the use of radioactive glucose to render the brain's energy consumption—that is, the activity or passivity of any region—visible.

12. Wynne, Cromwell, and Matthysse, *The Nature of Schizophrenia.*

13. Scheflen, *Levels of Schizophrenia;* Kernberg, *Internal World and External Reality;* Schneider, *Die Theorie Piagets.* After I completed the manuscript of this book, another study appeared, H. Krüger and M. Bauer, *Die Schizophrenien* (Stuttgart: Enke, 1981), which also presents a broad survey of psychosocial and neurophysiological evidence and arrives at a number of conclusions similar to the ones presented here.

14. For the few cases which never go through an acute phase, but which are sometimes diagnosed as "schizophrenia simplex," a temporary condition recognizable as psychotic is a minimum requirement for the diagnosis to be made.

15. J. Gottesman and J. Shields, "A Critical Review of Recent Adoption, Twin, and Family Studies on Schizophrenia: Behavioral Genetic Perspectives," *Schizophrenia Bulletin*, 2 (1976), 360–398; quotation p. 389.

16. See the debate between Theodore Lidz and the geneticists in *Schizophrenia Bulletin*, 2 (1976).

17. Kety et al., "Studies of Adopted Individuals."

18. L. C. Wynne, M. T. Singer, and M. L. Toohey, "Communication of the Adoptive Parents of Schizophrenics," in *Schizophrenia 75*, ed. J. I. Jørstadt and E. Ugelstad (Oslo: University of Oslo Press, 1976), pp. 413–451. The family studies by P. Tienari point in the same direction; see *The Finnish Adoption Study*, in *Psychosocial Intervention in Schizophrenia*, ed. Helm Stierlin, L. C. Wynne, and M. Wirsching (Berlin and New York: Springer, 1983), pp. 21–34.

19. P. Tienari et al., "Interaction of Genetic and Psychosocial Factors in Schizophrenia," *Acta Psychiatrica Scandinavica*, 71, supp. 319 (1985), 19–30.

20. Ciompi and Müller, *Lebenslauf und Alter der Schizophrenen*, p. 151; Bleuler, *The Schizophrenic Disorders.*

21. R. Lempp, *Psychosen im Kindes- und Jugendalter: Eine Realitätsbezugsstörung* (Bern: Huber, 1973); Leopold Bellak, ed., *Psychiatric Aspects of Minimal Brain Dysfunction in Adults* (New York: Grune and Stratton, 1979); J. Keppler, R. Lempp, D. Pascheday, H. E. Rebmann, and R. Rupps, "Die Frühkindliche Anamnese der Schizophrenen," *Nervenarzt*, 50 (1979), 719–724.

22. S. A. Mednick. F. Schulsinger, and H. Schulsinger, "Schizophrenia in Children of Schizophrenic Mothers," in *Childhood Personality and Psychopathology: Current Topics*, ed. A. Davis (New York: Wiley, 1975), pp. 221–252.

23. See Spohn and Patterson, "Psychophysiology in Schizophrenia"; Kimling et al., "Neurological Deviations."

24. Bleuler, *The Schizophrenic Disorders*, pp. 110–114.

25. World Health Organization, *Schizophrenia: An International Follow-Up Study* (New York: Wiley, 1979).

26. Janzarik, *Dynamische Grundkonstellationen;* Huber, Gross, and Schüttler, *Schizophrenie*, pp. 61–62.

27. Wing, "Clinical Concepts of Schizophrenia," p. 10.

28. Scheflen, *Levels of Schizophrenia*, p. 18.

29. Wing, "Clinical Concepts of Schizophrenia," p. 23.

30. See Ciompi and Müller, *Lebenslauf und Alter der Schizophrenen*, pp. 155–156, 168–169, 208–209. See also J. S. Strauss, R. F. Kokes, R. Klorman, and J. L. Sacksteder, "Premorbid Adjustment in Schizophrenia: Concepts, Measures, and Implications," *Schizophrenia Bulletin*, 3 (1977), 182–244.

31. Ciompi and Müller *Lebenslauf und Alter der Schizophrenen*, p. 72.

32. Kurt Schneider, *Klinische Psychopathologie*, 3d ed. (Stuttgart: Thieme, 1950), p. 138.

33. J. K. Wing, J. E. Cooper, and N. Sartorius, *The Description and Classification of Psychiatric Symptoms: An Instruction Manual for the PSI and Catego System* (London: Cambridge University Press, 1974).

34. Wing, "Clinical Concepts of Schizophrenia," p. 4.

35. Some authors have begun to suspect that different disease processes are at work in the two sets of symptoms and refer to positive symptoms as "syndrome I" and chronic or negative symptoms as "syndrome II"; T. J. Crow, "Molecular Pathology of Schizophrenia: More than One Disease Process?" *British Medical Journal*, 280 (1980), 66–68.

36. Wing, "Clinical Concepts of Schizophrenia," p. 5.

37. Scheflen, *Levels of Schizophrenia*.

38. Conrad, *Die beginnende Schizophrenie*, p. 160 (Conrad's emphasis).

39. Wing, "Clinical Concepts of Schizophrenia," p. 6.

40. See especially J. K. Wing and G. W. Brown, *Institutionalism and Schizophrenia* (London: Cambridge University Press, 1970).

41. G. W. Brown and J. L. T. Birley, "Crisis and Life Changes and the Onset of Schizophrenia," *Journal of Social Health and Social Behavior*, 9 (1968), 203–214; W. P. Dohrenwendt and G. Egri, "Recent Stressful Life Events and Episodes of Schizophrenia," *Schizophrenia Bulletin*, 7 (1981), 12–23.

42. See Gerald Caplan, *Principles of Preventive Psychiatry* (New York: Basic Books, 1964); G. F. Jacobson, "Programs and Techniques of Crisis Interven-

tion," in *American Handbook of Psychiatry,* ed. S. Arieti (New York: Basic Books, 1974), II, 810–825.

43. William Sargant, *Battle for the Mind* (New York: Doubleday, 1957).

44. Conrad, *Die beginnende Schizophrenie,* p. 51.

45. Ibid., p. 53.

46. P. Hartwich, *Schizophrenie und Aufmerksamkeitsstörungen* (Berlin and New York: Springer, 1980), pp. 18–19.

47. See Watzlawick, Beavin, and Jackson, *Pragmatics of Human Communication,* p. 49.

48. Wing, "Clinical Concepts of Schizophrenia," pp. 7–8.

49. In the fields of psychology and biology (and possibly in many other places), time is not something objective and immutable, like mathematical time, but rather a series of (rhythmic) events. "Events create time," one might say; without a rhythm of events time would not exist. Even modern physicists have reached this conclusion. See I. Prigogine and I. Stengers, *Order Out of Chaos: Man's New Dialogue with Nature* (Boulder, Colo.: New Science Library, 1984); K. G. Denbigh, *Three Concepts of Time* (Berlin and New York: Springer, 1981). A change in the events that "create time" can change subjective experience in a fundamental way. We are familiar with the way "time stands sill" when nothing is happening, and the way "time flies" when we are enjoying ourselves. It is no doubt for this reason that young people "have" and experience a different time from the old, and similar differences exist between "primitive" and "civilized" people, and between human beings in general and animals.

50. See L. P. Binswanger, *Einführung in die Probleme der allgemeinen Psychologie* (Berlin: Springer, 1922). See also Luc Ciompi, "Über abnormes Zeiterleben bei einer Schizophrenen," *Psychiatria et Neurologia,* 142 (1962), 100–121.

51. P. Matussek, "Wahrnehmung, Halluzination und Wahn," in *Psychiatrie der Gegenwart: Grundlagen und Methoden der klinischen Psychiatrie,* ed. H. W. Gruhle, R. Jung, W. Mayer-Gross, and M. Müller (Berlin: Springer, 1963), p. 51.

52. D. L. Rosenhan, "On Being Sane in Insane Places," *Science,* 179 (1973), 250–258.

53. Matussek, "Wahrnehmung," p. 51.

54. Schneider, *Die Theorie Piagets,* pp. 23–24.

55. J. J. Jaynes, *The Origins of Consciousness in the Breakdown of the Bicameral Mind* (Boston: Houghton Mifflin, 1976).

56. Scheflen, *Levels of Schizophrenia,* pp. 7, 47.

57. Bateson, *Mind and Nature,* pp. 104–105.

58. E. Jantsch, "Dissipative Strukturen: Ordnung durch Fluktuation," *Neue Zürcher Zeitung,* November 26, 1975, pp. 55–56; "Anwendung der Theorie dissipativer Strukturen," *Neue Zürcher Zeitung,* December 3, 1975, pp. 45–46. See also Prigogine and Stengers, *Order Out of Chaos;* P. F. Dell and H. A. Goolishan, "Ordnung durch Fluktuation: Eine evolutionäre Epistemologie für menschliche Systeme," *Familiendynamik,* 6 (1980), 104–122.

59. Jantsch, "Dissipative Strukturen" and "Anwendung der Theorie dissipativer Strukturen."

60. The word *positive* in this connection does not imply a value; it is used in the purely descriptive cybernetic sense of *increasing* a circular reaction, in contrast to negative feedback, which decreases or weakens a reaction.
61. Searles, "The Effort to Drive the Other Person Crazy," pp. 3–4.
62. Stierlin, *Von der Psychoanalyse zur Familientherapie,* pp. 87, 133.
63. Anonymous, "First Person Account: Problems of Living with Schizophrenia," *Schizophrenia Bulletin,* 7 (1981), 196–197.
64. Bellak, Hurvich, and Gedimann, *Ego Functions in Schizophrenics, Neurotics, and Normals.*
65. See especially J. Monod, *Le hasard et la nécessité: Essai sur la philosophie naturelle de la biologie moderne* (Paris: Seuil, 1970); Jean Piaget, *The Equilibration of Cognitive Structures* (Chicago and London: University of Chicago Press, 1985); Bateson, *Mind and Nature;* Prigogine and Stengers, *Order Out of Chaos.*
66. Ciompi, "Ist die chronische Schizophrenie ein Artefakt?"
67. Huber, Gross, and Schüttler, *Schizophrenie.*
68. See especially Ciompi, "Ist die chronische Schizophrenie ein Artefakt?" where I refer both to the literature and to our own clinical studies.
69. See C. Mundt, W. Radu, and E. Gluck, "Computertomographische Untersuchungen der Liquorräume an chronisch schizophrenen Patienten," *Nervenarzt,* 51 (1980), 743–748.
70. Krüger et al., *Die Schizophrenie,* pp. 42, 232.
71. Cf. Wing and Brown, *Institutionalism and Schizophrenia.*
72. Luc Ciompi, C. Agué, and H. P. Dauwalder, "Ein Forschungsprogramm zur Rehabilitation psychisch Kranker. II. Querschnittsuntersuchung einer Population von chronischen Spitalpatienten," *Nervenarzt,* 49 (1978), 232–238.
73. K. Ernst, "Neurotische Residualzustände und endogene Residualzustände," *Archiv der Psychiatrie und Neurologie,* 203 (1962), 61–84.
74. Bleuler, *The Schizophrenic Disorders,* pp. 333–334.
75. Ciompi and Müller, *Lebenslauf und Alter der Schizophrenen,* pp. 151–152.
76. S. S. Kety, D. Rosenthal, P. H. Wender, and F. Schulsinger, "The Types and Prevalence of Mental Illness in the Biological and Adoptive Families of Adopted Schizophrenics," in *The Transmission of Schizophrenia,* ed. D. Rosenthal and S. Kety (Oxford: Pergamon Press, 1968), pp. 345–362.
77. Luc Ciompi, H. P. Dauwalder, and C. Agué, "Ein Forschungsprogramm zur Rehabilitation psychisch Kranker. III. Längsschnittuntersuchungen zum Rehabilitationserfolg und zur Prognostik," *Nervenarzt,* 50 (1979), 366–378.
78. Ciompi and Müller, *Lebenslauf und Alter der Schizophrenen,* p. 82.
79. Luc Ciompi, "Gedanken zu den therapeutischen Möglichkeiten einer Technik der provozierten Krise," *Psychiatria Clinica,* 10 (1977), 96–101.
80. Ciompi, Dauwalder, and Agué, "Forschungsprogramm zur Rehabilitation."
81. Luc Ciompi, "Organo- oder Soziogenese? Beiträge neuerer Langzeituntersuchungen zur Frage der Aetiologie der Schizophrenie," in *Biologische Psychiatrie: Fortschritte psychiatrischer Forschung,* ed. H. Beckmann (Stuttgart and New York: Thieme, 1982), pp. 38–47; see also Manfred Bleuler, "Einzelkrankheiten in der Schizophreniegruppe?" in *Schizophrenie: Stand und Entwicklungstendenzen der Forschung,* ed. G. Huber (Stuttgart and New York: Schattauer, 1981).

82. See S. Hoyer, "Veränderungen von Hirndurchblutung und Hirnstoffwechsel bei verschiedenen Formen endogener Psychose," in *Biologische Psychiatrie,* ed. H. Beckmann (Stuttgart: Thieme, 1982); M. S. Buchsbaum, D. H. Ingvar, R. Kessler, R. N. Waters, et al., "Cerebral Glucography with Positron Tomography: Use in Normal Subjects and in Patients with Schizophrenia," *Archives of General Psychiatry,* 39 (1982), 151–159.

7. Consequences for Therapy

1. Bleuler, *The Schizophrenic Disorders,* p. 362.
2. See, for example, G. E. Hogarty, S. C. Goldberg, N. R. Schooler, and the Collaborative Study Group, "Drug and Socio-Therapy in the Aftercare of Schizophrenic Patients," *Archives of General Psychiatry,* 28 (1973), 54–64, and 31 (1974), 603–608; G. L. Paul and R. J. Lentz, *Psychosocial Treatment of Chronic Mental Patients: Milieu versus Learning Programs* (Cambridge, Mass.: Harvard University Press, 1977).
3. E. H. Erikson, *Identity, Youth, and Crisis* (New York: Norton, 1968).
4. Luc Ciompi, "How to Improve the Treatment of Schizophrenics: A Multicausal Illness Concept and Its Therapeutic Consequences," in *Psychosocial Intervention in Schizophrenia: An International View,* ed. Helm Stierlin, L. C. Wynne, and M. Wirsching (New York: Springer, 1983).
5. Ciompi, Dauwalder, and Agué, "Forschungsprogramm zur Rehabilitation. III," pp. 366–378.
6. L. R. Mosher, A. Reifman, and A. Menn, "Characteristics of Non-Professionals Serving as Primary Therapists for Acute Schizophrenics," *Hospital and Community Psychiatry,* 24 (1973), 391–396.
7. See M. Jones, *Beyond the Therapeutic Community* (New Haven: Yale University Press, 1968). See also A. J. Spandoni and I. A. Smith, "Milieu Therapy in Schizophrenia," *Archives of General Psychiatry,* 20 (1969), 547–551.
8. E. Heim, E. Johnson, C. Lilienfeld, H. Stauffacher, and P. Wirz, "Application of the Principles of the Therapeutic Community with the Participation of Schizophrenics," in Jørstadt and Ugelstad, *Schizophrenia 75.*
9. C. M. Anderson, "A Psycho-Educational Model of Family Treatment for Schizophrenia," and R. N. Liberman, J. R. H. Falloon, and R. A. Aitchison, "Multiple Family Therapy for Schizophrenia" (Papers presented at the Seventh International Symposium for Schizophrenia Psychotherapy, Heidelberg, 1981).
10. Even worse conditions still exist in places. As late as 1980 I visited the psychiatric wards of a hospital with over 2,000 beds in a large and modern European city; these wards contained beds covered with wire superstructures in which the schizophrenic patients were locked, like birds in cages. All attempts to abolish them had been defeated by the stubborn resistance of the orderlies.
11. Recently there has even been a trend to turn over the task of providing care and support for the dying, which ought to be a self-evident human task, to specialists, called "thanatologists"!
12. See, for example, L. R. Mosher, A. Z. Menn, and S. Matthews, "Soteria:

Evaluation of a Home-Based Treatment for Schizophrenics," *American Journal of Orthopsychiatry,* 45 (1975), 455–467; S. M. Matthews, M. T. Roper, L. R. Mosher, and A. Z. Menn, "A Non-Neuroleptic Treatment for Schizophrenia: Analysis of the Two-Year Post-Discharge Risk of Relapse," *Schizophrenia Bulletin,* 5 (1979), 322–333.

13. L. R. Mosher, and S. J. Keith, "Psychosocial Treatment: Individual, Group, Family, and Community Support Approaches," *Schizophrenia Bulletin,* 6 (1980), 10–41.

14. Personal account. See also P. Polak and M. Kirby, "A Model to Replace Psychiatric Hospitals," *Journal of Nervous and Mental Disease,* 162 (1976), 13–22.

15. See C. Müller, "Die Entwicklung vom Grossspital zur gemeindenahen Psychiatrie: Ein Beispiel," *Nervenarzt,* 47 (1976), 295–299; Ciompi, Agué, and Dauwalder, "Forschungsprogramm zur Rehabilitation. II," pp. 232–238.

16. Ciompi, Dauwalder, and Agué, "Forschungsprogramm zur Rehabilitation. III."

17. M.-C. Imfeld, "Berufliche Rehabilitation ehemaliger psychiatrischer Patienten: Konstruktion einer Beobachtungsskala für Arbeitsverhalten" (Licensing paper, University of Bern, 1977); J. Drezdowicz-Parizek, "Konstruktion einer Schätzskala zum Sozialverhalten" (Licensing paper, University of Bern, 1980).

18. Such a form of organization has proved very successful in a western sector of Switzerland containing rural areas and some towns, with a total population of about 90,000. See Müller, "Entwicklung vom Grossspital"; idem, *Psychiatrische Institutionen* (Berlin and New York: Springer, 1980). This form of health care has the inestimable advantage that personnel and funds can be transferred from one unit to another within the area without difficulty, whereas otherwise problems of rivalry and jurisdiction inevitably develop between "competing" institutions.

19. Most schizophrenics have not the vaguest idea of their financial circumstances; this fact alone keeps them at some remove from reality. They are often denied access to their own money (such as pensions) for entirely unjustified reasons.

20. The first and most important question which used to be asked of every stranger but which is now often forgotten in our anonymous modern world was "Where do you come from?" This question at once creates a sense of warmth, contact, and identity and, if it is followed by more precise questions about exact locations, neighborhoods, milieu, and the like, almost always *provides a wealth of information relevant to therapy.

21. See also Ciompi, "How to Improve Treatment."

22. This is presumably connected with a specifically *temporal* aspect of every metaphorical representation: such a representation is already a condensation of a diachronic event into something synchronic, and thus it comes very close to a synchronic or achronic internal schema.

23. M. Sechehaye, "La réalisation symbolique: Nouvelle méthode de psychothérapie appliquée à un cas de schizophrénie," *Revue suisse de Psychologie Appliquée,* supp. 12 (1947).

24. H. Leuner, *Guided Affective Imagery with Children and Adolescents,* trans. W. A. Richards (New York: Plenum Press, 1983); first published as *Katathymes Bilderleben* (Stuttgart: Thieme, 1970).

25. Selvini Palazzoli et al., *Paradox and Counterparadox,* pp. 84–86.

26. Watzlawick, Beavin, and Jackson, *Pragmatics of Human Communication,* p. 54.

27. Ibid., pp. 120–121.

28. See Guntern, *First Symposium on Transformation,* pp. 71–72.

29. M. H. Erickson and E. L. Rossi, "Varieties of Double Bind," *American Journal of Clinical Hypnosis,* 17 (1975), 143–147.

30. Jay Haley, *Uncommon Therapy: The Psychiatric Techniques of Milton H. Erickson, M.D.* (New York: Norton, 1973); E. L. Rossi, ed., *Collected Papers of Milton H. Erickson,* 4 vols. (New York: Halsted Press, 1980). See also R. Bandler and J. Grinder, *Patterns of the Hypnotic Techniques of Milton H. Erickson,* 2 vols. (Cupertino, Calif.: Meta, 1975).

31. See Selvini Palazzoli et al., *Paradox and Counterparadox.*

32. Sigmund Freud, "Psycho-Analysis" (1926), *Standard Edition,* XX, 265.

33. Selvini Palazzoli et al., *Paradox and Counterparadox,* p. 137.

34. See, for example, the case of the ten-year-old psychotic boy Ernesto, who, as therapy revealed, was attempting with his bizarre behavior to replace his grandfather. The death of this grandfather three years before had left a serious gap in the family equilibrium. The paradoxical prescription of just this grandfather's role finally broke the spell; ibid., pp. 78–80.

35. The phenomenon of equilibrium is central to both systems; it appears likely that this is somehow the point at which they meet, or the point at which one is transformed into the other.

36. G. Benedetti, "Entwicklungen in der Psychotherapie der Schizophrenie," *Schweizer Archiv der Neurologie, Neurochirurgie und Psychiatrie,* 128 (1981), 177–181.

37. See, for example, D. H. Malan, *A Study of Brief Psychotherapy* (Springfield, Ill.: Thomas, 1963).

38. S. Viderman, *La construction de l'espace analytique* (Paris: Denoël, 1970).

39. The term *conscious* here includes not only hypnotic but also other unusual states of awareness.

40. S. Freud, *New Introductory Lectures on Psycho-Analysis* (1933), *Standard Edition,* XXII, 80.

41. Haley, *Uncommon Therapy,* pp. 120–148.

42. Ibid., p. 147.

43. Bandler, and Grinder, *Hypnotic Techniques of Erickson,* I, 139–140.

44. Paul and Lentz, *Psychosocial Treatment.* S. C. Goldberg, N. R. Schooler, G. E. Hogarty, and M. Roper, "Prediction of Relapse in Schizophrenic Outpatients Treated by Drug and Sociotherapy," *Archives of General Psychiatry,* 34 (1977), 171–184.

45. C. Vaugh and J. P. Leff, "The Measurement of Expressed Emotion in the Families of Psychiatric Patients," *British Journal of Social and Clinical Psychology,* 15 (1976), 157–165.

Index